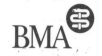

OXFORD MEDICAL PUBLICATIONS

Paediatric Surgery

General Oxford Specialist Handbooks

A Resuscitation Room Guide
Addiction Medicine
Perioperative Medicine, 2e
Postoperative complications, 2e

Oxford Specialist Handbooks in Anaesthesia

Cardiac Anaesthesia
Neuroanaesthesia
Obstetric Anaesthesia
Paediatric Anaesthesia

Oxford Specialist Handbooks in Cardiology

Adult Congenital Heart Disease
Cardiac Catheterization and Coronary Intervention
Echocardiography
Fetal Cardiology
Heart Failure
Hypertension
Nuclear Cardiology
Pacemakers and ICDs

Oxford Specialist Handbooks in End of Life Care

End of Life Care in the Intensive Care Unit
End of Life Care in Nephrology

Oxford Specialist Handbooks in Neurology

Epilepsy
Parkinson's Disease and Other Movement Disorders
Stroke Medicine

Oxford Specialist Handbooks in Paediatrics

Paediatric Endocrinology and Diabetes
Paediatric Dermatology
Paediatric Gastroenterology, Hepatology, and Nutrition
Paediatric Haematology and Oncology
Paediatric Nephrology
Paediatric Neurology
Paediatric Radiology
Paediatric Respiratory Medicine

Oxford Specialist Handbooks in Psychiatry

Child and Adolescent Psychiatry
Old Age Psychiatry

Oxford Specialist Handbooks in Radiology

Interventional Radiology
Musculoskeletal Imaging

Oxford Specialist Handbooks in Surgery

Cardiothoracic Surgery
Hand Surgery
Hepatopancreatobiliary Surgery
Neurosurgery
Operative Surgery, 2e
Oral and Maxillofacial Surgery
Otolaryngology and Head and Neck Surgery
Paediatric Surgery
Plastic and Reconstructive Surgery
Renal Transplantation
Surgical Oncology
Urological Surgery
Vascular Surgery

Oxford Specialist Handbooks in Surgery
Paediatric Surgery

Edited by

Mark Davenport

Consultant Paediatric Surgeon,
King's College Hospital,
London, UK

and

Agostino Pierro

Nuffield Professor of Paediatric Surgery and
Head of Surgery Unit,
UCL Institute of Child Health and Great Ormond Street
Hospital for Children NHS Trust, London, UK

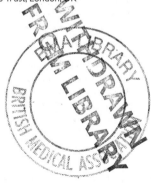

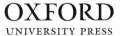

OXFORD
UNIVERSITY PRESS

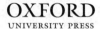

OXFORD
UNIVERSITY PRESS

Great Clarendon Street, Oxford OX2 6DP

Oxford University Press is a department of the University of Oxford.
It furthers the University's objective of excellence in research, scholarship,
and education by publishing worldwide in

Oxford New York

Auckland Cape Town Dar es Salaam Hong Kong Karachi
Kuala Lumpur Madrid Melbourne Mexico City Nairobi
New Delhi Shanghai Taipei Toronto

With offices in

Argentina Austria Brazil Chile Czech Republic France Greece
Guatemala Hungary Italy Japan Poland Portugal Singapore
South Korea Switzerland Thailand Turkey Ukraine Vietnam

Oxford is a registered trade mark of Oxford University Press
in the UK and in certain other countries

Published in the United States
by Oxford University Press Inc., New York

British Library Cataloguing in Publication Data
Data available

Library of Congress Cataloging in Publication Data
Oxford handbook of emergencies in clinical surgery

Typeset by Cepha Imaging Private Ltd., Bangalore, India
Printed by L.E.G.O S.p.A.

ISBN 978–0–19–920880–7

10 9 8 7 6 5 4 3 2 1

Contents

Foreword

This specialist handbook will be greatly used by trainees in Paediatric Surgery and all General Surgeons with an interest in children's surgery. In addition, trainers will be able to crosscheck their teaching material with the wealth of information to be found here. The two editors, Professors Davenport and Pierro, are to be congratulated on producing a text which is uniform and easily accessible throughout the book.

The British Association of Paediatric Surgery is very pleased to endorse this handbook, which will complement the other lengthier textbooks. Indeed, many of our members have contributed chapters on surgical topics but the book's value is greatly enhanced by the non-surgical chapters on topics related to the clinical practice of children's surgery. The care of our patients demands a team approach and an awareness of the family's situation and needs.

This is a most welcome addition to the series of Oxford Specialist Handbooks which include Paediatrics and other surgical specialities. I wish it every success.

David Drake
President of the British Association of Paediatric Surgeons (2008–2010)

Acknowledgements

The Editors wish to thank all the individual contributors for their diligence, knowledge, and experience. Our efforts have been directed at achieving consistency and harmony so that the whole appears to be more than the sum of its parts. Any mistakes, inconsistencies, or errors are, of course, solely ours.

Mark Davenport would like to thank colleagues at King's (senior and junior) for valued criticism and appreciation of its contents; and dedicates his contribution to Keren and Georgie.

Contributors

Niyi Ade-Ajayi
(Chapter 4—Umbilical anomalies and Limb ischaemia)
Consultant Paediatric Surgeon,
King's College Hospital,
London, UK

Manit Arya
(Chapter 6—Testicular tumours)
Senior Fellow in Urology,
University College Hospital,
London, UK

Hashim Uddin Ahmed
(Chapter 6—Testicular tumours)
MRC Clinical Research Fellow
and SpR Urology,
Division of Surgical and
Interventional Sciences,
University College London, UK

C. Martin Bailey
(Chapter 11—Otorhinolaryngology)
Consultant ENT Surgeon,
Department of Paediatric
Otolaryngology,
Great Ormond Street Hospital
for Children, London, UK

Caterina Silvia Barbàra
*(Chapter 3—Fluid balance,
Chapter 1—Nutrition in the
surgical patient)*
Clinical Research Fellow,
Surgery Unit,
Institute of Child Health
and Great Ormond Street
Hospital for Children,
London, UK

David Burge
(Chapter 4—Vomiting)
Consultant Paediatric Surgeon,
Wessex Regional Centre for
Paediatric Surgery,
Southampton General Hospital,
UK

Yair Cadena González
*(Chapter 8—Undescended testes
and Acute scrotum)*
Pediatric Urologist,
Fundación Cardio Infantil,
Bogotá, Colombia

Mara Cananzi
*(Chapter 4—Gastrointestinal
bleeding)*
Clinical Research Fellow,
Surgery Unit,Institute of Child
Health and Great Ormond Street
Hospital for Children,
London, UK

Mieke Cannie
*(Chapter 2—Fetal diagnosis –
magnetic resonance imaging)*
Department of Radiology,
CHU Brugmann,
Bruxelles, Belgium

Emma Carrington
*(Chapter 4—Persistent hyperinsuli-
naemic hypoglycemia of infancy)*
Academic Clinical Fellow in
Paediatric Surgery, UCL Institute
of Child Health and Great
Ormond Street Hospital for
Children NHS Trust,
London, UK

D.C.G. Crabbe
*(Chapter 5—Head and neck
lesions, Chest wall deformities,
Mediastinal tumours, Empyema,
and Oesophageal problems
(miscellaneous))*
Consultant Paediatric Surgeon,
Leeds General Infirmary, UK

Sarah Creighton
(Chapter 11—Gynaecology)
Consultant in Gynaecology,
University College Hospital,
London, UK

K Cross
Fellow in Paediatric Surgery,
Institute of Child Health and Great
Ormond Street Hospital,
London, UK

JI Curry
(Chapter 1—The neurologically
impaired child, Chapter 4—Pyloric
stenosis)
Consultant Neonatal and
Paediatric Surgeon,
Great Ormond Street Hospital
for Children, London, UK

Mark Davenport
(Chapter 10—Introduction and
Renal Transplantation, Chapter 9—
Abdominal injury, Burns, and Blast
injury, Chapter 7—Conventional
surgery, Chapter 3—Infant statistics,
Infant milk, and Neonatal antibiotics,
Chapter 6—Glossary of oncology
and genetics, Chapter 8—Renal
anomalies, Chapter 2—Lung anomalies, Chapter 1—Evidence-based
medicine, and Antibiotics and children, Chapter 4—Gastrointestinal
bleeding, Jaundice, Parenchymal lung
anomalies, Oesophageal atresia,
Intestinal atresia, Meconium ileus,
peritonitis, and plug, Exomphalos,
Biliary atresia and Sacrococcygeal
teratomas, Chapter 5—Dysphagia,
Jaundice, Cervical node infection
(uncommon causes), Oesophageal
substitution, Choledochal malformations, Gall bladder disease
and gallstones, Portal hypertension, The pancreas, The spleen,
Intussusception, Appendicitis, Short
bowel syndrome, and Abdominal
wall hernias)

Carl Davis
(Chapter 3—Fluid balance and
Extracorporeal membrane
oxygenation (ECMO))
Consultant Paediatric &
Neonatal Surgeon,
The Royal Hospital for
Sick Children,
Glasgow, UK

Paolo De Coppi
(Chapter 11—Congenital
vascular anomalies,
Chapter 4— Gastrointestinal
bleeding, Malrotation and
volvulus and Meconium ileus,
peritonitis, and plug)
Senior Lecturer and Consultant
Paediatric Surgeon,
UCL Insitute of Child Health and
Great Ormond Street Hospital for
Sick Children NHS Trust,
London, UK

Jan Deprest
(Chapter 2—Congenital diaphrag-
matic hernia and Fetal surgery)
Department of Obstetrics and
Gynaecology,
UZ Gasthuisberg,
Leuven, Belgium

Evelyn Dykes
(Chapter 9—General
Considerations, Thoracic injury,
Abdominal injury, Burns and
Blast injury)
Associate Postgraduate Dean
(North of Scotland),
Centre for Health Science,
Old Inverness, UK

Simon Eaton
(Chapter 1—Nutrition in the
surgical patient, Chapter 3—Fluid
balance and Extracorporeal mem-
brane oxygenation (ECMO))
Senior Lecturer in Paediatric
Surgery and Metabolic
Biochemistry,
UCL Institute of Child Health, and
Great Ormond Street Hospital for
Children NHS Trust,
London, UK

Anne Greenough
(Chapter 3—Newborn respiratory disease, Causes of respiratory
distress, Investigations of respiratory
distress, Differential diagnosis of
respiratory distress, and Treatment
of respiratory distress)

Head, King's College London
School of Medicine, Regional
Neonatal Intensive Care Centre,
King's College Hospital,
London, UK

Nigel Hall
(Chapter 7—Conventional surgery)
SpR in Paediatric Surgery,
Southampton General Hospital,
Southampton, UK

John Harper
(Chapter 11—Congenital vascular
anomalies)
Professor of Paediatric
Dermatology,
Institute of Child Health
and Great Ormond Street
Hospital for Sick Children,
London, UK

Keith Holmes
(Chapter 6—Rhabdomyosarcoma)
Consultant Paediatric Surgeon,
St George's Hospital,
London, UK

Khalid Hussain
Consultant Paediatric
Endocrinologist,
Great Ormond Street Children's
Hospital NHS Trust and UCL
Institute of Child Health,
London, UK

Saidul Islam
(Chapter 4—Exomphalos)
Clinical Fellow, Department of
Paediatric Surgery,
Kings College Hospital, London, UK

Jacques Jani
(Chapter 2) Harris Birthright
Research Centre for Fetal
Medicine,
King's College Hospital Medical
School,
London, UK

Paul R V Johnson
(Chapter 5—Intussusception,
Meckel's diverticulum,
and Duplications)

Reader in Paediatric Surgery,
University of Oxford;
Consultant Paediatric Surgeon,
John Radcliffe Hospital,
Oxford, UK

Niall Jones
(Chapter 5—Bariatric surgery)
Consultant Paediatric Surgeon,
The Royal London Hospital,
London, UK

Loshan Kangesu
(Chapter 11—Cleft lip and palate
and Congenital vascular anomalies)
Consultant in Plastic Surgery
St Andrews, Chelmsford and Great
Ormond Street Hospital,
London, UK

Simon E Kenny
(Chapter 4—Failure to pass meco-
nium, Chapter 5—Vomiting, Foreign
bodies, and Constipation)
Consultant Paediatric Surgeon /
Urologist and Honorary Senior
Lecturer in Child Health,
Royal Liverpool Children's
NHS Trust, Liverpool, UK

A Kate Khoo
(Chapter 4—Necrotizing entero-
colitis and Hirschsprung's disease)
Research Fellow, Surgery Unit,
UCL Institute of Child Health, and
Great Ormond Street Hospital for
Children NHS Trust,
London, UK

Edward Kiely
(Chapter 6—Neuroblastoma)
Consultant in Paediatric Surgery,
Great Ormond Street Hospital,
London, UK

Lara Kitteringham
(Chapter 4—Parenchymal lung
anomalies and Foregut duplication
cyst)
Consultant Paediatric and
Neonatal Surgeon,
Wessex Regional Centre for
Paediatric Surgery,
Southampton General Hospital, UK

Tom Kurzawinski
(Chapter 5—Thyroid surgery)
Consultant Pancreatic and
Endocrine Surgeon,
University College NHS Trust and
Great Ormond Street Hospital,
London, UK

Graham Lamont
(Chapter 5—Inflammatory bowel
disease)
Consultant in Paediatric Surgery,
Royal Liverpool Children's
Hospital, UK

Katie Lancaster
(Chapter 11—Cleft lip and palate
and Congenital vascular anomalies)
SpR Plastic Surgery,
St Andrews Centre for Burns
and Reconstuctive Surgery,
Chelmsford, UK

Victor Larcher
(Chapter 1—Ethics, Consent, and
Withdrawal of treatment)
Consultant in Paediatrics and
Clinical Ethics,
Great Ormond Street Hospital,
London, UK

Melissa Lees
(Chapter 11—Cleft lip and palate)
Consultant in Clinical Genetics,
Great Ormond Street Hospital
NHS Trust; Honorary Senior
Lecturer, Institute of Child Health,
London, UK

Keith J Lindley
(Chapter 5—The pancreas)
Consultant / Hon Reader in
Paediatric Gastroenterology,
UCL Institute of Child Health and
Great Ormond Street Hospital for
Children NHS Trust,
London, UK

Emily Livesey
(Chapter 4—Jaundice)
Research Fellow,
Department of Paediatric Surgery,
Kings College Hospital, UK

Pedro-Jose Lopez E.
(Chapter 8—Undescended testes
and Acute scrotum)
Paediatric Urologist,
Hospital Exequiel Gonzalez Cortes
& Clinica Alemana,
Santiago, Chile

Paul D. Losty
(Chapter 4—Diaphragm eventra-
tion, Chapter 7—Intestinal tumours,
Teratoma, and Soft tissue tumours,
Chapter 5—Rectal prolapse)
Professor of Paediatric Surgery,
Division of Child Health,
The Royal Liverpool Children's
Hospital (Alder Hey),
University of Liverpool, UK

Gordon Mackinlay
(Chapter 5—Gastro-oesophageal
reflux, Chapter 7—Laparoscopic
fundoplication and Thoracoscopy)
Consultant Surgeon,
Royal Hospital for Sick Children,
Edinburgh, UK

Padraig S J Malone
(Chapter 8—Urinary obstruction)
Consultant Paediatric Urologist,
Southampton University Hospitals
NHS Trust, Southampton, UK

Sean Marven
(Chapter 4—Gastroschisis)
Consultant Paediatric Surgeon,
Sheffield Children's Hospital, UK

Paul May
(Chapter 11—Neurosurgery)
Consultant Paediatric
Neurosurgeon,
Royal Liverpool Childrens Hospital
NHS Trust, Liverpool, UK

H. Fiona McAndrew
(Chapter 8—Varicocele, Phimosis
and paraphimosis, and Prune belly
syndrome)
Consultant Paediatric Urologist,
Regional Department of Paediatric
Urology, Alder Hey Children's
Hospital, Liverpool, UK

Alastair Millar
(Chapter 10—Liver and Intestinal Transplantation, Chapter 6—Liver tumours)
Professor of Paediatric Surgery, University of Cape Town and Red Cross Children's Hospital Cape Town, South Africa

Mary Montgomery
(Chapter 1—Transport of the sick child)
Paediatric Intensivist, Children's Acute Transport Service for North Thames & The Royal Brompton Hospital, UK

Felim Murphy
(Chapter 6—Endocrine tumours)
Consultant in Paediatric Urology, Department of Paediatric Surgery, St George's Hospital, London, UK

Imran Mushtaq
(Chapter 6—Wilms' tumour, Testicular tumours, and Endocrine tumours, Chapter 8—Hypospadias, Disorders of sex development, and Urinary tract stones)
Consultant in Paediatric Surgery, Great Ormond Street Hospital, London, UK

Kypros Nicolaides
(Chapter 2) Director Harris Birthright Research Centre for Fetal Medicine, King's College Hospital London, UK

Alp Numanoglu
(Chapter 10—Liver Transplantation)
Principal Specialist Paediatric Surgeon, Red Cross Children's Hospital, Rondebosch, Cape Town, Senior Lecturer, School of Adolescent and Child Health, University of Cape Town, South Africa

Modupe Odelola
(Chapter 4—Umbilical anomalies and Limb ischaemia)
Clinical Fellow, King's College Hospital London, UK

Bruce Okoye
(Chapter 6: Rhabdomyosarcoma)

Evelyn Ong
(Chapter 4—Assessment of the surgical neonate and Resuscitation)
Research Fellow, UCL Institute of Child Health and Great Ormond Street Hospital for Children NHS Trust

Sara Paramalingham
(Chapter 1—The neurologically impaired child, Chapter 4—Pyloric stenosis)
Research Fellow, Kings College Hospital, London, UK

Emma Parkinson
(Chapter 8—Bladder exstrophy)
Specialist Registrar Paediatric Surgery, King's College Hospital, London, UK

Shailesh Patel
(Chapter 1—Day-case surgery and Pre-assessment)
Consultant Paediatric Surgeon, King's College Hospital, London, UK

Catherine Peters
(Chapter 8—Disorders of sex development)
Specialist Registrar in Paediatric Endocrinology, Great Ormond Street Hospital, London, UK

Mark Peters
*(Chapter 1—and
Chapter 3—Intensive care)*
Consultant Paediatric &
Neonatal Intensivist,
Great Ormond Street Hospital
for Children, London; Research
Lead, Critical Care Group-Portex
Unit, UCL Institute of Child
Health, London, UK

Agostino Pierro
*(Chapter 7—Minimal access
surgery and Laparoscopic
inguinal hernia repair (infants),
Chapter 6—Neuroblastoma,
Chapter 4—Necrotizing ente-
rocolitis, Hirschsprung's disease,
Anorectal malformation, and
Persistent hyperinsulinaemic
hypoglycemia of infancy)*

Michael Prendergast
*(Chapter 3—Newborn respira-
tory disease, Causes of respiratory
distress, Investigations of respiratory
distress, Differential diagnosis of
respiratory distress, and Treatment
of respiratory distress)*
Neonatal Clinical Research Fellow,
King's College Hospital, London, UK

Prem Puri
(Chapter 8—Vesicoureteral reflux)
Consultant Paediatric Surgeon &
Director of Research,
Children's Research Centre,
Our Lady's Children's Hospital,
Dublin, Ireland

Derek Roebuck
*(Chapter 1—Vascular access
and Radiology)*
Consultant Interventional
Radiologist,
Great Ormond Street Hospital,
London, UK

Timothy Rogers
(Chapter 6—Lymphomas)
Consultant Paediatric Surgeon,
Bristol Royal Hospital for Children,
Bristol, UK

Ori Ron
*(Chapter 7—Minimal access
surgery and Laparoscopic
inguinal hernia repair (infants),
Chapter 6—Neuroblastom,
Chapter 4—Anorectal malformation,
Chapter 5—Abdominal
wall hernias)*
Research Fellow,
Great Ormond Street Hospital
for Children NHS Trust, UCL
Institute of Child Health and
London, UK

Andreas Roposch
(Chapter 11—Orthopaedics)
Consultant and Reader in
Orthopaedic Surgery,
Great Ormond Street Hospital
for Children and Institute of
Child Health, London, UK

Sonia Salas-Valverde
*(Chapter 6—Intestinal tumours
and Teratoma, Chapter 5—Rectal
prolapse)*
Consultant Pediatric Surgeon,
The National Children's Hospital,
University of Costa Rica,
San Jose, Costa Rica

Mahesh S. Sharma
*(Chapter 10—Cardiac
Transplantation)*
Consultant Pediatric Cardiac
Surgeon,
The Children's Heart Institute,
Methodist Children's Hospital,
San Antonio, USA

Lucilla Sharp
(Chapter 5—The spleen)
Clinical Fellow,
Department of Paediatric Surgery,
Kings College Hospital,
London, UK

CK Sinha
*(Chapter 5—Jaundice and
Choledochal malformations)*
Department of Paediatric Surgery,
Kings College Hospital,
London, UK

Marlene A. Soma
(Chapter 11—Otorhinolaryngology)
ENT Clinical Fellow,
Great Ormond Street Hospital,
London, UK

Richard Spicer
*(Chapter 6—General principles, UK
oncology survival statistics, Surgical
complications of oncological treat-
ment, and Lymphomas)*
Consultant Paediatric Surgeon,
Royal Hospital for Sick Children,
Bristol, UK

Henrik Steinbrecher
(Chapter 8—Urinary obstruction)
Consultant Pediatric Urologist,
Southampton University Hospital,
Southampton, UK

Ian Sugarman
*(Chapter 5—Abdominal distension
and masses and Gastrointestinal
bleeding)*

Nada Sudhakaran
*(Chapter 4—Malrotation and
volvulus)*
Specialist Registrar,
Great Ormond Street Hospital for
Children NHS Trust,
London, UK

Mike Sury
*(Chapter 1—Anaesthesia and
Analgesia)*
Consultant Paediatric Anaesthetist,
Great Ormond Street Hospital
for Children, London, UK

Victor T Tsang
*(Chapter 10—Cardiac
Transplantation)*
Consultant Cardiothoracic
Surgeon,
Great Ormond Street Hospital,
London, UK

Catalina Valencia
*(Chapte(r 2—Spina bifida/hydroce-
phalus)*
Research Fellow,
Harris Birthright Research Centre
for Fetal Medicine,
King's College Hospital
London, UK

Gregor Walker
*(Chapter 3—Extracorporeal mem-
brane oxygenation (ECMO))*
Consultant Paediatric Surgeon,
Yorkhill Hospital, Glasgow

Robert Yates
(Chapter 11—Cardiology)
Consultant Paediatric Cardiologist,
Great Ormond Street Hospital,
London, UK

George G Youngson
*(Chapter 1—Sepsis,
Chapter 5—The acute abdomen)*
Professor of Paediatric Surgery
and Consultant Paediatric Surgeon,
Department of Paediatric Surgery,
Royal Aberdeen Children's
Hospital, Aberdeen, UK

Augusto Zani
*(Chapter 4—Meconium ileus, peri-
tonitis, and plug)*
Research Fellow, Surgery Unit,
UCL Institute of Child Health, and
Great Ormond Street Hospital
for Children NHS Trust,
London, UK

Symbols and abbreviations

ABC	airways, breathing, and circulation
ABG	arterial blood gases
ACT	activated clotting time
ACTH	adrenocorticotrophic hormone
ADPKD	autosomal dominant polycystic kidney disease
A&E	accident and emergency
AFP	alpha feto protein
AHA	American Heart Association
ALT	alanine transaminase
ALTE	acute life-threatening event
AMH	anti-Müllerian hormone
ANOVA	analysis of variance
AP	acute pancreatitis
AP	anteroposterior
APC	adenomatous polyposis coli
APLS	Advanced Paediatric Life Support
APTR	activated partial thromboplastin ratio
ARDS	acute respiratory distress syndrome
ARM	anorectal malformation
ARR	absolute risk reduction
5-ASA	5-aminosalicylic acid
ASA	American Society of Anesthesiologists
ASD	atrial septal defect
ASIS	anterior superior iliac spine
AST	aspartate aminotransferase
ATLS	Advancd Trauma Life Support
AV	arteriovenous
AVSD	atrioventricular septal defect
AXR	abdominal x-ray
BAPS	British Association of Paediatric Surgeons
BASM	biliary atresia splenic malformation
BMI	body mass index
BMT	bone marrow transplant
BNR	bladder neck resection
BOO	bladder outlet obstruction
BP	blood pressure

BPD	bronchopulmonary dysplasia
BSA	body surface area
BUDT	bilateral undescended testes
BXO	balanitis xerotica obliterans
CAH	congenital adrenal hyperplasia
CAM	cystic adenomatoid malformation
CBD	common bile duct
CCAM	congenital cystic adenomatoid malformation
CCF	congestive cardiac failure
CCLG	Children's Cancer and Leukaemia Group
CD	Crohn's disease
CDH	congenital diaphragmatic hernia
CF	cystic fibrosis
CFTR	cystic fibrosis transmembrane conductance regulator
CHAOS	congenital high airway obstruction syndrome
CHD	congenital heart disease
CLP	cleft lip and palate
CM	choledochal malformation
CMP	cardiomyopathy
CMV	cytomegalovirus
CNS	central nervous system
CO	cardiac output
COG	Children's Oncology Group
COP	cyclophosphamide, prednisolone
COPADM	cyclophosphamide, vincristine, prednisolone, doxorubicin, methotrexate
COPDAC	cyclophosphamide, vincristine, prednisolone, dacarbazine
COPP	cyclophosphamide, prednisolone, procarbazine, vincristine
CP	cleft palate
CPAP	continuous positive airway pressure
CPB	cardiopulmonary bypass
CPR	cardiopulmonary resuscitation
CRP	C-reactive protein
CSAG	Care Standards Advisory Group
CT	chemotherapy
CT	computed tomography
CVP	central venous pressure
CVS	chorionic villous sampling
CXR	chest x-ray
DDH	developmental dysplasia of the hip
DHEAS	dehydroepiandrosterone sulphate

DIC	disseminated intravascular coagulation
DJ	duodenojejunal
DMSA	dimercaptosuccinic acid
DNAR	do not attempt resuscitation
DOT	directly observed therapy
DSD	disorders of sexual differentiation
DSRCT	desmoplastic small round cell tumour
EBV	Epstein–Barr virus
ECG	electrocardiogram
ECMO	extracorporeal membrane oxygenation
EEC	ectrodactyly, ectodermal dysplasia, clefting syndrome
EEG	electroencephalography
EF	ejection fraction
EGF	epidermal growth factor
ELBW	extremely low birth weight
ELS	extralobar sequestration
ELSO	Extracorporeal Life Support Organization
ENT	ear, nose and throat
EPLS	European Paediatric Life Support
ERCP	endoscopic retrograde cholangiopancreatography
ESR	erythrocyte sedimentation rate
ESRF	end-stage renal failure
ESWL	extracorporeal shock wave lithotripsy
ET	endotracheal
EUA	examination under anaesthesia
EXIT	ex utero intrapartum treatment
FAP	familial adenomatous polyposis
FAST	focal abdominal sonography in trauma
FBC	full blood count
FDG	[18F]-fluorodeoxyglucose
FETO	fetoscopic endoluminal tracheal occlusion
FFP	fresh frozen plasma
FLACC	face, legs, activity, cry, consolability
FMTC	familial medullary thyroid carcinoma
FiO_2	fraction of inspired oxygen
FISH	fluorescent in-situ hybridization
α-FP	alpha-feto protein
FSH	follicle-stimulating hormone
GA	general anaesthetic
GCS	Glasgow Coma Scale
GCSF	granulocyte colony-stimulating factor

GFR	glomerular filtration rate
GGT	gamma-glutamyl transferase
GI	gastrointestinal
GIA	gastrointestinal anastomosis
GIST	gastrointestinal stromal tumour
GLP	glucagon-like peptide
GOJ	gastro-oesophageal junction
GOR	gastro-oesophageal reflux
GORD	gastro-oesophageal reflux disease
GP	general practitioner
G&S	group and save
GTN	glyceryl trinitrate
GTT	glucose tolerance test
GU	genitourinary
GVHD	graft versus host disease
Hb	haemoglobin
HBV	hepatitis B virus
HCC	hepatocellular carcinoma
HCG	human chorionic gonadotrophin
HCV	hepatits C virus
HD	Hirschsprung's disease
HFOV	high-frequency oscillatory ventilation
HGF	hepatocyte growth factor
5-HIAA	5-hydroxyindoleacetic acid
HIV	human immunodeficiency virus
HL	Hodgkin's lymphoma
HLA	human leucocyte antigen
HLHS	hypoplastic left heart syndrome
HPB	hepatoblastoma
HR	heart rate
H_2RA	H_2 receptor antagonist
HVA	homovanillic acid
IBD	irritable bowel disease
ICD	International Classification of Diseases
ICP	intracranial pressure
ICU	intensive care unit
I&D	incision and drainage
IE	infective endocarditis
IF	intestinal failure
IFALD	intestinal failure-associated liver disease

Ig	immunoglobulin
IH	intrahepatic
IL	interleukin
ILS	intralobar sequestration
IM	intramuscular
iNO	inhaled nitric oxide
INPC	International Neuroblastoma Pathology Classification
INR	international normalized ratio
INSS	International Neuroblastoma Staging System
IO	inferior oblique/intraosseus
ISSVA	International Society for Study of Vascular Anomalies
ITP	idiopathic thrombocytopenic purpura
IUGR	intrauterine growth restriction
IV	intravenous
IVA	ifosfamide, vincristine, actinomycin D
IVADo	IVA + doxorubicin
IVC	inferior vena cava
IVU	intravenous urogram
KHE	kaposiform haemangioendothelioma
LAGB	laparoscopic adjusted gastric band
LCPD	Legg–Calve–Perthes disease
LDH	lactate dehydrogenase
LFT	liver function tests
LHR	lung-to-head circumference ratio
LHRH	luteinizing hormone-releasing hormone
LLQ	left lower quadrant
LOH	loss of heterozygosity
LOS	lower oesophageal sphincter
LR	likelihood ratio
LRYGB	laparoscopic Roux-en-Y gastric bypass
LST	life-sustaining treatment
LUQ	left upper quadrant
MAP	mean airway pressure
MAS	minimal access surgery
MAS	meconium aspiration syndrome
MCDK	multicystic dysplastic kidney
MCT	medium-chain triglycerides
MCUG	micturating cystourethrogram
MEN	multiple endocrine neoplasia
MI	meconium ileus

MIBG	meta-iodobenzylguanidine
MIP	megameatus intact prepuce
MMR	measles, mumps, and rubella
MR	mitral regurgitation
MRA	magnetic resonance angiography
MRCP	magnetic resonance cholangiopancreatography
MRI	magnetic resonance imaging
MRSA	meticillin-resistant *Staphylococcus aureus*
MRV	magnetic resonance venography
MVA	motor vehicle accident
MW	molecular weight
NAI	non-accidental injury
NBM	nil by mouth
NCA	nurse-controlled analgesia
NEC	necrotizing enterocolitis
NF	neurofibromatosis
NG	nasogastric
NGT	nasogastric tube
NHL	non-Hodgkin's lymphoma
NICE	National Institute for Health and Clinical Excellence
NICH	non-involuting congenital haemangioma
NICU	neonatal intensive care unit
NNT	number needed to treat
NPV	negative predictive value
NSAID	non-steroidal anti-inflammatory drug
NSAP	non-specific abdominal pain
NSF	National Service Framework
NTB	nosocomial tracheobronchitis
NTM	non-tuberculous mycobacteria
OA	oesophageal atresia
OEIS	omphalocele, exstrophy of the bladder, imperforated anus, and spinal defects
OEPA	oncovin, etoposide, prednisolone, adriamycin
OG	orogastric
OGD	oesophagogastroduodenoscopy
17-OHP	17-hydroxyprogesterone
OIS	organ injury scaling
OPSI	overwhelming post-splenectomy infection
$PaCO_2$	pressure of arterial carbon dioxide
PaO_2	pressure of arterial oxygen

PAPP-A	pregnancy-associated placental protein A
PC	pectus carinatum
PCA	patient-controlled analgesia
PCA	post-conceptional age
PCNA	percutaneous nephrolithotomy
PCR	polymerase chain reaction
PDA	patent ductus arteriosus
PDA	personal digital assistant
PDS	polydiaxonone
PDS	polydioxone suture
PE	pectus excavatum
PE	physical education
PEEP	positive end expiratory pressure
PEG	percutaneous endoscopic gastroscopy
PET	positron emission tomography
PH	pulmonary hypertension
PHHI	persistent hyperinsulinaemic hypoglycaemia of infancy
PI	pectus index
PICC	peripherally inserted central catheter
PICU	paediatric intensive care unit
PIE	pulmonary interstitial emphysema
PIP	peak inspiratory pressure
PN	parenteral nutrition
PNAC	parenteral nutrition-associated cholestasis
PNET	primitive neuroectodermal tumour
PONV	postoperative nausea and vomiting
PPD	purified protein derivative
PPHN	persistent pulmonary hypertension of the newborn
PPI	proton pump inhibitor
PPV	patent processus vaginalis
PPV	positive predictive value
PR	parental responsibility
PRETEXT	pretreatment extent
PSARP	posterior sagittal anorectoplasty
PT	parathyroid
PTC	percutaneous transhepatic cholangiography
PTLPD	post-transplant lymphoproliferative disorder
PUJ	pelvi-ureteric junction
PUJO	pelvi-ureteric junction obstruction
PUV	posterior urethral valves

r	Pearson correlation coefficient
RBC	red blood cell
RCCA	right common carotid artery
RCPCH	Royal College of Paediatrics and Child Health
RCT	randomized controlled trial
RDS	respiratory distress syndrome
RICH	rapidly involuting congenital haemangioma
RIF	right iliac fossa
RIJV	right internal jugular vein
RLQ	right lower quadrant
RMS	rhabdomyosarcoma
ROC	receiver operator curve
RR	relative risk
RRR	relative risk reduction
RT	radiotherapy
rtPA	recombinant tissue plasminogen activator
RT-PCR	reverse transcription polymerase chain reaction
RUQ	right upper quadrant
SaO_2	arterial oxygen saturation
SB	small bowel
SBA	serum bile acid
S/C	subcutaneous
SCA	sickle cell anaemia
SCFE	slipped capital femoral epiphysis
SD	standard deviation
SIADH	syndrome of inappropriate antidiuretic hormone secretion
SIOP	International Society of Paediatric Oncology
SIRS	systemic inflammatory response syndrome
SLE	systemic lupus erythematosus
SMA	superior mesenteric artery
SMV	superior mesenteric vein
SNP	single nucleotide polymorphism
SPA	supra-pubic aspiration
STEP	serial transverse enteroplasty
SVC	superior vena cava
SvO_2	venous saturation of oxygen
T_3	tri-iodothyronine
T_4	thyroxine
TGA	transposition of great arteries
TIP	tubularized incised plate

TNF	tissue necrosis factor
TOF	tracheo-oesophageal fistula
tPA	tissue plasminogen activator
TSH	thyroid-stimulating hormone
TTN	transient tachypnoea of the newborn
UC	ulcerative colitis
UDT	undescended testis
U&E	urea and electrolytes
UPDGT	uridine diphosphate glucuronyltransferase
URTI	urinary tract infection
US	ultrasound
USS	ultrasound scan
URA	unilateral renal agenesis
URTI	upper respiratory tract infection
UTI	urinary tract infection
UVJ	ureterovesical junction
VA	veno-arterial
VA	ventriculoatrial
VAT	video-assisted thoracoscopy
VATER	vertebral and ventricular septal defects, anal atresia, tracheo-oesophageal fistula, renal anomalies, radial dysplasia
VID	vitello-intestinal duct
VLBW	very low birth weight
VMA	vanillylmandelic acid
VP	ventriculoperitoneal
VPI	velopharyngeal incompetence
VRE	vancomycin-resistant enterococci
VSD	ventricular septal defect
VUJ	vesico-ureteric junction
VUJO	vesico-ureteric junction obstruction
VUR	vesico-ureteral reflux
VV	veno-venous
WBC	white blood cells (count)
WT	Wilms' tumour

Introduction

British Association of Paediatric Surgeons

This is an organisation founded in November 1953 by surgeons with the declared aim of 'setting the standards of care of paediatric surgical practice in the UK'. It has become an international family with a worldwide membership of about 800 full members. A number of roles can be identified, including

- Leadership and standard setting,
- Academic and scientific promotion of paediatric surgery,
- Fostering international relationships between like-minded surgeons.

President of BAPS

This is a post elected by the council to serve for a two-year period.

Denis Browne (1892–1967)

Australian surgeon, who entered surgical practice at the Hospital for Sick Children, Great Ormond Street, London in 1926. One of the first surgeons to concentrate exclusively on the surgery of children, making many original contributions in gastrointestinal, orthopaedic, ENT and plastic surgery. He was elected the first president of the BAPS.

Previous incumbents

Denis Browne	1953–57	John Scott	1983/84
Isabella Forshall	1957/58	Duncan Forrest	1985/86
David Waterston	1960/61	Joe Cohen	1987/88
Robert Zachary	1962/63	John Atwell	1989/90
James Mason Brown	1964	Dan Young	1991/92
Wallace Dennison	1965/66	Sean Corkery	1993/94
Peter Paul Rickham	1967/68	Edward Guiney	1995/96
Frederick Robarts	1969/70	Lewis Spitz	1997/98
Andrew Wilkinson	1971/72	Leela Kapila	1999/2000
Harold Nixon	1973/74	David Lloyd	2001/02
James Lister	1975/76	Peter Raine	2003/04
John Bentley	1977/78	Victor Boston	2005/06
Ambrose Jolleys	1979/80	Ray Fitzgerald	2007/08
Barry O'Donnell	1981/82	David Drake	2009/10

Congresses

Traditionally host centres are shared between the British Isles and the European mainland.

Recent annual congress venues			
Leeds	1992	London	2001
Manchester	1993	Cambridge	2002
Rotterdam	1994	Estoril, Lisbon	2003
Sheffield	1995	Oxford	2004
Jersey	1996	Dublin	2005
Istanbul	1997	Stockholm	2006
Bristol	1998	Edinburgh	2007
Liverpool	1999	Salamanca	2008
Sorrento	2000	Graz	2009

Address

British Association of Paediatric Surgeons
The Royal College of Surgeons
35-43 Lincoln's Inn Fields
London WC2A 3PE

Office: Kate Billington, Wendy Rees

President: Mr David Drake, president@baps.org.uk
Hon Secretary/Treasurer: Mr Richard Stewart honsec@baps.org.uk

Email for general information: adminsec@baps.org.uk
Tel: +44 (0)20 7869 6915; fax: +44 (0)20 7869 6919

Literature of paediatric surgery

Journal of Pediatric Surgery

Published by Elsevier Inc
Current editor-in-chief – Jay Grosfeld, with regional editors including Mark
Davenport (British Isles), Juan Tovar (European mainland) and TM Miyano
(Asia)
Website http://www.jpedsurg.org/home

Editorial Office

Department of Surgery
JW Riley Hospital for Children
702 Barnhill Dr, Suite 2500
Indianapolis, IN 46202, USA

Pediatric Surgery International

Published by Springer Berlin/Heidelberg
Editors-in-chief – Prem Puri (Dublin) and Arnold Coran (Michigan, USA)
Website http://www.springerlink.com/content/101176
On-line submission https://www.editorialmanager.com/psi/

European Journal of Pediatric Surgery

Published by Thieme Medical Publishers Inc. Stuttgart and New York
Editor in Chief – Benno Ure (Hannover)
Website http://www.thieme.de/fz/ejps/index.html
On-line submission http://mc.manuscriptcentral.com/ejps

Seminars in Pediatric Surgery

Quarterly reviews, organised by a guest editor, using invited reviewers.
Published by Elsevier Inc.
Editor-in-Chief Jay Grosfeld
Website http://www.sempedsurg.org

General considerations

Ethics

What is ethics?

The term is sometimes used to refer to a set of rules or principles that distinguish between right and wrong. However there is not often one single 'right' way to do something. Ethics provides a means of evaluating and choosing between different, often competing options. Ethics also describes a field of study that examines the standards of right and wrong.

Where do ethical values come from?

- Religion, but ethics is not confined to or connected with a particular religion or religion in general.
- Social norms, but standards of behavior in society can deviate from what is ethical.
- The law often incorporates ethical standards, but not all laws are ethical.

Personal sense of right and wrong, based on religious beliefs, habit, cultural educational and family background, experiences, professional code etc, but not universally accepted.

How do ethical dilemmas arise?

- Application of clinical facts alone cannot determine actions.
- There is disagreement about the right course of action.
- Application of moral principles conflict.
- The law is ambivalent or silent.

Ethical conflicts require professionals to make value judgments to resolve them

How do we make ethical decisions?

- Distinguishing facts from values
- Applying moral theory
- Conforming to ethical values
- Respecting appropriate laws

Relevant moral theories

Utilitarian

Concerned with outcomes of actions. An action is morally right if it is useful in maximizing welfare or preferences of those involved. 'The greatest good for the greatest number.'

Deontological

Based on duty: a rational determination of what one *ought* to do. Implies that what *ought to be done can* be done.

Moral laws apply to everyone equally and treat human beings as being of intrinsic worth, hence obligation to respect autonomy.

Rights

Justifiable moral claims made by others that entail actions or forbearance. Negative rights have greater moral force, e.g. right not to be killed. Special rights exist, e.g. those between parents and their children.

Moral basis of medicine and surgery

All treatments should be in the patient's best interests and professionals have the following duties:

- to do more good than harm (sustain life, improve health, prevent disease)
- to respect patients' autonomy to the extent they can exercise it
- to do both fairly and justly, and to appropriate standards.

Box 1.1 Prima facie moral principles

The term 'prima facie' means that in any specific situation where there is a clash between different principles we have to decide in the light of those circumstances which principle is the most important.

- **Beneficence:** the duty to do good to patients, i.e. to act in their best interests, must be balanced against respecting their preferences.
- **Non-maleficence:** the duty to cause patients no net harm.
- **Respect for autonomy:** the duty to respect the patient's right to make their own free and informed decisions about their lives.
- **Justice.** The duty to distribute limited resources fairly and without discrimination on morally irrelevant grounds.

Plus **scope**, i.e. considering to whom and how widely the principles should be applied in given circumstances.

Further reading

Hope T, Savulescu J Hendrick J. *Medical Ethics and Law: the core curriculum*. London: Churchill Livingstone, 2003.

Sokol DK, Bergson G. *Medical Ethics and Law: surviving the wards and passing exams*. London: Trauma Publishing, 2000.

Consent

Definition

Consent is the patient's voluntary agreement to treatment or examination or other aspects of health care. Obtaining consent respects patients' right to make free, autonomous choices. It is a dynamic process and may be verbal or written and can be witnessed. To be valid, consent must be adequately informed, given by a person who is competent to do so and obtained voluntarily

Children (under 18 years) and consent

The legal age of consent to treatment is 16 years, but younger children may give legally valid consent to treatment provided that they have the understanding to do so ('Gillick' competence in English law). Children who are over 16 but under 18 may be unable to refuse treatment that is in their best interests and which is intended to prevent death or serious harm, even if they are 'Gillick' competent.

Information

The information that should be disclosed about a procedure includes its nature (what it entails), purpose (what it is intended to achieve), risks, and side-effects and alternatives (including non-treatment) and should be sufficient to enable a reasonable person to decide whether to have it performed.

Complex or risky procedures require specific patient-targeted information and adequate time for its assimilation.

Competence

Competence is task specific and involves the ability to understand, believe and retain information, and to use it to make the relevant decision. Some children achieve this before the legal age of consent to treatment. Clinicians have the responsibility for assessing competence and a general duty to enhance it by providing children with information in a form and at a pace that they can comprehend.

Voluntariness

The ability of children and parents to make free choices may be compromised by fear, stress or circumstance, e.g. the need to deliver urgent treatment. Parents and competent children have the right to withdraw their consent for investigations and treatment not yet completed, but clinicians may challenge this if it is not in the child's best interests. In intransigent disputes, social services intervention and/or legal advice may be necessary.

Consent givers

A child's assent or agreement should be obtained and non-urgent procedures deferred if refusal is persistent. In children who lack capacity, valid consent may be provided by individuals with legal parental responsibility (PR):
- mothers
- fathers
  - if married to the mother at the time of birth
  - if they have acquired PR by court order or parental responsibility agreement

- if their name appears on the birth certificate (England, Wales and N Ireland, with effect from December 2003)
- authorized carers, e.g. school teachers
- legally appointed guardians
- local authorities (if the child is under care order etc).

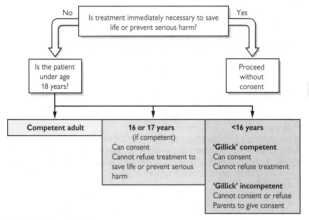

Fig. 1.1 Pathway for Consent

NB Victoria Gillick, after whom this point of law is named, campaigned against giving minors consent over their treatment (in her case, contraception).

Further reading

Department of Health. *Good Practice in Consent Implementation Guide: consent to examination or treatment.* London: Department of Health, 2001.

Hope T, Savulescu J, Hendrick J. *Medical Ethics and Law: the core curriculum.* London: Churchill Livingstone, 2003.

Larcher V. Consent, competence and confidentiality. In: Viner R] (ed). ABC of adolescence. *British Medical Journal* 2005;**330**:353–6.

Withdrawal of treatment

All members of the child health team in partnership with parents have the duty to act in the best interests of children by offering treatment that sustains life and restores health. However, there may be circumstances in which treatments, including cardiopulmonary resuscitation (CPR), sustain life but fail to restore health, impose more burdens than benefits, and hence are no longer in the child's best interests. When this occurs it may be ethical and legal to consider the withdrawal of life-sustaining treatment (LST)

Specific situations in which discussion of withholding/withdrawing LST may occur are:

- **brain stem death** where established criteria are agreed by two physicians in the usual way
- **permanent vegetative state** in which two physicians conclude that the child's failure of interaction or response to the outside world (sustained as a result of cerebral insults, e.g. trauma hypoxia, will not recover)
- **no chance** when treatment delays death but does not relieve suffering
- **no hope** when treatment can prolong life but only at the expense of an unacceptable degree of physical or mental impairment, or the outcome is such that the child has no prospect of future self-directed activity or social interaction
- **unbearable** where, in the face of progressive irreversible illness, further treatment cannot be borne by the child and/or family

Decision making

- Where there is uncertainty about outcomes, the child's life should be safeguarded until they can be resolved as far as possible; some may remain.
- Decisions should be based on best evidence and may require independent second opinions.
- Professional/parental disputes over best interests require multidisciplinary review, mediation and/or ethical review.
- Adequate time should be available to reach consensus.
- Decisions to withdraw LST always require provision of palliative care to alleviate symptoms and to provide support and comfort for those involved.
- Courts are the final arbiters of best interests **if disputes persist**.

Non-resuscitation orders

CPR is medical treatment and should be in the patient's best interests. Its use may be inappropriate when:

- attempting CPR will be unsuccessful
- there is no benefit in restarting heart and breathing because
  - there will only be brief extension of life
  - of the likely severity of side-effects
- expected benefits are outweighed by burdens.

Decisions about non-resuscitation in children (DNAR orders) should be explicit and made in partnership with parents. Where no DNAR order exists, CPR should be given in accordance with established clinical practice.

Further reading

Royal College of Paediatrics and Child Health. Withholding or Withdrawing Life Sustaining Treatment in Children: a framework for practice (2nd edn). London: Royal College of Paediatrics and Child Health, 2004.

Royal College of Physicians. The vegetative state – guidance on the diagnosis and management. A report of a working party of the Royal College of Physicians. *Clin Med* 2003;**3**:249–54.

Task Force for the Determination of Brain Stem Death in Children. Guidelines for the determination of brain stem death in children. *Ann Neurol* 1987;**21**:616–7.

Evidence-based medicine

Hierarchy

Table 1.1 Hierarchy of evidence

Level	Summary
I	Randomized controlled trial
II	Cohort study
III	Case-control study
IV	Case series
V	Expert opinion

Evaluation of randomized controlled trial (RCT)

Although uncommon in paediatric surgical practice, this is the epitome of evidence-based medicine. Questions that should be addressed are:
- randomization? – ideal is computer-generated, less ideal is randomization based on unit numbers, day of week etc
- are all patients the same at entry? – statistically tested for demographic homogeneity
- were groups treated equally, after randomization? Did the intervention group get more tests, better follow-up etc
- were all patients randomized actually followed up?
- were assessments or observers 'blinded' to treatment group? i.e. use of placebo.

Presentation of results

Relative risk (RR) = risk of outcome (treatment)/risk (control)

Absolute risk reduction (ARR) = risk (treatment) − risk (control)

Relative risk reduction (RRR) = 1 − RR

Number needed to treat (NNT) = 1/ARR

Box 1.2 Example: RCT of postoperative steroids in biliary atresia ($n = 100$)

End-point – need for liver transplant at 2 years is 40% in steroid group and 50% in placebo

$$RR = 0.4/0.5 = 80\%$$

$$ARR = 0.4 - 0.5 = 10\%$$

$$RRR = 1 - RR = 20\%$$

$$NNT = 1/ARR = 10 \text{ (to avoid one liver transplant at 2 years)}$$

- Whether the results have precision requires testing. Use 95% confidence intervals and if there is overlap, then this implies it is not significant.
- Finally – does it matter? Many drugs trials are performed where the end-point has no real clinical meaning or relevance.

Type I (α) error – usually set at $P = 0.05$
- Rejecting a null hypothesis when it is actually true

Type II (β) error
- Rejecting the alternative hypothesis when it is actually true – typically because the sample size is too small

Sample size calculation
There are three elements to this calculation: (i) α, the probability of detecting a false effect, usually set at 5%; (ii) β, the power, i.e. the probability of actually detecting a real effect, typically 80–90%; (iii) the estimated absolute risk reduction (by the treatment).

$$\text{Number in each arm} = \alpha \times \beta/ARR^2$$

Meta-analysis

This is a way of determining the 'average' from a number of studies, and works by 'pooling' data. The elements within must contain a Test for Heterogeneity (i.e. are the component studies broadly similar) and illustration of the synthesized results. Typically this in the form of a Forest Plot (odd name with no clear affiliation, but certainly not Dr Forest), where the X axis is indicative of the odds ratio of the 'result' and the individual studies are plotted along the Y axis.

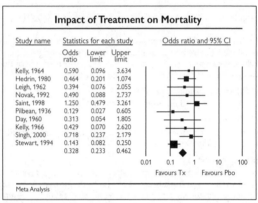

Fig. 1.2 Impact of treatment on mortality. Reproduced with permission from Biostat, Inc. Forest plot created using the program Comprehensive Meta-Analysis (www.meta-analysis.com)

The lines indicate the confidence interval for each study, while the squares area of each square implies its statistical weighting. The summary diamond at the bottom is the conclusion of the analysis.

Statistically speaking

How to describe a population

Typically, if enough can be measured, biological values have a 'normal' distribution and can be expressed as an index of central tendency (mean) and a spread around this mean (standard deviation, SD).

- 68% of the population will lie within ± 1 SD, and 95% will lie within ± 2SD.

Some types of data, do not conform to these characteristics and can be termed *non-parametric or non-normal*, and are best described with medians and a range (or interquartile range). It is usually less wasteful of data if they can be shown to have a normal distribution, and this feature can be tested statistically (e.g. Shapiro–Wilk test). If this assumption of normality cannot be made, then non-parametric tests should be used to compare values.

Is there a significant difference here?

Groups from normal population
Comparison of means
- Two unrelated groups – t test (also known as Student t test)
- Two related groups (e.g. before or after drug) – paired t test

Comparison of means from >2 groups – analysis of variance (ANOVA)

Groups from non-normal population
Comparison of medians
- two unrelated groups – Mann–Whitney U test
- two related groups – Wilcoxon rank-sum test

Comparison of medians from >2 groups – Kruskal–Wallis test

Groups are categorical (e.g. yes/no; alive/dead)
If data can be arranged as a simple 2 x 2 grid, then variation from expected can be tested using a Chi squared (X^2) test (needs ≥5 in each cell). A Fisher exact test can be used if there are small numbers in each cell.

For ≥3 or more categories (e.g. low, medium, high expression), then an extended X^2 (r x c) test can be used for variation from expected, or where a trend is seen.

Is there an association or correlation?

This is a different concept from above, and is looking for a *relationship* between two (or more) features/variables. Initial assessment should be based on a scatter plot. The degree of the relationship is measured as the **Pearson correlation coefficient (r)**, which varies between −1 (i.e. perfect inverse correlation) and +1 (i.e. perfect correlation). If either of the variables are non-parametric then there is an equivalent coefficient **(Spearman r_S or Kendall τ)**. A line (of regression) is often drawn on the scatter plot to suggest a measured relationship. This can be used to calculate from one value to the other.

How useful is my diagnostic test?

Simply showing that two groups have statistically different means doesn't mean that this is the basis for a discriminatory or diagnostic test between them. For this process then the concept of 'cut-off' needs to be addressed.

Receiver operator curve (ROC)
This is a graph of all sensitivities and specificities for every possible 'cut-off' value. The furthest point or shoulder of the plotted curve is then regarded as the best choice for cut-off value. Using this value, you can then estimate how good the test is with these concepts (Fig. 1.3).

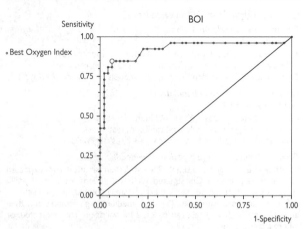

Fig. 1.3 ROC curve of value of best oxygen index (BOI) in prognosis of congenital diaphragmatic hernia. The shoulder (o) suggest best combination of both high sensitivity and specificity. Actival value for cut-off not shown.

Table 1.2

	Condition +ve	Condition –ve
Test +ve	A (i.e. true positive)	B (i.e. false positive)
Test –ve	C (i.e false negative)	D (i.e. true negative)

Using Table 1.2:

$$\text{Sensitivity} = \frac{A}{A+C}$$

$$\text{Sensitivity} = \frac{D}{B+D}$$

$$+\text{ve predictive value} = \frac{A}{A+B}$$

$$-\text{ve predictive value} = \frac{C}{C+D}$$

Likelihood ratio (LR)

This statistic tells us how much the test changes the 'odds' of the disease being present. It can be expressed as LH+, i.e. likelihood of a positive test, or LH–, i.e. likelihood of a negative test.

$$LH+ = \frac{\text{sensitivity}}{(1 - \text{specificity})}$$

$$LH- = \frac{(1 - \text{specificity})}{\text{specificity}}$$

Worked example: CRP in acute appendicititis

100 acute abdomens – 25 have appendicitis (although you don't know that at the outset). The test is CRP elevation (must have preset level, i.e. cut-off, say >20 mg/l). If matrix is as shown in Table 1.3:

Table 1.3 CRP as discriminator in appendicitis

	Appendix +ve	Appendix –ve
CRP +ve	21 (i.e. true positive)	9 (i.e. false negative)
CRP –ve	4 (i.e. false positive)	66 (i.e. true negative)

$$\text{Sensitivity} = \frac{21}{21} + 4 = 84\%$$

$$\text{Specificity} = \frac{66}{66} + 9 = 88\%$$

$$\text{PPV} = \frac{21}{21} + 9 = 70\%$$

$$\text{NPV} = \frac{66}{4} + 66 = 94\%$$

$$LH+ = \frac{0.84}{1} - 0.88 = 7$$

$$LH- = 1 - \frac{0.84}{0.88} = 0.18$$

A high LH+ (arbitrarily >10) implies a good test, and conversely a very low LH– (arbitrarily <0.1) implies a good test for excluding disease. As you can see – CRP lies in the pretty useless group!

Further reading

Centre for Evidence Based Medicine. Real-time calculator for determination of the above concepts: http://www.cebm.utoronto.ca/practise/ca/statscal/

The Cochrane Collaboration produces various systematic reviews on a range of surgical topics: http://www.cochrane.org/index.htm

Lewis S, Clarke M. Forest plots: trying to see the wood and the trees. *BMJ* 2001;**322**:1479–80. (Explanation and illustrations of Forest plots) http://www.bmj.com/cgi/content/full/322/7300/1479

Transport of the sick child

Transport includes not only transport between hospitals but also intra-hospital journeys (e.g. to the x-ray or CT department).

Factors to consider

Is transport necessary?
- Can images be sent electronically or by taxi for a specialist opinion?
- Can the surgeon travel to the patient for assessment?
- Is tele-conferencing available?

Timing of transport
- Is the transport time critical?
- Local emergency surgery with secondary transport post-operatively?

Team composition
- Trained transport team
- Local team
  - medical grade/specialty/experience
  - nurse grade/specialty/experience

Communication
- Paramount to have safe transport
- Vital to include everyone in the loop – all local team members, receiving unit, transport team, and parents
- Include full documentation

Parents
- Try to ensure they stay with the child
- Will need to get consent for operation – this may be best done at the receiving centre or by telephone
- Make a note of their telephone numbers
- Are they aware of destination, contact details, and is transport arranged?

Safety
- Reduce need for emergency driving with good preparation
- Restrain all personnel in the rear compartment of the ambulance
- Restrain the patient securely
- Restrain all equipment

Management (ABC principles)

Airway
- Self-maintained? (Likely to remain self-maintained for the journey?)
- What is the likelihood of sudden deterioration?

If there is doubt about adequacy of the airway, it is safer to place a formal airway as a semi-elective controlled procedure (doing this in CT/corridor/lift/ambulance is much more difficult!)

Breathing
- Adequacy likely to be maintained?
- Pain relief/diaphragmatic splinting
- Shock/capillary leak? (Likely to develop pulmonary oedema?)

If breathing is compromised or likely to become so, placement of formal airway and ventilation should be performed prior to transfer (doing this in CT/corridor/ambulance is much more difficult!)

> Try to support the newborn with TOF/OA disorder without intubation, and if intubated use the lowest pressures possible and treat as a time-critical emergency – insufflation of the stomach can lead to perforation.

Circulation
- Sufficiently resuscitated?
- Likely to need more fluid – sepsis, ongoing losses
- What fluid? – crystalloid/colloid/blood/blood products
- IV access sufficient and working? – peripheral/intraosseus/central?
- Will there be a need for inotropes or vasopressors? – drawn up/ attached
- Pumps with sufficient battery life?
- Long extensions in place?

Disability and other
- Pain relief adequate?
- Sedation and muscle relaxant in sufficient quantities for journey
- Maintenance and replacement fluids in sufficient quantity
- Blood glucose maintained – likely to be maintained for length of journey?
- GCS – adequate to maintain airways and breathing and likely to remain so?
- Maintenance of normothermia – cover exposed areas, burns/ omphalocele with cling film to reduce heat and moisture loss
- Large-bore NG/OG tube or Replogle in situ and on free drainage

Checklist (Table 1.4)
Use this to ensure nothing is forgotten in the heat of the moment! It is useful to have a checklist of equipment in the transport kit, and a checklist of any additional equipment that might be required. Battery life of pumps should be checked and ambulance 12 V socket adapters carried if necessary. Amount of oxygen and/or other medical gases that will be required should also be checked prior to transfer.

Table 1.4 Pre-departure checklist

Airway/breathing	CXR checked
	ABG post placement on transport ventilator
	Humidivent/viral filter
	End-tidal CO_2
	Oxygen/air available in sufficient quantity
	Airway/drug bag
	Ambubag
	Secondary bagging oxygen
Circulation	Appropriate BP/circulation monitoring
Drugs/fluids	Sufficient and working IV access
Sedation	Sedation, analgesia, paralysis
Other	NGT – free drainage
	Chest drains on Heimlich valve
	Equipment packed
	Mobile phone/PDA
Paperwork/communication	Consultant informed and plan agreed
	Maternal blood if surgical neonate
	Receiving unit contacted – estimated time of arrival
	CXR, CT scans and notes copied

Anaesthesia

General considerations

Compared with adults, infants and small children have a higher resting metabolic rate and oxygen consumption. Respiratory exchange and cardiac output are therefore increased also. Furthermore, the pulmonary oxygen reserve is reduced, and consequently failure to oxygenate results in rapid hypoxia. The airway is narrowest at the cricoid ring and may be damaged permanently by a tracheal tube that is too large. Minor tracheal damage or laryngeal oedema may cause stridor or obstruction.

Hepatic and renal function may be immature and extracellular fluid is increased so that pharmacokinetics and dynamics are altered. Relative blood volume is highest in infants (95–100 mL/kg). Vasoconstriction is slower but is effective so that blood pressure can be preserved in hypo-volaemic shock (absent peripheral pulses and cool skin). Blood loss must be assessed and managed carefully. Body surface area in proportion to mass is increased, causing vulnerability to hypothermia. All of the problems above are greatest in infancy especially in neonates and preterm (or ex-preterm) infants.

Pre-operative assessment (coincident medical disease)

- **Cardiac** – approximately 5% of children have cardiac murmurs and their cause should, ideally, be defined before elective surgery. It is acceptable to anaesthetize children (not infants) who have a quiet early systolic murmur without a definite cardiac diagnosis, provided they are well and have a normal oxygen saturations and no other signs such as radiation of the murmur or a thrill (cardiac enlargement due to aortic stenosis or cardiomyopathy may be detected on CXR or ECG). Cardiomyopathy, pulmonary hypertension and aortic stenosis require referral to a specialist centre because they are associated with a high mortality from anaesthesia.
- **Airway** – major difficulty with airway management should be anticipated with some syndromes (e.g. Pierre–Robin, Goldenhar and Treacher–Collins syndromes). Children with mucopolysaccharidoses (e.g. Hurler's or Hunter's syndrome) also have particularly difficult airways and will need careful assessment.
- **Cerebral palsy** – such children have difficulties with reflux, seizures, positioning during surgery, communication, and assessment of pain.
- **Sickle cell disease** – these children may need pre-operative blood transfusion or intravenous fluids for rehydration before major surgery, but not usually for minor body surface procedures.
- **Diabetic patients** – these should be co-managed by an endocrinologist and the patient scheduled first on the operating list.

Coincident fever and URTI

Upper respiratory infections are common and are associated with increased respiratory complications (laryngospasm and hypoxia), particularly if the trachea has been intubated. Postponement of elective surgery should be considered for 4 weeks if the child has a high fever (>38°C), purulent secretions, or signs of collapse or consolidation. Fever of any cause may justify postponement. Vaccination is neither a contraindication to nor a reason for a delaying anaesthesia.

Screening blood tests are rarely required for routine non-major surgery in normal children. Investigations should be appropriate to the disease.

Latex allergy

Typically seen in children with spina bifida (~18%) and children who have had repeated surgical interventions. Anaphylaxis provoked by latex gloves tends to occur slowly during surgery. Modern equipment is latex-free but special theatre precautions and planning are still required.

Risk and consent

Obtaining consent for a procedure must involve communicating the balance of *benefit versus risk*, and consequently it is standard practice in the UK for the surgeon to obtain written consent first and that verbal consent for anaesthesia by the anaesthetist is acceptable.

> The risk of death from anaesthesia alone is difficult to quantify but has been estimated at **1 in 185,000**.

The risk from additional anaesthetic procedures such as epidurals need a separate explanation by the anaesthetist.

The American Society of Anesthesiologists (ASA) scoring system is used widely to categorize risk (Table 1.5).

Table 1.5 ASA scoring system for risk evaluation

I	Fit and well
II	Mild non-limiting systemic disease
III	Limiting systemic disease
IV	Life-threatening systemic disease
V	Imminent risk of death

Fasting

The following guidelines are recommended to avoid aspiration of gastric contents related to anaesthesia:

- 6 h for solids and non-breast milk
- 4 h for breast milk
- 2–3 h for water or any clear fluid.

Most oral medications should be taken as usual with a small volume of water. Small infants should be first on routine operating lists to avoid distress from hunger.

Anxiety, behavioural problems, and premedication

Anxious or distressed children can be calmed with play therapy beforehand or with an anxiolytic or sedative. Midazolam (0.5 mg/kg orally) has a calming effect by 15 min. Some uncooperative children, often those who need repeated procedures or those with learning difficulties need extra planning and consideration.

Induction

Parents should be allowed to attend and calm their children at induction. An intravenous technique is the most rapid, and local anaesthetic creams reduce the pain of venepuncture. Sevoflurane is the least-unpleasant inhalational drug and causes unconsciousness in less than 2 min. Both techniques are equivalent in terms of safety and causing distress.

Recovery and postoperative care

There should be a dedicated paediatric recovery ward managed by specialist nurses. Airway obstruction is common. Agitation in children due to pain or delirium is a common problem that usually resolves within 10 minutes after awakening. Parents may help to calm their children. Extra or 'rescue' analgesia should be administered promptly before discharge to the ward. Postoperative nausea and vomiting (PONV) is common over the age of three years, and is associated with opioids, certain types of surgery (e.g. ENT, dental, gastrointestinal, and squint). The best anti-emetic drug combination may be ondansetron (100 microgram/kg 2–12 years, 4 mg >12 years), and dexamethasone.

Neonates and ex-preterm infants <60 weeks post-conceptional age are at risk of apnoeas for the first 12 h after anaesthesia.

Analgesia

General guidance and a review of the evidence are available on the Association of Paediatric Anaesthetists' website http://apagbi.org.uk/.

Assessment of pain

Experience has shown that pain-assessment tools help to ensure regular assessment and to encourage achievement of analgesia objectives. Older children can self-report using visual analogue pain scales such as the Wong–Baker FACES scale. In younger children, behavioural scales such as the FLACC (face, legs, activity, cry, consolability) scale and markers of sympathetic activation are used.

Multi-modal analgesia

Combinations of local anaesthesia and non-steroidal analgesia provide the best analgesia profile for minor surgery and help to minimize the dose of both drug types. If opioids are necessary, their doses and side-effects are also minimized.

Local anaesthesia

Skin infiltration

This is easy and often effective, ideally performed before surgery to reduce autonomic arousal during surgery. The safe dose must not be exceeded by any route of administration (Table 1.6).

Table 1.6 Local anaesthetic agents

	Duration of action	Maximum dose
Lidocaine	1–2 h	3 mg/kg (0.3 mL/kg of 1% solution)
Lidocaine (+ adrenaline)	2–4 h	7 mg/kg
Bupivacaine	4–12 h	2 mg/kg
Levobupivacaine (+/– adrenaline)	4–12 h	2 mg/kg (0.8 mL/kg of 0.25% solution)

Extradural analgesia

This can be lumbar, thoracic, or caudal. Single injections can be used during anaesthesia. Infusions through an indwelling catheter are effective for post-operative analgesia. Efficacy depends upon placement at the appropriate vertebral level. Common minor complications include urinary retention and motor weakness. Lumbar and thoracic extradural blocks (known as epidurals) can cause hypotension from vasodilatation. Neurological damage, by infection or haematoma, is rare.

Thoracic or lumbar extradurals can be technically difficult but usually provide excellent postoperative analgesia for extensive thoracic or abdominal surgery. Specialist nursing and support from a pain team are, however, needed. The addition of extradural opioids and other adjuncts increases analgesia.

Caudal extradural single injections are less technically difficult and are effective for minor lower abdominal and anogenital surgery. A catheter can be advanced from the sacral hiatus to infuse local anaesthetic to higher vertebral levels, for example to provide analgesia for thoracotomy in a neonate who has had a repair of oesophageal atresia.

Subarachnoid (spinal) anaesthesia
A much smaller volume of local anaesthetic, injected into the subarachnoid space causes dense anaesthesia of the lower nerve roots such that an awake infant may lie still for inguinal hernia repair lasting approximately one hour.

Individual nerve blockade
Blockade of individual nerves and nerve plexi (e.g. the brachial plexus) is effective depending on placement accuracy. Ultrasound is becoming accepted as the best method of effective needle placement.

Non-opioids
The combination of paracetamol (oral, IV, or rectal) with non-steroidal anti-inflammatory drugs (NSAIDS) such as ibuprofen (oral) or diclofenac (oral or rectal) is useful for mild to moderate pain. Regular use is *opioid sparing*. NSAIDs are contraindicated if there is a history of allergy, aspirin-sensitive asthma, low cardiac output, or renal failure. Gastrointestinal side-effects are rare in children.

Opioids
These are used for moderate to severe pain and in some chronic pain conditions. Respiratory depression in fully conscious children with standard doses is rare. Neonates and preterm infants may be sensitive. Other problems include PONV, constipation, tolerance, and dependence. Morphine is commonly used by infusion or by patient (PCA) or nurse (NCA) control; it is also available orally. Ketamine, added to a morphine is effective in controlling refractory pain.

Further reading
Bingham R, Lloyd Thomas A, Sury M. *Textbook of Paediatric Anaesthesia* (3rd edn). London: Hodder, 2007.

Marchant WA, Walker I. Anaesthetic management of the child with sickle cell disease. *Paediatr Anaesthes* 2003;**13**:473–89.

Intensive care

- On an intensive care unit (ICU), more-detailed monitoring and treatment can be provided than would normally be available on conventional wards.
- Most techniques used on intensive care are 'supportive' rather than 'curative'.
- Recovery from critical illness requires this supportive care, but also treatment of the underlying condition. Surgical conditions requiring intensive care exemplify this principle.

Essentials of ICU

Interventions are prioritised as support for – Airway, Breathing, and Circulation.

> Good ICU requires that simple procedures are done well i.e.
> **'right tube, right place, right time'.**

Airway

Indications (for artificial protection of airway)

- Risk of airway obstruction (malformation, facial, or laryngeal trauma/burns)
- Loss of airways reflexes (coma, lower cranial nerve dysfunction)
- Need for positive pressure ventilation (respiratory failure or planned major surgery)

Guidelines (for artificial protection of airway)

- Endotracheal tube (cuffed if >8years):
  - diameter (cm) = (age+ 4)/4
  - length (cm) = (age/2) + 12(oral) or +14 (nasal).
  - degree of ET leak that is acceptable depends on scenario but – *sicker patient, less leak.*

Anaesthesia and intubation should be carried out by the most experienced member of staff available. Gaseous induction if difficult airway anticipated (stridor, restricted jaw/neck movement, prominent upper teeth, small jaw, large tongue, large tonsils).

Choice of induction drugs can be complex but if stable one option is:
- fentanyl (2–4 microgram/kg) or morphine 0.1–0.2 mg/kg
- midazolam (0.1–0.2 mg/kg)
- atracurium (0.5–1.0 mg/kg).

Breathing

Indications for artificial ventilation

- Absent/ inadequate respiratory drive (anaesthesia/neuromuscular blockade, coma, e.g. post-head injury)
- Inadequate respiratory pump (failure to expand chest adequately due to chest wall malformation, traumatic flail-segment, neuromuscular disease etc)
- Inadequate gas exchange (adult RDS, newborn RDS, pneumonia, lung hypoplasia, or malformation)

Guidelines (for artificial ventilation)

- High pressure, volume, and oxygen concentrations cause lung injury (barotrauma). Therefore, aim to limit to the minimum required.
- Mean airway pressure (MAP) and fraction of inspired oxygen (F_iO_2) determine oxygenation (PaO_2).
- Minute ventilation (i.e. tidal volume x rate) determines carbon dioxide level ($PaCO_2$).

Suggested settings

- F_iO_2 < 0.6, tidal volume 4–7 mL/kg
- Peak inspiratory pressure (PIP) < 30 cmH$_2$O,
- Positive end expiratory pressure (PEEP) 4–8 cmH$_2$O

Aim for pH of 7.25–7.3 regardless of $PaCO_2$ (permissive hypercapnia), in the absence of pulmonary hypertension or concerns about cerebral blood flow (e.g. post-head injury).

Use PEEP to 'open the lung and keep it open'.

Often require neuromuscular blockade initially and when settings are high (e.g. PIP > 25 cmH$_2$O or when tolerating very high $PaCO_2$).

If FiO_2 > 0.6 and MAP > 16 cmH$_2$O needed for PaO_2 > 8 KPa, high-frequency oscillatory ventilation (HFOV) may offer an advantage.

Circulation

This is the major consideration in the intensive care of the surgical patient. There may be loss of blood during surgery or trauma, or redistribution of intravascular fluid following surgery or development of sepsis.

Indications (for circulation support)

There is no consensus about the ideal marker for inadequacy of the circulation ('shock'). However, hypotension is a late sign and resuscitation should not be delayed until a blood pressure fall.

Useful signs

Tachycardia, increased pulse pressure, prolonged capillary refill time, altered mental state, oliguria, acidosis, raised blood lactate. Central venous oxygen saturation appears to offer advantages as a guide for on-going resuscitation in septic shock and trauma.

Guidelines (for circulation support)

Fluid resuscitation is the key element of circulation support.

Inadequate circulation should be treated aggressively with volume expansion (aliquots of 20 mL/kg). This should be administered rapidly and repeated immediately if the response is inadequate. Falling heart rate and narrowing pulse pressure may be the early signs of fluid responsiveness. Colloid may offer an advantage in the context of sepsis, whereas normal saline is the fluid of choice in head trauma.

An inadequate response to aggressive fluid resuscitation should prompt rapid escalation of the treatment of shock with vasoactive drugs (e.g. as dopamine). International consensus guidelines recommend a hierarchy of such drugs (Fig. 1.4).

Maintainence

Critically ill children excrete free water poorly. Good humidification in modern ventilator circuits reduces insensible losses to low levels. Therefore fluid therapy must balance the risk of water overload and hyponatraemia with risk of intravascular fluid depletion.

A typical postoperative regimen for a child outside the neonatal period would be 60 mL/kg/day of 0.45% saline + 2.5% dextrose on day 0 and day 1. Colloid boluses can then be given if there is evidence of poor perfusion. Depending on fluid balance measurements, this might be increased to 80 mL/kg/day subsequently.

Communication

Effective intensive care requires clear lines of responsibility and communication between professionals and with families.

In most units, intensive care staff assume overall clinical responsibility for cases but actively involve specialist staff around relevant cases. Collaborative decision making in paediatric and especially neonatal surgery is fundamental.

All staff have a responsibility to consider the child's best interests at all times. On ICUs there is the constant challenge that technically possible treatment options may not always be in a child's interest due to a low probability of success, invasiveness, or a risk of an unacceptably low subsequent quality of life. Guidance from the RCPCH (2004) *Withholding or Withdrawing Life Sustaining Treatment in Children* (2nd edn) should be considered in such cases.

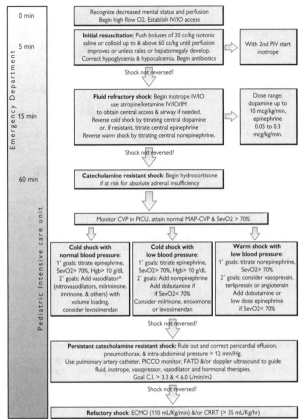

Fig 1.4 Stepwise management of hemodynamic support in infants and children. Taken from Carcillo et al. *Clinical practice parameters for hemodynamic support of pediatric and neonatal patients in septic shock* Care Med 2002;**30**:1365–78, with permission.

Sepsis

Introduction

Sepsis remains a leading cause of morbidity and mortality in children (e.g. 7% of all deaths among children in USA were sepsis related).

Definitions

- Sepsis = inflammation + evidence or suspicion of microbial invasion
- Severe sepsis = sepsis + organ dysfunction
- Septic shock = sepsis + hypotension despite adequate fluid resuscitation (After Goldsten *et al.* 2005).

In severe sepsis, organ dysfunction includes sepsis plus one of the following:
- Cardiovascular organ dysfunction
- Acute respiratory distress syndrome (ARDS)
- Or two or more organ dysfunctions (respiratory, renal, neurological, haematological, or hepatic)

In septic shock, infection is associated with hypotension in spite of an adequate fluid administration($\geq$40 mL/kg in 1h). Severe sepsis in childhood is often referred to as SIRS (paediatric systemic inflammatory response syndrome). The physiological variables change with age and age-specific interpretation of vital signs and laboratory data is required. SIRS must have two of the following four criteria, one of which must be abnormal temperature or leucocyte count.
- Core temperature >38.5°C or <36°C
- Tachycardia (HR > 2 SD for age)
- Tachypnoea (mean respiratory rate > 2 SD for age)
- Leucocyte count elevated or depressed for age or >10% immature cells

Septic shock can also can also be described as fluid refractory or inotrope refractory.

Three populations at risk

While health is no defence, and severe sepsis can complicate trivial wounds, inherent susceptibility to certain pathogens (e.g. *pneumococcus*) and certain genetic profiles (1b-511 homozygosity) are emerging. Susceptibility profiles might include:
- **Phagocytic defects,** e.g. chronic granulomatous disease, myeloperoxidase deficiency, leukocyte adhesion molecule deficiency
- **Primary** immunodeficiency
- **Acquired** immunodeficiency, e.g. cancer patients, transplant patients, post-splenectomy, HIV-1, HIV-2, steroids

Clinical features

Sepsis is a clinical diagnosis characterized by the classical triad of fever, tachycardia, and vasodilatation. Signs are highly variable and depend upon host resistance, the inoculum dose, and the subsequent response. Shock occurs before hypertension in children, and the following are clinical signs of septic shock:
- tachycardia and decreased peripheral pulses
- altered alertness

- flash capillary refill or capillary refill >2s
- mottled cool extremities
- decreased urine output.

The classical triad of septic shock includes:

- hypothermia or hyperthermia
- altered mental status
- peripheral vasodilatation (warm shock)/cool extremities (cold shock).

Pathophysiology

In children, septic shock is associated with severe hypotension (in adults it is associated with myocardial dysfunction and vasomotor paralysis) and children respond well to aggressive volume resuscitation (e.g. 60 mL/kg in the first hour). Oxygen delivery (not oxygen extraction) is a major determinant of prognosis.

Treatment

Antibiotics

The crucial element in effective treatment is prompt and appropriate empiric antimicrobial therapy guided by clinical diagnosis, susceptibility of patient (if any), and knowledge of local bacterial sensitivities. Early administration (<4 h from admission) reduces mortality and length of stay.

Intravenous fluids

The colloid versus crystalloid controversy is unresolved in children. Fluid is given in boluses of 20 mL/kg titrated against cardiac output (heart rate, urine output, capillary refill, level of consciousness), in an attempt to optimize perfusion pressure (mean arterial pressure – central venous pressure).

Oxygen delivery

Oxygen delivery = cardiac output (CO) x blood oxygen content

where,

Blood oxygen content = [Hb bound + dissolved in plasma]

$(1.36 \times Hb$ (in g/dl) $\times O_2$ saturation (as decimal)) + $(PaO_2 \times 0.0003)$
(NB: PaO_2 is relatively unimportant compared to O_2 saturation)

Monitoring

- Oximetry and ECG
- Blood pressure and temperature
- Urine output
- Plasma glucose and calcium
- CVP and intra-arterial monitoring should be used in fluid refractory shock. SVC oxygen saturation >70% is associated with good outcome. Pulmonary artery catheter placement is restricted to fluid refractory and dopamine refractory shock.

Vasopressor therapy
- Dopamine remains the first-line vasopressor
  - 2–5 microgram/kg/min ('renal dose', dopaminergic receptors)
  - 10–15 microgram/kg/min (+ve inotropic, β agonist)
- Dobutamine, selective β_1 agonist
  - 5–20 microgram/kg/min
- Adrenaline (epinephrine) acts on α and β_1 adrenergic receptors
  - 2 microgram/kg/min (starting), reducing to 0.1–1microgram/kg/min
- Noradrenaline (norepinephrine) acts on α (especially) and β receptors, and increases peripheral resistance, thereby countacting vasodilatation seen in sepsis
  - 0.05–1 microgram/kg/min

Some authors recommend low-dose adrenaline as the first-line choice for cold hypodynamic shock (10 microgram/kg/min) and noradrenaline for warm shock.

Vasodilator therapy
May be indicated in hypovolemic shock with high systemic vascular resistance. Newer agents (e.g. the phosphodiesterase inhibitors, amrinone and milrinone) are probably better than older agents (e.g. sodium nitroprusside). Inhaled nitric oxide may also be used in septic shock.

Steroid treatment
- 1–2 mg/kg or 50 mg IV hydrocortisone (controversial)

This has been suggested in children with adrenal insufficiency, catecholamine-resistant shock, history of steroid use, and purpura fulminans (widespread skin lesions associated with disseminated intravascular coagulation associated with meningococcal or streptococcal infection).

Other agents and modalities
Use of recombinant activated protein C (Xigris®), anti-TNFα and anti-lipopolysaccharide monoclonal antibodies have been reported, but there is a lack real evidence of efficacy in children. High-volume haemofiltration may also have a role.

Outcomes
Outcome is dependent on early aggressive treatment with mortality strongly associated with the number of failed organs.

Further reading

Carcillo JA, Fields AI. Clinical practice parameters for haemodynamic support of pediatric and neonatal patients in septic shock. *Crit Care Med* 2002;**30**:1365–78.

Goldstein B, Giroir B, Randolph A. International pediatric sepsis consensus conference: definitions for sepsis and organ dysfunction in pediatrics. *Pediatr Crit Care Med* 2005;**6**:2–8.

Watson RS, Carcillo JA, Linde- Zwirble WT *et al.* The epidemiology of severe sepsis in children in the USA. *Am J Respir Crit Care Med* 2003;**167**:695–701.

Antibiotics and children

> **Box 1.3 The discovery of penicillin**
>
> Credited to Alexander Fleming (1881–1955) working at St Mary's Hospital, London, who identified antibacterial properties of the fungus *Penicillium notatum*. in 1928. Howard Florey (1898–1968) and Ernst Chain (1906–1969) isolated and purified it. They shared the Nobel prize for medicine in 1945.

Penicillin-derived antibiotics (Box 1.3)

Benzyl penicillin – or G, parenteral only
Phenoxymethyl penicillin or V, oral only

Has limited indications nowadays, because of widespread resistance (due to β-lactamase). The only remaining organisms which retain sensitivity include *Streptococcal* spp., *Clostridial* spp. *Neissera* spp. and *Leptospira*. Thus the remaining indications focus on postnatal Gp B streptoccocci of maternal origin; treatment and prevention of tetanus, gas gangrene, and pneumococcal meningitis (not first-line) and pneumonia.

● Side effect: hypersensitivity (rashes – common, anaphylaxis <0.05%)

Ampicillin/amoxicillin

Extension of spectrum to include some common Gram –ve organisms (e.g. *E. coli* (50% are resistant), *H. influenzae* (15% are resistant). Indications include community-acquired pneumonia, otitis media, pharyngitis, and prophylaxis of endocarditis. Maculopapular rashes are common but are not regarded as hypersensitivity.

Flucloxacillin

Extension of spectrum to include *Staphylococcal* spp. and is acid stable. Indications include soft tissue infection, impetigo, endocarditis, osteomyelitis, Staphylococcal pneumonia etc.

Co-amoxiclav (amoxicillin–clavulanic acid combo)

Potent, broad-spectrum and popular for gastrointestinal surgical prophylaxis. Extends spectrum, because is no longer susceptible to β-lactamase, to include *Staphylococcal* spp., *E. Coli* and anaerobic organisms (e.g. *Bacteroides* spp.). Rare side-effect is cholestatic jaundice.

Antipseudomonal penicillins (e.g. ticarcillin, piperacillin)

Combinations of ticarcillin/clavulanate (Timentin®) and pipericillin and tazobactam (Tazocin®) are used in severe sepsis where pseudomonas a possibility.

Cephalosporins

Based on similar molecule to penicillin (~15% cross-sensitivity). Expressed in terms of generations. So current favourite, cefuroxime, is second generation, while ceftazidime and ceftriaxone are third generation. This tends to imply better activity against Gram −ve organisms at the expense of Gram +ve activity. Mostly parenteral but there are some that are orally available (e.g. cefuroxime axetil, cefalexin, cefradine etc).

Imipenem, meropenem,

These are carbapenems, with a broad spectrum including aerobic and anaerobic organisms. Imipenem is combined with cilastatin as Primaxin®.

Neomycin, gentamicin, netilmicin, amikacin

These are aminoglycosides; all are bacteriocidal and active against some Gram +ve and most Gram −ve organisms. Neomycin is highly toxic but not absorbed and is given orally to alter bowel flora for overgrowth states or as part of a bowel preparation regimen. Gentamicin is the aminoglycoside of choice for severe sepsis, typically involving Gram −ve bacteria (no anaerobic action). Typical side-effects include nephrotoxicity and ototoxicity. Avoid concurrent use with furosemide. Levels required (1 h peak 5–10 mg/L, pre-dose trough < 2mg/L – if multiple daily dose and <1 mg/L if single daily dose).

Erythromycin, clarithromycin, azithromycin

Examples of macrolide antibiotics with similar activity and spectrum to penicillin. Main use of erythromycin is in penicillin sensitivity, and main side effect is GI disturbance. The other two have prolonged half-lives (single daily dose), and activity against NTB.

MRSA antibiotics (vancomycin, teicoplanin, linezolid)

The first two are bacteriocidal glycopeptide antibiotics with broad-spectrum Gram +ve and −ve activity. Used in severe Staphylococcal sepsis. Vancomycin can be given orally as treatment for antibiotic-associated colitis or prophylaxis of NEC. Teicoplanin, has longer duration of action and given as once-daily dose. Linezolid is an oxazolidinone agent effective against MRSA and VRE.

Metronidazole

Active against anaerobic bacteria (e.g. B. fragilis) and protozoa. Common as treatment of, and prophylaxis for, GI sepsis, including Hirschsprung's enterocolitis. Rectal administration as effective as IV. GI side-effects common including nausea, and taste disturbance.

Anti-tuberculous chemotherapy

The current recommendations include a two-phase regimen, consisting of an initial three-drug protocol (two months) and then a more-prolonged two-drug protocol for up to six months in total.

The commonest medications used are rifampicin, isoniazid, pyrazinamide, and ethambutol. Typically these may be given as combinations (e.g. Rifater®) to sustain compliance. Rifampicin and isoniazide are the usual second-phase drugs. Side-effects are common, and some influence use in children (e.g. ethambutol is not recommended for young children because it can cause optic neuritis and the early symptoms may be missed). Rifampicin may cause orange-coloured urine and stain teeth.

Directly observed therapy (DOT) is mechanism to improve complicance, which is the main cause of treatment failure.

Table 1.7 Common antibiotic drug doses in children

	IV	Oral			Frequency
	(mg/kg)	1 m–2 years	2–6 years	6–12 years	
Penicillin G/V	25 mg	62.5 mg	125 mg	250 mg	qds
Amoxicilllin	20–30 mg	62.5 mg	250 mg	500 mg	tds
Co-amoxiclav	30 mg	0.25 mL/kg (125/31)	5 mL (125/31)	5 mL (250/62)	tds
Flucloxacillin	12.5–25 mg	62.5mg	125mg	250mg	qds
Cefuroxime	20 mg	10 mg/kg	125mg	250mg	tds
Ceftazidime	25 mg	–	–	–	tds
Ceftriaxone	50 mg	–	–	–	once daily
Meropenem	10 mg	–	–	–	tds
Gentamicin	2.5 mg	–	–	–	tds
	7 mg	–	–	–	once daily
Metronidazole	7.5 mg	7.5 mg/kg			tds
			250 pr	500 pr	
Erythromycin	12.5 mg	125 mg	250 mg	500 mg	qds
Vancomycin	15 mg	5 mg/kg	5 mg/kg	62.5 mg	tds
Teicoplanin	10 mg (dose 1–3), then 6 – once/day	–	–	–	bd

Abridged from BNF for Children 2006; www.bnfc.org/bnfc NB All IVs are mg/kg; all orals (unless stated) are mg.

Day-case surgery

History

Paediatric day surgery is not new! James Henderson Nicoll (1863–1921) reported on over 6000 cases of day surgery in infants (including cleft lip, pyloric stenosis, talipes, and inguinal hernia) in 1909 performed at the West Graham Street Dispensary, Glasgow.

> Physical and psychological recovery is quicker if children have a short time in hospital and return early to normal family life. Wherever possible, elective surgery in a day-care unit should be considered to avoid admission to hospital.

Environment

The highest standards and efficiency are more likely if a separate paediatric day ward is available. Elective cases should be scheduled on regular dedicated children's theatre lists. Otherwise children must be scheduled for the beginning of lists to facilitate day-case care and minimize pre-operative starvation.

The environment should be child and family friendly, with separate paediatric areas for holding bays and recovery.

Professional staff

Day-case sessions must be staffed by at least two registered children's nurses. Play specialists should be available. Where operations are performed in a day unit, there should be a named paediatrician available for liaison and immediate advice and cover.

The consultant surgeon is responsible for care of the child, although the assessment and conduct of day-case surgery may be undertaken by senior experienced trainees or other career grade surgeons.

An experienced paediatric-trained consultant anaesthetist must be present.

Supporting parents/carers

All children should have been pre-assessed, and the family appropriately prepared for surgery. A two-stage consent process should be in place. Parents should be allowed to accompany their child into the anaesthetic room and recovery area where possible. Starvation periods required are shown in Table 1.8.

Table 1.8 Starvation periods required before surgery

Type of feed	Starvation period (h)
Solids or milk	6
Breast milk	4
Clear fluids	2

Pre-operative care

Topical local anaesthetic cream such as EMLA® (leave for 1 h) or Ametop® (leave for 30 min), or inhalational induction of anaesthesia should be considered to minimize fear of needles.

Postoperative care

Carers should receive clear instructions on follow-up and written information on arrangements to deal with any postoperative emergency (including out-of-hours contact telephone numbers).

Units must have a pain-management policy including advice on pain assessment and management at home and the provision of 'take home' analgesia.

Additional standards for centres undertaking day-case children's surgery *without inpatient paediatrics* include:

- a surgeon experienced in the condition should undertake the surgery
- the surgeon must remain at the hospital until arrangements have been made for the discharge of all patients or (exceptionally) patients been transferred to the surgeon's base hospital
- at least one member of the team involved in treating day cases should hold the APLS/EPLS certificate, and other team members must have up-to-date basic skills for paediatric resuscitation
- at least one member of staff with up-to-date skills in basic paediatric life support should be present while the child is in the unit
- a neighbouring children's service should take formal responsibility for the children being managed in the unit, with agreed and robust arrangements in place for paediatric assistance and transfer if required.

Documentation

The pattern of day-case activity should be audited and regularly reviewed. Clinical governance requires units to develop standards, protocols and audit tools in order to monitor the quality of care. Ensuring that all patient care is clearly and fully documented prior to the child's discharge aids this process.

Indications

Suitability for day-case surgery will be dictated by the need for overnight stay in hospital for postoperative monitoring, pain relief, or care of drains or catheters.

Term infants (<46 weeks post-conceptional age (PCA)) and preterm infants (<60 weeks PCA); infants with anaemia or pre-existing chronic lung disease all need apnoea monitoring overnight following GA and would not be suitable for day surgery.

The following procedures are examples of those generally suitable for day-case surgery, although this may vary according to local protocol.

- Head and neck:
  - epidermoid/dermoid cyst excision
  - preauricular sinus/skin tag excision and pinnaplasty
  - ankyloglossia (tongue-tie) and ranula excision
  - lymph node excision
  - thyroglossal and branchial remnant excision

- Chest wall:
  - removal of Hickman line/Portacath
- Abdomen
  - OGD/oesophageal dilatation
  - hernia (umbilical, epigastric and inguinal)
  - hydrocoele and orchidopexy
- Genitalia
  - preputial stretch and preputioplasty and circumcision
  - minor hypospadias repair
  - cystoscopy
  - separation of labial adhesions
- Anus
  - proctosigmoidoscopy and colonoscopy
  - anal sphincter stretch and sclerotherapy for prolapse
  - fistulo-in-ano and perianal warts excision
- Laparoscopy
  - diagnostic for undescended testis
  - first-stage Fowler–Stephens orchidopexy
  - ligation of varicocoele
- Soft tissue/vascular
  - excision of skin naevi/pilomatrixoma/ebaceous cyst
  - haemangioma/lymphangioma/lipoma excision
- Limbs
  - ganglion excision and supernumerary digit excision
  - correction of ingrown toenails

Further reading

Department of Health. *Day Surgery – operational guide*. London: Department of Health, 2002.

Royal College of Nursing. *Children/Young People in Day Surgery*. London: Royal College of Nursing, 2002.

Royal College of Surgeons of England. *Surgery for Children: Delivering a First Class Service*. Report of the Children's Surgical Forum. London: Royal College of Surgeons of England, 2007. www.rcseng. ac.uk/publications/docs

Walter-Larsen S, Rasmussen LS. The former preterm infant and risk of post-operative apnoea: recommendations for management. *Acta Anaesthesiol Scand* 2006;**50**:888–93.

Pre-assessment

Pre-assessment is the process by which the child and family are prepared physically and psychologically for the child's journey from admission to discharge.

Pre-assessment facilitates a smoother patient- and family-orientated experience and begins before the child is admitted for surgery. It involves direct contact with the day ward and staff who will be looking after the family, as part of an organized pre-admission programme that incorporates many elements of the day-surgery process.

The clearly documented assessment should include:
- decision on fitness for anaesthetic (any concern should be discussed with a consultant paediatric anaesthetist)
- social history (who has parental responsibility for purposes of consent?)
- length of journey time to hospital – should be no longer than 1h
- measurement of weight (for drug dosages)
- baseline pulse oximetry
- pre-operative investigations such as sickle cell test
- explanation of pre- and postoperative care, including negotiation of level of parental involvement (family-centred care)
- assessment of the levels of child and parental anxiety regarding surgery/admission. If the child is very anxious, or phobic about hospitals or needles, sedative premedication or inhalational induction can be discussed.
- explanation of fasting times for surgery
- negotiation of date for surgery with parents, including the possibility of short-notice cancellation appointments
- explanation of what will happen on the day of admission (anaesthetic induction and surgery)
- discussion of pain management and demonstration of pain management tool
- explanation of after care at home (i.e. post-GA care and specific care and treatment, related to type of surgery)
- explanation of how long the child will need to be off school, and when able to return to normal activities, e.g. PE and swimming
- what follow-up appointments will be necessary?
- opportunity for family to ask questions
- informed two-stage consent for the whole experience.

All information should be supported in written form, for the family to refer to at home. A contact phone number should be given so that the family can resolve any questions or concerns that may arise after they have left the hospital.

A pre-operative telephone call, usually on the day before surgery, confirms the family is ready and the child fit and well for surgery. If unfit, a new date can be given at that time. The appointment can then be offered to parents who have expressed their availability to come in at short-notice.

Further reading

NHS Modernisation Agency. *National Good Practice Guidance on Pre-operative Assessment for Day Surgery.* London: Department of Health, 2002.

The neurologically impaired child

This group of children makes up a significant population of the paediatric surgical workload and can pose major medical, surgical, and ethical challenges.

Optimization of pre-operative status, with sound peri-operative principles and comprehensive postoperative care will maximize the chances of a good outcome.

Is the procedure necessary?

It is vital that these children are adequately investigated (but not over-investigated) to ensure that a surgical intervention or a concomitant procedures is actually required (e.g. is a feeding gastrostomy required, in addition, to fundoplication in a child with symptomatic gastro-oesophageal reflux?).

Medical

Multidisciplinary team approach:
- early involvement of all relevant teams pre-operatively (e.g. neurology for anti-epileptics review, respiratory for chest assessment, cardiology imaging if known cardiac anomaly, renal, and haematology)
- physiotherapy assessment
- dietician review

Surgical

Multidisciplinary team approach:
- surgeon
- anaesthetist
- other surgical specialties if joint procedure

Postoperative course

- Enable clear communication between surgeon and nursing team. Ensure appropriate analgesia and good pressure-area care.
- Involve physiotherapist to expedite mobilization and clear chest secretions.
- Maintain nutrition status.

Other issues

- Consent (ethical considerations, resuscitation orders)
- Maintain effective communication with parents, other members of team and other teams
- Early discharge planning
- Psychosocial support for child and parents (if appropriate).
- Community support (GP, local paediatric service, specialist nurse, community nurse)

Nutrition in the surgical patient

The optimum nutrition is oral enteral feeding, however, artificial enteral feeding or parenteral nutrition (PN) may be required if adequate oral feeds cannot be tolerated.

Artificial enteral feeding

Indications

- Immaturity of swallowing (e.g. prematurity)
- Delayed gastric emptying
- Gastroesophageal reflux
- Impaired intestinal motility
- Crohn's disease
- Neurological or metabolic co-morbidity
- Intensive care

Route

- Nasogastric, orogastric, or jejunal tubes
- Gastrostomy or jejunostomy tubes

Gastric feeding is preferred, and transpyloric feeds are restricted to patients who: (i) cannot tolerate gastric feeds; (ii) are at increased risk of aspiration; or (iii) have anatomical contraindications to gastric feeds. Combination oral and enteral feeds, and either bolus or continuous feeds are used depending on clinical condition and tolerance. In patients requiring long-term gastric tube feeding, a gastrostomy is advisable – open, laparoscopic or percutaneous endoscopic (PEG).

Enteral feeds are optimally breast or artificial formula milk for neonates and infants. A variety of other enteral formulae is available, including protein hydrolysates and modular feeds, and choice depends on age, nutritional status, fluid tolerance and underlying disease. The aim is to achieve an appropriate caloric intake for age (Table 1.9).

Complications

- Vomiting
- Mechanical – tube displacement, occlusion
- Perforation
- GI complications, such as reflux, aspiration pneumonia, dumping syndrome, and diarrhoea.
- Infection – of feed, tube, or gastrostomy/jejunostomy site.

Parenteral nutrition

Indications

- Post-operative ileus
- Mechanical obstruction/atresia
- Intestinal ischaemia
- Necrotizing enterocolitis
- Short bowel syndrome
- Other gastroenterological problems, e.g. malabsorption, intractable diarrhoea or vomiting, inflammatory bowel disease
- Respiratory co-morbidity

PN should be given for the shortest period of time possible and the proportion of nutrition given enterally increased as tolerated. Energy reserves are such that stable term infants can tolerate 3–4 days without enteral feeds, and older children 7–10 days, before starting PN, if it is anticipated that enteral nutrition may be resumed within this time. Premature neonates have smaller energy reserves and the time before introducing PN is much shorter.

Route

PN must be administered via centrally placed catheters (including peripherally inserted central catheters (i.e. PICC lines), surgically placed central catheters, or centrally-placed umbilical catheters), as peripheral administration gives significant risk of complications from hyperosmolar glucose. Central catheter choice depends on catheters already in place, and the length of time over which PN is anticipated.

PN should include:

- carbohydrate (up to 18 g/kg/day in infants <10 kg, up to 12 g/kg/day in older children)
- lipid emulsion (up to 3 g/kg/day)
- amino acids (up to 3 g/kg/day in infants, and 1.5–2.0 g/kg/day in older children)
- electrolytes
  - sodium 2–4 mmol/kg/day infants, 1–3 mmol/kg/day in children
  - potassium 0–3 mmol/kg/day
  - other electrolytes (chloride, calcium, phosphate) are very dependent on the clinical condition of the patient and technical pharmacy aspects of stability and compounding
- Vitamins – are added to PN, usually as commercial available mixtures (e.g. Vitlipid N® for fat-soluble vitamins and Solivito N® for water-soluble vitamins)
  - lipid-soluble vitamins – D, A, K, E
  - water-soluble vitamins (vitamin B complex, C, pantothenate, biotin and folic acid)
  - iron and trace elements (zinc, copper, manganese, selenium, fluoride, and iodide) are usually added to PN if longer than a few days' duration. Available as commercial mixtures (e.g. Peditrace®)
- water is necessary to decrease osmolality of the solution; the quantity depends on the fluid status of the patient
- glutamine – there has been much interest in the use of glutamine, which may decrease infective complications and speed recovery of full enteral function. It is not contained in current PN amino acid mixtures, but can be added to PN, or given as a separate infusion (e.g. Dipeptiven®).

The caloric requirement of a PN-fed patient is approximately 10–20% lower than that of enterally fed patients because stool and other losses are minimal. PN is usually given 24 h a day, but with a 4 h suspension of lipid infusion to allow triglyceride clearance.

Complications
- Mechanical catheter complications, e.g. thrombosis, incorrect position/ displacement etc
- Metabolic, e.g. hyperglycaemia or hypoglycaemia, hypertriglyceridaemia, electrolyte alterations
- Fluid overload, e.g. oedema, failure of closure of PDA
- Infection – catheter, bacterial translocation etc
- Cholestasis – requires long-term PN, and immature liver

Table 1.9 Suggested calorific intake in children

Age of child	Target caloric intake (kcal/kg/day)	
	Males	Females
Premature	110–120	110–120
0–1 month	113	107
1–3 months	100	97
3 months –1 year	80	80
1–4 years	82	78
5–8 years	73	70
9–13 years	64	58
14–18 years	53	47

Monitoring
Careful monitoring of patients on PN is mandatory. This is particularly important during the period over which PN is introduced. Full blood count, electrolytes, blood gases, urea/creatinine, glucose, calcium/phosphate, albumin, liver function tests (especially bilirubin), and cholesterol/triglycerides should all be monitored, together with vitamins and trace elements for long-term PN patients.

PN should not be a 'one size fits all' prescription, but individual tailoring is recommended, dependent on clinical status, monitoring results and introduction of enteral nutrition.

Further reading
Goulet O, Colomb V. Enteral nutrition. In: Guandalini S (ed). *Textbook of Pediatric Gastroenterology and Nutrition*. London: Taylor and Francis, 2004, pp539–54.

Goulet O, Hunt J et al. Koletzko B et al. Guidelines on paediatric parenteral nutrition. ESPGHAN, ESPEN, ESPR. *J Pediatr Gastroenterol Nutr* 2005;**41**(Suppl 2): S1–S87.

Vascular access

Peripheral cannulae

In most children, 22-gauge cannulae are adequate, 24-gauge in infants. The dorsum of the non-dominant hand is the most common site, but the palmar aspect of the wrist, long saphenous vein (anterior to the medial malleolus), lateral aspect of the foot, scalp veins, and the antecubital fossa are also useful. Cannulae at the latter two sites are difficult to fix. Venous distension can be achieved by a tourniquet (or assistant), heating with a warm towel, application of glyceryl trinitrate patch, hanging the limb over the side of the bed, or asking the child to clench his or her fist. Cold-light fibreoptic transillumination may also facilitate puncture. Cutdown to a peripheral vein is rarely necessary. Cannulae are inappropriate for long-term access or for infusion of certain drugs.

Umbilical vein access

This is usually easy in the first days of life. The vein is larger and has a thinner wall than the arteries, and is usually found at the 12 o'clock position.

Peripherally inserted central venous catheters (PICCs)

Neonatal long lines (2–3 Fg) can be threaded to a central position through a peripheral cannula. The tip should be left outside the pericardial reflection to decrease the risk of tamponade. In older children, 3–6 Fg PICCs are usually inserted through a peel-away sheath in an upper limb vein. The tip should be left in the superior vena cava or upper right atrium.

Central vein puncture

Internal jugular veins are the best site with ultrasound-guided puncture replacing the landmark technique and cut-down. Potential advantages include safety, success rate and ease of training.

Central venous access devices

Short catheters

These include temporary haemodialysis catheters and are inserted directly over a guidewire, when the expected duration of use is less than about ten days.

Hickman (Broviac) catheters (e.g. 2.7–12 Fg)

These have one to three lumens, and are tunnelled to a remote exit site. A tissue ingrowth cuff decreases the risks of accidental removal and infection. The tip should be left in the upper right atrium. This seems to reduce the risk of thrombosis without causing tamponade (unlike neonatal long lines), and allows for growth.

Long-term haemodialysis catheters

These are similar to above, but have two lumens with offset openings.

Venous port devices

These have a central venous catheter connected to a subcutaneous reservoir, which is accessed with a non-coring needle. Ports are less restrictive for the child, and infection is less common than with Hickman catheters.

Complications

Significant procedural complications are rare when ultrasound is used (Fig 1.5):

- exit site and wound infections (~1% of procedures)
- catheter-related bacteriaemia – depends on the indication for insertion, ~1 per 1000 catheter days. Treatment is with intravenous antibiotics (according to sensitivities from blood culture) but catheter removal maybe required
- blocked catheters – may be treated with alteplase, recombinant tissue plasminogen activator, 2 mg/2mL/two doses – ~80% success) or urokinase, e.g. 5–10,000 u/2mL.

Alternative venous access methods

These include use of collateral veins, recanalization of occluded veins, and surgical insertion into the right atrium. In emergencies, an intraosseous needle can be inserted into the tibia. In extreme emergency, the superior sagittal sinus can be punctured in an infant with an open anterior fontanelle.

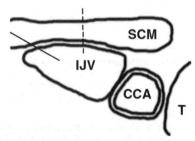

Fig. 1.5 Ultrasound-guided puncture. Transverse section of the right neck as viewed from below (i.e. as seen with ultrasound). Small high-frequency (>7 MHz) linear array probes are essential in children. The right internal jugular vein (IJV) is lateral to the right common carotid artery (CCA). It is less circular in cross-section and has a thinner wall. If in doubt, Doppler ultrasound (colour or pulsed wave) can be used. The vein can be punctured from an anterolateral (solid line) or anterior (dotted line) approach. SCM = sternocleido mastoid

Further reading

Blaney M, Shen V, Kerner JA et al. Alteplase for the treatment of central venous catheter occlusion in children: results of a prospective, open-label, single-arm study (The Cathflo Activase Pediatric Study). *J Vasc Interv Radiol* 2006;**17**:1745–51.

Radiology

X-ray techniques

Plain radiographs

These are most useful for evaluation of the lungs and bones. In the abdomen, plain films are often regarded as the best first imaging test, particularly for bowel obstruction or perforation, but are gradually being replaced for some indications such as necrotizing enterocolitis, and are already obsolete for others, such as abdominal masses.

Contrast studies

These remain useful for some purposes, including evaluation of swallowing or neonatal bowel obstruction, and in children with suspected malrotation. The standard radio-opaque contrast medium for GI studies is barium sulfate suspension. This is cheap and has no systemic absorption. It should not be used if there is a significant risk of perforation, as it causes chemical peritonitis, but aspiration into the airway is safe in small quantities. Various preparations of water-soluble (iodinated) contrast are available. Isotonic or near-isotonic preparations are used for both upper- and lower-GI studies. Significant systemic absorption can occur in neonates. High iso-molality contrast (Gastrografin®) can be used to treat meconium ileus, but care should be taken to avoid hypovolaemia due to fluid shift into the bowel. It should not be used for upper GI studies as aspiration can cause severe pulmonary oedema. Air (or carbon dioxide) can be used as negative (or double) contrast. Air insufflation is commonly used for reduction of intussusception.

Computed tomography (CT)

This is often used for chest and abdominal imaging in children, but its use is limited by radiation dose considerations. CT is the most accurate imaging technique for evaluation of the lungs. Multidetector CT technology has reduced the need for sedation or anaesthesia for scanning in children.

Ultrasound techniques

Sonography is increasingly important in paediatric imaging because of its portability, patient acceptability and lack of adverse effects. Although it is rarely useful for lung disease it has applications in the neck, mediastinum, body wall and pleura, abdomen, and pelvis and limbs. It is particularly useful for solid organs, where it may be complementary to other cross-sectional techniques. Doppler techniques allow accurate estimation of the direction and velocity of blood flow.

Magnetic resonance imaging (MRI)

Future technical developments are likely to increase the use of MRI for body imaging at the expense of CT and nuclear medicine. MRI does not use ionizing radiation and therefore does not increase the risk of the child developing cancer in the future. The soft tissue contrast is superior to that of CT. Various imaging sequences are available, depending on the clinical indication. T_1-weighted images show fat, recent haemorrhage and contrast agents containing gadolinium as high signal (bright). T_2-weighted images show fat, most body fluids and tissue with a high water content (i.e. most important pathology) as high signal. In addition to standard cross-sectional images, MRI can generate renal function studies, cholangiograms, and numerous other applications.

Nuclear medicine

The role of nuclear medicine is slowly changing. Already some of the standard scintigraphic techniques such as bone and renal scans are being replaced by MRI. Labelled red cell or white cell scans are still useful in some children, as is the pertechnetate scan for suspected Meckel's diverticulum. Future growth in nuclear medicine is likely to occur in functional imaging, particularly positron emission tomography (PET) with [^{18}F]-fluorodeoxyglucose (FDG), which detects the dependency of certain cells on anaerobic glycolysis, and is therefore highly sensitive (but not 100% specific) for malignancy.

Radiation risk

Children are particularly sensitive to ionizing radiation, and most expect to have a long life in which to develop cancer, which is the most important adverse effect of diagnostic x-ray exposure. The radiation doses of the various investigations vary significantly between children of different sizes and at different centres, but approximate values are given in the Table 1.10. In general, paediatric centres are better at minimizing the dose given to children. Estimates of risk of fatal cancer induction are uncertain.

Table 1.10 Dosage equivalents

Test	Effective dose (mSv)	Equivalent in chest x-rays	Lifetime risk of fatal malignancy
Wrist x-ray	0.001	0.1	1×10^{-7}
Frontal chest x-ray	0.01	1	1×10^{-6}
Voiding cystogram	2	200	2×10^{-4}
Barium meal	3	300	3×10^{-4}
CT chest	2–3	200–300	2.5×10^{-4}
CT abdomen and pelvis	3–5	300–500	4×10^{-4}
Nuclear medicine bone scan	4	400	4×10^{-4}
FDG-PET	10	1000	1×10^{-3}

Fetal medicine

Fetal screening

Fetal chromosomal abnormalities are found in about 1 in 300 pregnancies. The most common is trisomy 21, which accounts for about half of the cases. The other common abnormalities are trisomies 18 and 13.

Screening for chromosomal defects:

Every pregnant woman carries a risk that her fetus has a chromosomal defect. In order to calculate an individual patient-specific risk, it is necessary to take into account the background or a priori risk, which depends on maternal age, and multiply this by a series of factors or likelihood ratios, which depend on the results of a series of screening tests carried out during the course of the pregnancy.

In the first-trimester of pregnancy, chromosomally abnormal pregnancies are associated with the sonographic finding of increased subcutaneous accumulation of fluid in the neck region (nuchal translucency, Fig. 2.1) and the biochemical finding of altered maternal serum concentration of the placental products of free ß-human chorionic gonadotropin (β-HCG) and pregnancy associated placental protein-A (PAPP-A).

In the second-trimester, many chromosomally abnormal fetuses have sonographically detectable defects, such as diaphragmatic hernia, oesophageal atresia or exomphalos, and altered concentrations of maternal serum free ß-HCG, estriol, and alpha feto protein (AFP).

Screening by a combination of maternal age, fetal nuchal translucency and serum free ß-HCG and PAPP-A at 11–13 weeks of gestation identifies about 90% of major chromosomal abnormalities at a screen-positive rate of 5%. With second-trimester biochemical screening the detection rate is about 65% at a screen-positive rate of 5%. The performance of screening by ultrasound alone has not been investigated systematically.

Diagnosis of chromosomal defects

This requires cytogenetic analysis:
- **chorionic villous sampling** (CVS) – obtained from the placenta at 11–13 weeks
- **amniocentesis** – from amniotic fluid obtained at 16–20 weeks
- **cordocentesis** from fetal blood obtained usually > 20 weeks.

In each case a needle is introduced through the maternal abdomen into the uterus under ultrasound guidance.

The risk of miscarriage from each of these invasive tests is around 1%.

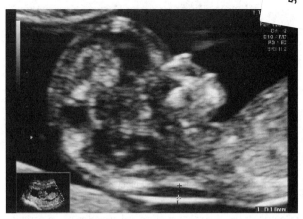

Fig. 2.1 Sagittal section of fetal head and neck. Crosses indicate increased nuchal translucency.

Fetal diagnosis – magnetic resonance imaging

Prenatal ultrasound with its wide availability, general acceptance, low cost and real-time properties remains the screening investigation of choice in fetal medicine. Interest in prenatal magnetic resonance imaging (MRI) is rising because of the absence of known biological risks and the recent availability of fast imaging sequences allowing superb contrast resolution in imaging the fetal brain but also other soft tissue structures.

The indications for fetal MRI are expanding. At present, specific indications for fetal MRI are threefold as itemized under the following headings.

Fetal brain abnormalities

Abnormalities such as mild lateral cerebral ventriculomegaly (transverse diameter of 10–12 mm). Fetal MRI provides additional information in nearly 6% of cases with isolated ventriculomegaly as diagnosed by ultrasound, half of them being cell migration and organization disorders, and the other half are cavitations of the white matter, agenesis of the corpus callosum, intraventricular haemorrhage and anomalies of the posterior fossa.

Congenital diaphragmatic hernia

MRI allows measurement of total fetal lung volume in the prediction of pulmonary hypoplasia in CDH. Fetal lungs are filled with fluid and easily seen on MRI because of the contrast with the surrounding structures (Fig. 2.2). MRI can visualize both the ipsilateral and contralateral lungs and measure these reliably, whereas with ultrasound it is not possible to examine the ipsilateral lungs in nearly half of the cases. Whether the prediction of postnatal outcome is superior by MRI rather than by the simple measurement on two- or three-dimensional ultrasound still needs further investigation. MRI should therefore be limited to referral centres conducting research for such indications.

Postmortem fetal MRI

This is another gradually expanding indication. In nearly half of the cases of fetal death, parents decline conventional necropsy to save the integrity of their child. Postmortem autopsy is an acceptable alternative since it provides comparable diagnostic utility to that obtained by necropsy for most organs such as the brain, skeleton, thoracic organs except the heart, abdominal organs except the pancreas, ureters, bladder, and genitals. It can also be particularly useful for the central nervous system where practical difficulties with handling unfixed tissues arise.

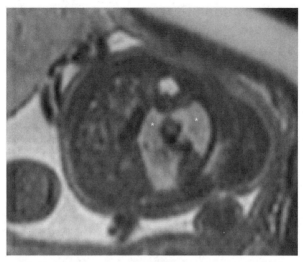

Fig. 2.2 T$_2$-weighted MR image in an axial view of a left-sided congenital diaphragmatic hernia at 29 weeks and 2 days of gestation clearly showing both lungs (*) due to the difference in contrast with the surrounding structures.

Cardiac anomalies

Abnormalities of the heart and great arteries are the most common congenital abnormalities. In general, about half are either lethal or require surgery, and half are asymptomatic.

Incidence

Cardiovascular abnormalities are found in 5–10 per 1000 live births and in about 30 per 1000 stillbirths.

Aetiology

The aetiology of heart defects is heterogeneous and probably depends on the interplay of multiple genetic and environmental factors, including maternal diabetes mellitus or collagen disease, exposure to drugs such as lithium, and viral infections such as rubella. Specific mutant gene defects and chromosomal abnormalities account for less than 5% of the patients. Heart defects are found in more than 90% of fetuses with trisomy 18 or 13, 50% of those with trisomy 21, and 40% of those with Turner's syndrome, deletions, or partial trisomies involving a variety of chromosomes.

When a previous sibling has had a congenital heart defect, in the absence of a known genetic syndrome, the risk of recurrence is about 2%, and with two affected siblings the risk is 10%. When the father is affected, the risk for the offspring is about 2%, and if the mother is affected the risk is about 10%.

Reliability of prenatal diagnosis

Echocardiography has been successfully applied to the prenatal assessment of fetal cardiac function and structure, and has led to the diagnosis of most cardiac abnormalities. Studies from specialist centres report the diagnosis of about 90% of defects. However, the majority of such studies refer to the prenatal diagnosis of moderate to major defects in high-risk populations.

Screening for cardiac abnormalities

The main challenge in prenatal diagnosis is to identify the high-risk group for referral to specialist centres. The indications include congenital cardiac defects in one of the parents or previous pregnancies, maternal diabetes mellitus, or ingestion of teratogenic drugs. However, more than 90% of fetuses with cardiac defects are from families without such risk factors. A higher sensitivity is achieved by examination of the four-chamber view of the heart at the routine 20-week scan; screening studies have reported the detection of about 30% of major cardiac defects. Recent evidence suggests that a higher sensitivity (more than 50%) can be achieved by referral for specialist echocardiography of patients with increased nuchal translucency at 11–13 weeks.

Lung anomalies

The most common fetal lung lesions are congenital diaphragmatic hernia, pleural effusions, congenital cystic adenomatoid malformation (CAM) (Fig. 2.3), pulmonary sequestration (PS) and congenital high airway obstruction syndrome (CHAOS).

In CHAOS, due to laryngeal and/or tracheal atresia, the massively enlarged lungs result in cardiac and superior mediastinal compression with secondary progressive hydrops and fetal or neonatal death. Inevitably, in the majority of antenatally diagnosed cases the parents choose the option of pregnancy termination. In the few cases where therapeutic interventions were undertaken either prenatally or during delivery by EXIT, some of the babies survived. However, these babies often have other serious abnormalities such as Fraser syndrome or chronic respiratory morbidity and in most of the reported cases there are no data on long-term prognosis.

In pulmonary sequestration, a portion of lung parenchyma is directly supplied by an aberrant branch of the aorta rather than by a branch of the pulmonary artery. In the vast majority of cases there is no obvious connection with the tracheo-bronchial tree. Ultrasound examination demonstrates a uniformly echogenic lesion with or without an associated pleural effusion, and with colour Doppler it is possible to visualize the systemic arterial blood supply arising from the aorta. In the cases with no pleural effusions expectant management is associated with excellent survival, and in about half of the fetuses the lesion regresses antenatally with, perhaps, no need for postnatal surgery. In the cases with pleural effusions the condition may progress to hydrops and perinatal death. Effective antenatal intervention is provided by occlusion of the feeding vessel at the hilus of the tumour by ultrasound-guided laser coagulation or the injection of a sclerosant agent.

In CAM, prenatal diagnosis is based on the demonstration of a uniformly hyperechogenic mass (microcystic), echo-free cysts (macrocystic), or a multicystic tumour with echogenic stroma (mixed type), usually involving one lobe of the lungs. The macrocystic and mixed types usually persist throughout pregnancy and necessitate postnatal thoracotomy and lobectomy. Cases with a large cyst causing a major mediastinal shift can be treated successfully by placement of a thoraco-amniotic shunt.

In the case of microcystic CAM with no hydrops, the survival rate is more than 95% without the need for antenatal intervention. In about half of the cases there is antenatal resolution of the hyperechogenic lesion, usually at around 32 weeks of gestation. In about 70% of these cases with antenatal resolution, no lesion can be demonstrated postnatally and it is possible that at least in some of these the underlying cause may not be CAM but rather a transient bronchial tree obstruction with retention of mucoid fluid distal to the obstruction. In contrast, in more than 95% of cases with prenatal persistence of the hyperechogenic lesion, postnatal imaging confirms the presence of CAM.

In CAM with hydrops managed expectantly, the babies usually die before or after birth. Open fetal surgery with lobectomy could improve survival, but such treatment has not been accepted widely because it is highly invasive for the mother. The extent to which the less-invasive approach of ultrasound-guided laser coagulation of the vascular supply to the tumour could improve survival, merits further investigation.

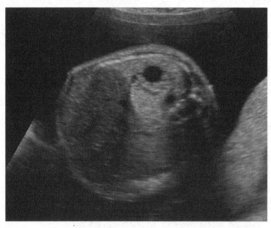

Fig. 2.3 Fetus at 26 weeks of gestation. Axial view demonstrating a congenital diaphragmatic hernia and a macrocystic congenital cystic adenomatoid malformation of the contralateral lung.

Congenital diaphragmatic hernia

This is a simple defect in the diaphragm that leads to impaired lung development. The condition, which is sporadic with unknown etiology, is found in 1 in 4000 births. In about half of the cases, there are associated structural, chromosomal or syndromic anomalies (e.g. Pallister–Killian, Fryns). In isolated CDH fetuses, non-survivors usually succumb to the consequences of pulmonary hypoplasia and pulmonary hypertension.

Ultrasound screening allows diagnosis of CDH prior to birth. The prenatal prediction of pulmonary hypoplasia and consequently of postnatal survival relies on the two-dimensional measurement of the lung-to-head area circumference ratio (LHR) and intrathoracic position of the liver (Fig. 2.4).

In fetuses with LHR < 1.0 and intrathoracic liver, survival rate in expectantly managed cases is less than 10%. In such cases, prenatal intervention is an option.

Criteria for *in utero* intervention
- Isolated CDH
- LHR < 1.0 and the liver herniated into the thorax

Fetoscopic endoluminal tracheal occlusion (FETO)
- Performed under local or regional anesthesia.
- Intramuscular injection is given to the fetus, containing pancuronium (0.2 mg/kg), atropine (20 microgram/kg), and fentanyl (15 microgram/kg).
- An endoscope is introduced through the maternal abdomen into the uterus, then over the fetal tongue into the oropharynx and then through the vocal cords into the trachea (Fig. 2.5).
- A detachable latex balloon is inflated to 0.8 mL and left in situ from about 26 to 34 weeks of gestation.

Reversal of tracheal occlusion
- Achieved by fetal tracheoscopy, or by *in utero* ultrasound-guided balloon puncture.
- In case of advanced labour and premature birth before balloon removal, the balloon can be removed either by tracheoscopy after clamping of the umbilical cord or punctured with a 20G needle inserted through the neck in the midline just under the cricoid cartilage.
- *Ex utero* intrapartum therapy (EXIT) is another alternative but has a high maternal morbidity.

Results
Postnatal survival rates after FETO is about 50% and the rate depends on the pre-FETO lung size as assessed by LHR (Fig. 2.4).

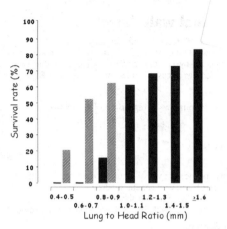

Fig. 2.4 Survival rate according to the fetal lung-area-to-head circumference ratio in expectantly managed fetuses with isolated left-sided diaphragmatic hernia with intra-thoracic herniation of the liver (black bars). Same with FETO (shaded bars).

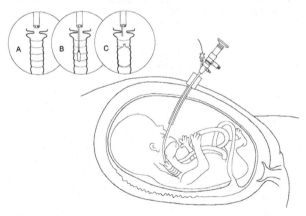

Fig. 2.5 Schematic illustration of the FETO procedure: through a small cut in the mother's abdomen, a small camera is introduced into the mouth of the unborn baby and a balloon is delivered in the trachea.

Abdominal wall defects

At 8–10 weeks, all fetuses demonstrate herniation of the mid-gut in the base of the umbilical cord, and retraction into the abdominal cavity is normally completed by 11 weeks and 5 days. There are four types of abdominal wall defects as discussed under the following headings.

Exomphalos

This results from failure of regression of the mid-gut into the abdominal coelom.

Incidence
- 1 in 4000 births

Aetiology
- Majority are sporadic with a recurrence risk less than 1%.
- May be associated with genetic syndromes.
- Trisomy 13 or 18 is found in about 50% of cases.
- Possible association with Beckwith–Wiedemann syndrome.

Prenatal diagnosis
Diagnosis is based on the demonstration of the mid-line anterior abdominal wall defect, the herniated sac with its visceral contents, and the umbilical cord insertion at the apex of the sac.

Prognosis
- This is a correctable malformation and survival mainly depends on the presence of associated anomalies.
- In isolated cases, survival after surgery is about 90%.

Gastroschisis

Results from evisceration of the intestine through a small abdominal wall defect located just lateral and usually to the right of an intact umbilical cord (Fig. 2.6).

Incidence
- 1 in 4000 births

Aetiology:
- This is a sporadic condition of unknown aetiology.
- Associated anomalies are rare.

Prenatal diagnosis
Diagnosis is based on the demonstration of the normally situated umbilicus and the herniated loops of intestines, which are free-floating and widely separated.

Prognosis
- Postoperative survival is about 90%.
- Mortality is usually the consequence of short gut syndrome.

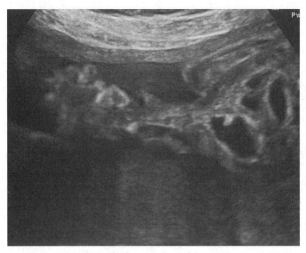

Fig. 2.6 Fetus at 23 weeks of gestation. Image of a gastroschisis demonstrating herniated loops of intestine, free-floating in the amniotic fluid.

Body stalk anomaly

This is characterized by the presence of a major abdominal wall defect, severe kyphoscoliosis and a rudimentary umbilical cord.

Incidence
- 1 in 10,000 births

Aetiology
- This is a sporadic abnormality which may be caused by early amnion rupture with amniotic band syndrome.

Prenatal diagnosis:
- The US features are a major abdominal wall defect, severe kyphoscoliosis, and a short umbilical cord.

Prognosis
- This is a lethal abnormality.

Bladder and cloacal exstrophy

Bladder exstrophy is a defect of the caudal fold of the anterior abdominal wall and can lead to the exposure of the posterior bladder wall when the defect is large. In cloacal exstrophy, both the urinary and gastrointestinal tracts are involved. Cloacal exstrophy, also referred to as OEIS complex, is the association of an omphalocele, exstrophy of the bladder, imperforate anus, and spinal defects such as meningomyelocele.

Incidence
- 1 in 30,000 births for bladder exstrophy
- 1 in 200,000 births for cloacal exstrophy

Aetiology
- Both bladder and cloacal exstrophy are sporadic abnormalities.

Prenatal diagnosis
The diagnosis is suspected when, in the presence of normal amniotic fluid, the fetal bladder is not visualized, and an echogenic mass is seen protruding from the lower abdominal wall, in close association with the umbilical arteries. In cloacal exstrophy, the findings are similar to bladder exstrophy, but a posterior anomalous component (myelomeningocele) is present.

Prognosis
With aggressive reconstructive bladder, bowel, and genital surgery, survival is more than 80%. Although it has been suggested that gender re-assignment to females should occur, psychological follow-ups of such patients suggest that both males and females with this condition are capable of a normal lifestyle with normal intelligence.

Gastrointestinal anomalies

Polyhydramnios is always present in obstructions involving the upper part of the gastrointestinal tract, and therefore prenatal diagnosis is relatively easy. In contrast, in obstructions of the lower part of the gastrointestinal tract, amniotic fluid volume is normal or even decreased in case of imperforate anus with associated urinary anomalies, and prenatal diagnosis can be difficult.

Oesophageal atresia and tracheoesophageal fistula

- Incidence: 1 in 3000 births.
- Mainly sporadic. Trisomies 18 or 21 are found in about 20% of cases
- May be part of the VATER association (vertebral and ventricular septal defects, anal atresia, tracheo-oesophageal fistula, renal anomalies, radial dysplasia and single umbilical artery).
- Prenatal diagnosis is unusual even in the presence of polyhydramnios, (usually after 25 weeks).
- Survival depends on gestation at delivery and the presence of associated anomalies. For babies with an isolated OA/TOF, born after 32 weeks, when an early diagnosis is made, avoiding reflux and aspiration pneumonitis, postoperative survival is more than 95%.

Duodenal atresia

- Incidence: 1 in 5000 births.
- Mainly sporadic. In some cases, there is an autosomal recessive pattern of inheritance. In nearly half of the cases, there are associated abnormalities including trisomy 21, skeletal defects, gastrointestinal abnormalities, cardiac and renal defects.
- Prenatal diagnosis is based on the demonstration of the characteristic 'double bubble' appearance of the dilated stomach and proximal duodenum, commonly associated with polyhydramnios (Fig. 2.7).
- Survival after surgery in cases with isolated duodenal atresia is more than 95%.

Intestinal obstruction

- Incidence: 1 in 2000 births.
- In about half of the cases, there is small bowel obstruction and in the other half anorectal atresia.
- Mainly sporadic. However in multiple intestinal atresia, familial cases have been described (typically lethal). Associated abnormalities and chromosomal defects are otherwise rare.
- Associated defects such as genitourinary, vertebral, cardiovascular, and gastrointestinal anomalies are found in about 80% of cases of anorectal atresia,
- Prenatal diagnosis of obstruction is usually made quite late in pregnancy (after 25 weeks), as dilatation of the intestinal lumen is slow and progressive. Polyhydramnios is common, especially with proximal obstructions. In anorectal atresia, prenatal diagnosis is usually difficult because the proximal bowel may not demonstrate significant dilatation and the amniotic fluid volume is usually normal.

- Survival depends on gestation at delivery, the presence of associated anomalies and site of obstruction. For babies with an isolated obstruction, born after 32 weeks and requiring a resection of only a short segment of bowel, survival is more than 95%.

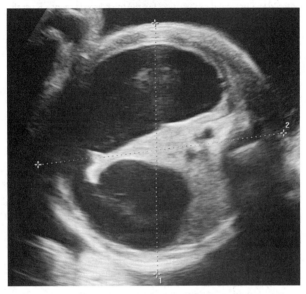

Fig. 2.7 Fetus at 37 weeks of gestation. Axial view demonstrating a duodenal atresia with the charachteristic 'double bubble' appearance of the dilated stomach and proximal duodenum.

Abdominal masses

Renal tract anomalies or dilated bowel are the most common cause. Additionally, cystic structures may arise from the biliary tree, ovaries, mesentery, or uterus. The correct diagnosis of these abnormalities may not be possible by ultrasound examination, but the most likely diagnosis is usually suggested by the position of the cyst, its relationship with other structures, and the normality of other organs.

Ovarian cysts

These tend to occur after 25 weeks of gestation. The majority of cysts are benign and resolve spontaneously in the neonatal period. Potential complications include development of ascites, torsion, infarction, or rupture. Prenatally, the cysts are usually unilateral and unilocular, although, if the cyst undergoes torsion or haemorrhage, the appearance is complex or solid. Obstetric management should not be changed, unless an enormous or rapidly enlarging cyst is detected or there is associated polyhydramnios; in these cases, prenatal aspiration may be considered.

Mesenteric or omental cysts

Mesenteric or omental cysts may represent obstructed lymphatic drainage or lymphatic hamartomas. Antenatally, the diagnosis is suggested by the finding of a multiseptate or unilocular, usually midline, cystic lesion of variable size; a solid appearance may be secondary to hemorrhage. Antenatal aspiration may be considered in cases of massive cysts resulting in thoracic compression.

Hepatic cysts

Hepatic cysts are typically located in the right lobe of the liver. They are quite rare and result from obstruction of the hepatic biliary system. They appear as unilocular, intrahepatic cysts, and they are usually asymptomatic, although rarely may show complications such as infections or hemorrhages.

Intestinal duplication cysts

These are quite rare, and may be located along the entire gastrointestinal tract. They sonographically appear as tubular or cystic structures of variable size. They may be isolated or associated with other gastrointestinal malformations. Differential diagnosis includes other intra-abdominal cystic structures and also bronchogenic cysts, adenomatoid cystic malformation of the lung, and pulmonary sequestration. Thickness of the muscular wall of the cysts and the presence of peristalsis may facilitate the diagnosis.

Sacrococcygeal teratoma

These are found in ~1 per 40,000 births. The condition is sporadic but some cases are familial, with autosomal dominant inheritance. They usually appear solid or mixed solid and cystic. Most teratomas are extremely vascular. The tumours may be entirely external, partially internal and partly external, or mainly internal. Polyhydramnios is frequent, and this may be due to direct transudation into the amniotic fluid and to fetal polyuria, secondary to the hyperdynamic circulation, which is the consequence of arteriovenous shunting. Similarly, high-output heart failure leading to hepatomegaly, placentomegaly and hydrops fetalis can occur.

Sacrococcygeal teratoma is associated with a high perinatal mortality (about 50%), mainly due to the preterm delivery (the consequence of polyhydramnios) of a hydropic infant requiring major neonatal surgery. Prenatal intervention with laser or sclerosant agents has been used to occlude the vascular supply to the tumour in cases of polyhydramnios and evidence of fetal heart failure.

Obstructive uropathy

The term 'obstructive uropathy' encompasses a wide variety of different pathological conditions characterized by dilatation of part or all of the urinary tract. When the obstruction is complete and occurs early in fetal life, renal hypoplasia and dysplasia ensue. On the other hand, where intermittent obstruction allows for normal renal development, or when it occurs in the second half of pregnancy, hydronephrosis will result and the severity of the renal damage will depend on the degree and duration of the obstruction. Dilatation of the fetal urinary tract frequently, but not absolutely, signifies obstruction. Conversely, a fetus with obstruction may not have any urinary tract dilatation.

Hydronephrosis

Varying degrees of pelvicalyceal dilatation are found in about 1% of fetuses. Mild hydronephrosis or pyelectasia is defined by the presence of an anteroposterior diameter of the pelvis of >5 mm at 15–19 weeks, >8 mm at 20–29 weeks, and >10 mm at 30–40 weeks. Transient hydronephrosis may be due to relaxation of smooth muscle of the urinary tract by the high levels of circulating maternal hormones and resolves in the neonatal period. In about 20% of cases, there may be an underlying ureteropelvic junction obstruction or vesicoureteric reflux that requires postnatal follow-up and possible surgery.

Moderate hydronephrosis, characterized by an anteroposterior pelvic diameter of more than 10 mm and pelvicalyceal dilatation, is usually progressive, and in more than 50% of cases surgery is necessary during the first 2 years of life.

Pelvi-ureteric junction obstruction

In 80% of cases, the condition is unilateral. Prenatal diagnosis is based on the demonstration of hydronephrosis in the absence of dilated ureters and bladder. The degree of pelvicalyceal dilatation is variable and, occasionally, perinephric urinomas and urinary ascites may be present. Postnatally, renal function is assessed by serial isotope imaging studies and, if there is deterioration, pyeloplasty is performed.

Vesico-ureteric junction obstruction

This is characterized by hydronephrosis and hydroureter in the presence of a normal bladder. The dilated ureter is tortuous, localized between the renal pelvis, which is variably dilated, and the bladder, which is of normal morphology and dimensions. The aetiology is diverse, including ureteric stricture or atresia, retrocaval ureter, vascular obstruction, valves, diverticulum, ureterocele, and vesicoureteral reflux.

Vesicoureteric reflux

This is suspected when intermittent dilatation of the upper urinary tract over a short period of time is seen on ultrasound scanning. Occasionally, in massive vesicoureteric reflux without obstruction, the bladder appears persistently dilated because it empties but rapidly refills with refluxed urine. Primary megaureter can be distinguished from VUJ obstruction by the absence of significant hydronephrosis.

Urethral obstruction

Urethral obstruction can be caused by urethral agenesis, persistence of the cloaca, urethral stricture or posterior urethral valves. Posterior urethral valves (PUV) occur only in males and are the commonest cause of bladder outlet obstruction. The condition is sporadic and is found in about 1 in 3000 male fetuses. With PUV, there is usually incomplete or intermittent obstruction of the urethra, resulting in an enlarged and hypertrophied bladder with varying degrees of hydroureter, hydronephrosis, a spectrum of renal hypoplasia and dysplasia, oligohydramnios, and pulmonary hypoplasia. In some cases, there is associated urinary ascites from rupture of the bladder or transudation of urine into the peritoneal cavity.

Fetal therapy for obstructive uropathy

Encouraged by the results of animal studies and on the assumption that unrelieved obstruction causes progressive renal and pulmonary damage, several investigators in the 1980s performed *in utero* decompression of the urinary tract in the human. Although these techniques demonstrated the feasibility of intrauterine surgery, they did not provide conclusive evidence that such intervention improves renal or pulmonary function beyond what can be achieved by postnatal surgery. It is possible that, in a few selected cases, intrauterine intervention may be beneficial.

Spina bifida/hydrocephalus

Spina bifida

The neural arch, usually in the lumbosacral region, is incomplete with secondary damage to the exposed nerves.

Incidence
● ~1 in 1000 births

Aetiology
● Unknown in the majority of cases
● Chromosomal abnormalities
● Genetic syndromes
● Maternal diabetes mellitus
● Ingestion of teratogens (e.g. anti-epileptic drugs)

Prenatal diagnosis (Fig 2.8)

Diagnosis of spina bifida requires the systematic examination of each neural arch from the cervical to the sacral region, both transversely and longitudinally. In the transverse scan the normal neural arch appears as a closed circle with an intact skin covering, whereas in spina bifida the arch is 'U'-shaped and there is an associated bulging meningocele (thin-walled cyst) or myelomeningocele. The extent of the defect and any associated kyphoscoliosis is best assessed in the longitudinal scan. The diagnosis of spina bifida has been greatly enhanced by the recognition of associated abnormalities in the skull and brain. These abnormalities are secondary to the Arnold–Chiari malformation, and include frontal bone scalloping ('lemon sign'), and obliteration of the cisterna magna with either an 'absent' cerebellum or abnormal anterior curvature of the cerebellar hemispheres (banana sign). A variable degree of ventricular enlargement is present in virtually all cases of open spina bifida at birth, but in only about 70% of cases in the mid-trimester.

Prognosis

Surviving infants are often severely handicapped, with paralysis in the lower limbs and double incontinence. Postnatal neurological outcome depends on site of vertebral lesion and the degree of ventriculomegaly.

Fetal therapy

The rationale behind fetal intervention in the treatment of myelomeningocele is to correct the structural defect at a time when significant neuronal damage has either not yet occurred or still has the potential to be reversed. There is some experimental evidence from animal studies that *in utero* closure of myelomeningocele may reduce the risk of handicap because the amniotic fluid in the third trimester is thought to be neurotoxic.

Fetal surgery in the human, involving hysterotomy and the insertion of a patch over the spinal lesion, has not prevented paralysis or incontinence but may have reduced the severity of associated hindbrain herniation and hydrocephalus. These two cerebral afflictions provide a major source of additional lifelong morbidity and impaired cognitive function. A NIH-funded multicentre prospective randomized clinical trial to investigate these issues is underway.

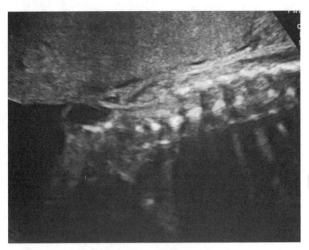

Fig. 2.8 Fetus at 25 weeks and 5 days. Sagittal view at the level of the lower spine demonstrating a spina bifida.

Hydrocephalus

Definition

Hydrocephalus is defined as a pathological increase in the size of the cerebral ventricles with lateral ventricle diameter of 10 mm or more.

Prevalence

This is the most frequent fetal brain anomaly, with a prevalence of ~1 per 1000 live births. Ventriculomegaly is found in ~1% of pregnancies at the 18–23-week scan. Therefore, the majority of fetuses with ventriculomegaly do not develop hydrocephalus.

Aetiology

This is unknown in most but includes:
- chromosomal abnormalitie and genetic syndromes
- intrauterine haemorrhage
- congenital infection
- central nervous system structural defects, e.g. agenesis of the corpus callosum, anomalies of the posterior fossa, aqueduct stenosis, spina bifida.

Diagnosis

Fetal hydrocephalus is diagnosed by US by the demonstration of abnormally dilated lateral cerebral ventricles. Certainly before 24 weeks, and particularly in cases of associated spina bifida, the head circumference may be small rather than large for gestation. A transverse scan of the fetal head at the level of the cavum septum pellucidum will demonstrate the dilated lateral ventricles (defined by a diameter of ≥10 mm). The choroid plexuses, which normally fill the lateral ventricles, are surrounded by fluid. A distinction is usually made between ventriculomegaly (diameter of the posterior horn 10–15 mm) and hydrocephalus (diameter > 15 mm).

Prognosis

This depends on the presence of other defects and the severity of ventricular dilation. Other malformations, commonly spina bifida, are found in ~50% of cases. In cases of isolated ventriculomegaly the rate of developmental impairment is about 15% if the atrial ventricle width is 13–15 mm and about 50% if the width is more than 15 mm.

Fetal therapy

There is some experimental evidence that *in utero* cerebrospinal fluid diversion may be beneficial. However, earlier attempts to treat hydrocephalic fetuses by ventriculo-amniotic shunting have been abandoned because of poor results, mainly because of inappropriate selection of patients. In isolated cases, it is possible that intrauterine drainage may be beneficial if serial ultrasound scans demonstrate progressive ventriculomegaly.

Fetal surgery

The widespread use of high-resolution ultrasound allows for a more accurate and earlier diagnosis of congenital anomalies. Some of these are amenable for surgical correction, the vast majority being best managed after birth. In a limited number of conditions, however, *in utero* surgery may save the life of the fetus or prevent permanent damage. This can be by correction of the malformation, arresting the progression of the disease, or by treating temporarily some of the immediately life-threatening effects of the condition, leaving more definitive treatment for after birth.

Criteria for fetal surgery

An international consensus, endorsed by the International Fetal Medicine and Surgery Society has been reached on the criteria and indications for fetal surgery:
- accurate diagnosis and staging possible, with exclusion of associated anomalies
- natural history of the disease is documented, and prognosis established
- currently no effective or too late postnatal therapy
- *in utero* surgery has been proven feasible in animal models, reversing deleterious effects of the condition
- interventions are done in specialized multidisciplinary fetal treatment centres within strict protocols, after fully informed consent of both mother and partner.

Techniques of fetal surgery

In some centres, mainly in the USA, open fetal surgery has been used for the treatment of diaphragmatic hernia, cystic adenomatoid malformation of the lungs, myelomeningocoele, and sacrococcygeal teratoma. The technique involves the administration of general anaesthesia to the mother, laparotomy and hysterotomy for exposure of the fetus, and then operative repair of the defect in a similar way as in postnatal life. This approach, which is highly invasive with considerable risks to the mother, has now been largely abandoned.

The most commonly used approaches for fetal intervention involve the introduction of an endoscope or cannulas through the maternal abdomen into the uterus, after either local or epidural anaesthesia. Endoscopy is used to guide the introduction of a fetal endotracheal balloon in cases of diaphragmatic hernia and for laser coagulation of communicating placental vessels in cases of monochorionic pregnancies presenting with severe twin-to-twin-transfusion syndrome. Cannulas are used for the insertion of shunts between the fetal thorax or bladder and the amniotic cavity in cases of pleural effusions and obstructive uropathy, respectively, and for the coagulation of feeding vessels by laser in cases of sacrococcygeal teratomas or large extralobar sequestrations.

Neonatal medicine

Infant statistics

Definitions
- Neonate (1–28 days)
- Early-neonatal (1–7 days)
- Late-neonatal (8–28 days)
- Post-neonatal (29 days–1 year)
- Perinatal (variably defined – 7 days)

    Perinatal mortality rate = stillbirths + early neonatal deaths/all births
- Infant (up to 1 year)

Live births

Table 3.1 shows the numbers of live births in England, Wales, and Scotland. 1980–2003, Office for National Statistics

Table 3.1 Live births in England, Wales, and Scotland

Year	England	Wales	Scotland	Northern Ireland	Irish Republic
1980	618,371	37,357	68,892	28,582	74,064
1990	666,920	38,866	65,973	26,251	53,044
2000	572,826	31,304	53,076	21,512	54,789
2003	589,851	31,400	52,408	21,648	61,517

Proportion of live births
By birth weight
The proportion of live births by birth weight for England and Wales is shown in Table 3.2.

Table 3.2 Proportion of live births by birth weight for England and Wales

Birth weight (g)		% of live births	
		1983	2000
Low*	<2500	6.7	7.59
Very low	<1500	0.84	1.25
Extremely low	<1000	0.27	0.5

*ICD-9.

By gestational age
The proportion of live births by gestational age for Scotland are shown in
Table 3.3 (data are not available for England and Wales).

Table 3.3 Proportion of live births by gestational age for Scotland

Gestation at birth (weeks)	% of live births	
	1990	2002
24–27	0.3	0.3
28–31	0.7	0.8
32–36	5.3	6.2

Mortality rate
Mortality rates in England and Wales are shown in Table 3.4.

Table 3.4 Mortality rates per 1000 live births for England and Wales

Year	Neonatal	Post-neonatal	Infant
1970	12.3	5.9	18.2
2003	3.6	1.7	5.3

Classification of neonatal units
Table 3.5 shows the classification of neonatal units in the UK.

Table 3.5 Classification of neonatal units in the UK (British
Association of Perinatal Medicine, 2001)

		Nurse-to-infant ratio	
Level 1	Special care	1:4	±resident medical staff
Level 2	High-dependency care	1:2	medical staff often shared
Level 3	Intensive care	1:1	separate medical staffing

Newborn respiratory disease

Respiratory distress is the most frequent indication for both neonatal intensive care unit admission and mechanical ventilation.

Signs of respiratory distress

Inspection

Tachypnoea

The normal respiratory rate of a newborn is ~40/min, and tachypnoea is defined as a rate of >60/min. Infants with RDS are tachypnoeic, as they have a reduced lung compliance and low lung volume and their work of breathing is reduced by shallow, fast breathing. Infants with TTN have isolated tachypnoea with rates up to 120/min in the first 6 h, which resolves within 24–72 h.

Grunting

This is a sign of atelectasis and classically occurs in infants with untreated RDS. It is produced by expiration through a partially closed glottis, as the infant attempts to maintain functional residual capacity by delaying the escape of air from the lungs during expiration.

Dyspnoea

This reflects an increased work of breathing. In the neonate, the major respiratory muscle is the diaphragm and the rib cage is compliant. Affected infants have intercostal and subcostal recession, sternal retraction and flaring of the alae nasi. Those signs are seen in untreated RDS, MAS and pulmonary air leak.

Cyanosis

This becomes apparent when the arterial oxygen tension falls below 40 mmHg (5.3 kPa). Infants with pulmonary hypertension remain cyanosed even when high inspired oxygen concentrations are administered.

Chest wall

The chest can appear barrel-shaped in infants with TTN or MAS. In ventilated infants with a tension pneumothorax, there may be reduced chest wall movement on the affected side.

Palpation

Mediastinal shift

A tension pneumothorax can result in lateral displacement of both the trachea and cardiac apical impulse

Abdominal distension

This may occur in a tension pneumothorax as a result of downward displacement of the diaphragm

Palpable liver

This occurs in infants with hyperinflated lungs, for example TTN or MAS, due to downward displacement of the diaphragm.

Auscultation

There may be a marked reduction in air entry in RDS, or widespread sticky crepitations and occasional rhonchi in MAS. In pleural effusion, breath sounds are absent on the affected side, which is dull to percussion. In PPHN, the second heart sound is often single and loud because of the high pulmonary artery pressure and there may also be a soft systolic murmur of tricuspid incompetence.

Congestive heart failure leads to tachycardia, hypotension, gallop rhythm, systolic murmur, hepatosplenomegaly, crepitations, and peripheral oedema and can occur in MAS and pulmonary haemorrhage. The characteristic murmer in patent ductus arteriosis is a continuous 'machinery' murmur in the pulmonary area, an active precordium and/or bounding pulses.

Causes of respiratory distress

Transient tachypnoea of the newborn (TTN)

This occurs in 5 per 1000 births at term, because of delay in clearance of fetal lung fluid. Most common in infants delivered by Caesarean section without labour.

Respiratory distress syndrome (RDS)

Occurs in ~1% of infants and results from immaturity of the lungs, particularly the surfactant synthesizing systems. Surfactant is a complex mixture of phospholipids and four surfactant proteins A–D that reduces surface tension, stabilizes the alveoli, and prevents atelectasis and transudation of fluid. The incidence of RDS is inversely proportional to gestational age at birth, and contributing factors include sex (M:F = 1:1.7, as androgen delays maturation of surfactant), race (Caucasian > African infants), Caesarean section, birth depression, maternal diabetes (insulin delays surfactant maturation), and genetic predisposition.

Pulmonary airleaks

About 1% of all newborns develop airleaks, but only 10% are symptomatic. Although pneumothoraces can occur immediately after birth as a complication of resuscitation or due to the high transpulmonary pressure swings generated during the first breaths, they are more commonly a complication of respiratory disease or respiratory support.

Meconium aspiration syndrome (MAS)

Meconium staining of the amniotic fluid occurs in 8–20% of pregnancies, and 5% of infants born through meconium-stained fluid develop MAS. It is a disease of term, particularly post-term, infants. Meconium plugs can act as a ball-valve, resulting in gas trapping and overdistension. Meconium is a chemical irritant causing pneumonitis and it predisposes to pulmonary infection due to its organic nature, and inhibits surfactant production.

Pulmonary hypertension

This is characterized by disproportionately severe hypoxaemia to the degree of respiratory distress. It may be primary or secondary to infection, pulmonary hypoplasia, drug treatment in pregnancy, or congenital heart disease.

Pulmonary haemorrhage

This occurs most commonly in very low birth weight infants who have heart failure because of large pulmonary blood flow secondary to a patent ductus arteriosus (PDA). Pulmonary haemorrhage also occurs in infants who have severe birth depression, sepsis, fluid overload, and/or clotting abnormalities.

Pulmonary hypoplasia

This can occur as a primary disorder, but more commonly is secondary to other conditions which adversely affect the intrathoracic cavity (e.g. congenital diaphragmatic hernia), amniotic fluid volume (e.g. premature and prolonged rupture of the membranes), or fetal breathing movements (e.g. neuromuscular disorders).

Pleural effusions

These are uncommon in the neonatal period, with the incidence of primary fetal hydrothorax being 1 per 15,000 pregnancies. Pleural effusions diagnosed antenatally are often associated with chromosomal or congenital abnormalities; postnatally, pleural effusions can occur as a consequence of bacterial infection or haemothorax due to trauma.

Pneumonia

Early-onset (within four days of birth) pneumonia is acquired transplacentally or during labour or delivery; late-onset pneumonia usually occurs in ventilated prematurely born infants.

Bronchopulmonary dysplasia

This is diagnosed when infants are oxygen dependent beyond 28 days. It has a multifactorial aetiology including predisposition by premature birth and/or abnormal antenatal lung growth and then exposure to insults such as high levels of supplementary oxygen or baro/volutrauma

Further reading

Kinsella JP, Greenough A, Abman SH. Bronchopulmonary dysplasia. *Lancet* 2006;**367**:1421–31.

Rubaltelli FF, Bonafe L, Tangucci M, Spagnolo A, Dani C. Epidemiology of neonatal acute respiratory disorders. A multicenter study on incidence and fatality rates of neonatal acute respiratory disorders according to gestational age, maternal age, pregnancy complications and type of delivery. Italian Group of Neonatal Pneumology. *Biol Neonate* 1998;**74**:7–15.

Investigations of respiratory distress

Chest radiograph

Unless the infant's condition dictates otherwise, the first chest xray should be taken at least four hours after delivery to allow time for lung fluid to be resorbed.

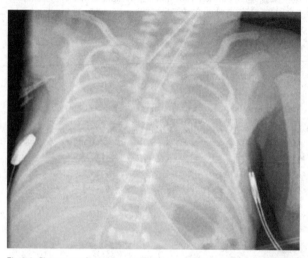

Fig. 3.1 Chest x-ray of an infant with RDS demonstrating fine granular opacification and air bronchograms.

Typically infants with RDS show diffuse bilateral, fine granular opacification with an air bronchogram, where the airfilled bronchi stand out against the atelectatic lungs. (Fig. 3.1)

Transient tachypnoea of the newborn

In TTN, chest x-ray shows hyperinflation, fluid in the fissures, and prominent perihilar vascular markings.

Pneumothorax

If small, pneumothorax can be recognized by differences in translucency of the two lung fields; a large pneumothorax is indicated by a lack of lung markings and collapsed lung (a non-compliant lung may not collapse). If the pneumothorax is under tension, the diaphragm is everted with bulging of the intercostal spaces and mediastinal shift. (Fig. 3.2).

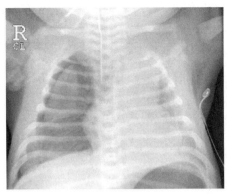

Fig. 3.2 Right-sided pneumothorax in a ventilated infant. The non-compliant lung has not collapsed, there is difference in the translucency of the two lung fields and bulging of the intercostals spaces on the right.

Pneumomediastinum

This appears as a halo of air adjacent to the heart borders; gas can be seen completely surrounding the heart if there is a pneumopericardium.

Pulmonary haemorrhage

If large, haemorrhage will result in a 'white out' of the lung fields with just an air bronchogram visible; lobar consolidation is seen if it is less severe.

Pulmonary hypertension (PH)

The radiographic changes may be minimal in primary PH, and in secondary PH the chest x-ray appearance will be that of the underlying lung disease.

Pleural effusion

If large, pleural effusion results in a 'white out' on the affected side with depression of the diaphragm; small effusions collect in the most dependent parts and present as a rim of fluid around the lateral chest wall or diaphragm.

Meconium aspiration syndrome

There are widespread patchy infiltrations with overexpansion and small pleural effusions in the early stages; by 72 h, in severe cases, there is bilateral opacification due to pneumonitis and interstitial oedema. Air leaks are common (Fig. 3.3).

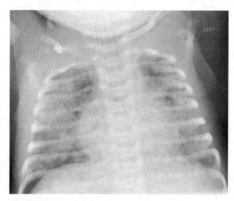

Fig. 3.3 Infant with MAS showing with coarse bilateral shadows and a small right-sided airleak.

Pulmonary hypoplasia

The chest wall is disproportionately small with respect to the abdomen and the chest may be bell-shaped (Fig. 3.4).

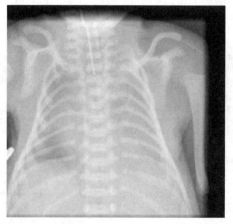

Fig. 3.4 Pulmonary hypoplasia – note the bell-shaped chest and large heart: thoracic cavity ratio.

Pneumonia

This may present as lobar or segmental consolidation, atelectasis or diffuse haziness or opacification. Infants with group B streptococcal septicaemia can have a chest x-ray appearance indistinguishable from that of RDS (Fig. 3.5).

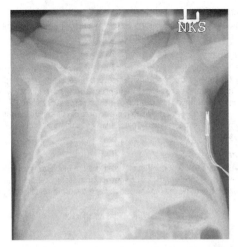

Fig. 3.5 Infant with pneumonia with complete opacification of the right lung.

Bronchopulmonary dysplasia (BPD)

BPD was previously characterized by hyperinflation, interstitial shadows representing fibrosis, and cystic translucencies; infants with new BPD have small-volume, hazy lung fields.

> **Transillumination** with an intense beam from a fibreoptic light can identify abnormal air collections due to a pneumothorax by an increased transmission of light on the involved side. Pulmonary interstitial emphysema (PIE), however, can give the same appearance.

Blood gas and pH measurement

Infants with RDS will have hypoxaemia and a respiratory acidosis; this will be complicated by a metabolic acidosis if the infant is infected or hypotensive. Hypoxaemia disproportionate to the chest x-ray abnormalities and a discrepancy between pre- and post-ductal PaO_2 indicates pulmonary hypertension

Microbiology

Sepsis is an important differential diagnosis of respiratory distress; therefore blood and gastric aspirates obtained on admission to the neonatal unit should be cultured and blood cultures obtained from infants who deteriorate while receiving neonatal intensive care. Culture of respiratory secretions can help to inform the choice of antibiotics, but bacterial growth may represent colonization.

Haematology

In sepsis, there can be a raised or low white cell count, thrombocyto-paenia and/or coagulation abnormalities.

Biochemistry

Renal function may be impaired in infants with respiratory distress, particularly those who are hypotensive because of sepsis or birth depression. Serum albumin levels are often low in prematurely born infants with RDS, but albumin infusion does not improve their respiratory status. All babies have a raised unconjugated bilirubin in the first days after birth; it is important to monitor levels regularly, particularly in infants at increased risk of haemolysis.

Echocardiography

This enables exclusion of congenital heart disease in a hypoxaemic infant. In pulmonary hypertension, the right ventricular systolic pressure can usually be estimated from the maximum velocity of a tricuspid regurgitant jet.

Differential diagnosis of respiratory distress

Early respiratory distress

Prematurely born infants

RDS is the most likely diagnosis particularly if the mother did not receive antenatal corticosteroids. The infant, however, may have congenital pneumonia (risk factors include chorioamnionitis and premature and prolonged rupture of the membranes). Of course, RDS and pneumonia can co-exist. If the mother has had a Caesarean section without labour then the infant may have TTN in addition to RDS; retained lung fluid will result in a chest x-ray appearance resembling severe RDS, but this will resolve rapidly as the lung fluid is reabsorbed. Premature and prolonged rupture of the membranes and any cause of oligohydramnios are risk factors for pulmonary hypoplasia; affected infants may also have limb contractures and Potter's facies.

Infants born at term

MAS should be considered if there has been meconium staining of the amniotic fluid and/or birth depression; affected infants are usually postmature and have dry, flaky skin and meconium-stained skin, nails and umbilical cord. Pulmonary hypertension is more common in infants who have suffered birth depression, and affected infants will be hypoxic but, unless there is co-existing respiratory disease, not have a raised CO_2; it is important to exclude cyanotic congenital heart disease in such babies. Asphyxia predisposes to pulmonary haemorrhage; affected infants will be hypotensive and blood-stained fluid may well up the trachea. Pneumothorax should be suspected in any infant who has required resuscitation at birth and in any ventilated infant who suddenly deteriorates. Isolated pleural effusions sufficient to cause neonatal respiratory distress will usually have been diagnosed, if not treated, antenatally. Early respiratory distress can occur as a result of a neuromuscular disorder such as congenital myotonic dystrophy; there may be a history of reduced fetal movements and polyhydramnios due to poor fetal swallowing. Similarly, infants with spinal muscular atrophy can present with respiratory distress; classically affected infants are weak and areflexic with gracile ribs on chest x-ray. The diagnosis is confirmed by genetic studies.

Late-onset respiratory distress

The most common cause, particularly in infants with BPD, is nosocomial pneumonia and will be associated with new chest x-ray changes. Infants with RDS may deteriorate because of heart failure due to a PDA, they are hypotensive with a low diastolic blood pressure and have an active precordium, a continuous or systolic murmur and bounding pulses. Aspiration pneumonia is most common in babies with structural malformations or neurological defects, but can occur in prematurely born infants who have poor coordination of sucking and swallowing.

Treatment of respiratory distress

Respiratory support

An absolute indication for intubation and positive pressure ventilation is a major apnoea with failure to respond promptly to bag and mask resuscitation. Relative indications include recurrent minor apnoeas, cerebral oedema due to hypoxic ischaemic encephalopathy, and worsening blood gases.

Inhaled nitric oxide (iNO)

This is the preferred pulmonary vasodilator for term born infants starting at a dose of 20 ppm, which is reduced over the first few hours to 5 ppm. Prior to starting iNO, lung volume should be optimized, an echocardiograph undertaken to rule out congenital heart disease, and any coagulation disturbance or thrombocytopenia corrected. iNO has a short duration of action, and rebound vasoconstriction and hypoxaemia can occur if withdrawn abruptly; therefore, precautions need to be taken, for example if the baby requires endotracheal suction.

Surfactant

This should be given to infants at risk of developing RDS, preferably within the first hour after birth. Natural surfactants are more effective than the older synthetic surfactants. Surfactant is usually administered as a bolus, but in MAS surfactant lavage is more effective.

Antibiotics

It is difficult to rule out sepsis as a cause of respiratory distress or co-existing; as a consequence all infants with respiratory distress should be screened for infection and given antibiotics until blood culture results are available. A combination of ampicillin or benzylpenicillin and gentamicin should be used, or a third-generation cephalosporin.

Blood pressure support

Unless the infant is fluid overloaded, first-line management of hypotension is either crystalloid or a blood transfusion, depending on the haemoglobin concentration. Inotropes should be started if hypotension persists; dopamine is more effective than dobutamine. Adrenaline (epinephrine) has both inotropic and chronotropic effects, but may cause renal and myocardial ischaemia and is best reserved for use when dopamine and dobutamine are insufficient.

Drainage of airleaks

Asymptomatic pneumothoraces do not require treatment, but the infant should be monitored until resolution. Nursing an infant in 100% oxygen favours resorption of the extra-alveolar gas, but should not be undertaken if there is a risk of retinopathy of prematurity. If the infant is symptomatic or the pneumothorax is under tension, then it must be drained. If the infant is *in extremis* and there is insufficient time for insertion of a chest drain, emergency drainage can be performed by needle aspiration using an 18-gauge butterfly needle. To insert a chest drain, local anaesthetic should be given and the drain inserted in the sixth intercostal space in the mid-axillary line and the tip angled retrosternally to achieve most effective drainage. The chest drain should be connected to an underwater seal (Heimlich valves are only used for transport) and a chest x-ray taken to determine the position of the tip of the drain. The drain should be left in position for 24 h after bubbling has ceased.

Drainage of effusions

Thoracocentesis by needle aspiration may be required to achieve effective ventilation and, if there is reoccurrence, a chest drain inserted to achieve continuous drainage; the tip of the drain is positioned to lie posteriorly.

Further reading

Finer NN, Barrington KJ. Nitric oxide for respiratory failure in infants born at or near term. *Cochrane Database Syst Rev* 2006;**4**:CD000399.

Soll RF, Blanco F. Natural surfactant extract versus synthetic surfactant for neonatal respiratory distress syndrome. *Cochrane Database Syst Rev* 2001;**2**:CD000144.

Soll RF, Dargaville P. Surfactant for meconium aspiration syndrome in full term infants. *Cochrane Database Syst Rev* 2000;**2**:CD002054.

Intensive care

Newborns and especially preterm neonates have a range of particular vulnerabilities that require special consideration on intensive care:

Fluid requirements – see page 94

Limited urinary concentrating capacity means neonates are especially vulnerable to both dehydration and fluid overload. Fluid allowance must consider age in days in addition to severity of illness and any surgery.

Pulmonary hypertension

The newborn must change from the feto-placental circulation (low pulmonary blood flow, high ductus arterosus flow) to the normal situation of falling pulmonary vascular resistance and closure of the ductus arterosus. Hypoxia, acidosis, and severe illness inhibit this change. Minimal handling and avoidance of pain contribute to falls in pulmonary vascular resistance.

Persistent pulmonary hypertension of the newborn (PPHN) describes children with low pulmonary blood flow, hypoxia, shock, and acidosis who have failed to make this adaptation readily. In some surgical conditions, especially congenital diaphragmatic hernia, this is the predominant problem leading to early cardiorespiratory failure.

Suggested treatment of pulmonary hypertension
- Good analgesia, sedation (and paralysis if required)
- Artificial ventilation (aim for pH 7.45–7.5 and PaO_2 > 8 KPa)
- Maintain mean arterial pressure >45–50 mmHg in term infant)
- Treat polycythaemia (aim for haematocrit ~ 0.4)
- Pulmonary vasodilators (best option inhaled nitric oxide at 20 ppm)
- If no progress consider referral for ECMO

Glycaemic control

Newborns are especially vulnerable to harmful neurological consequences of hypoglycaemia (<2.7 mmol/l). At risk-patients (preterm, sick, poor feeding, infant of diabetic mother) should be monitored and supplemental glucose given to avoid this.

Temperature control

Oxygen consumption rises rapidly outside of a narrow thermoneutral range. Careful control of temperature is a key element of neonatal (especially preterm) care.

Fluid balance

Maintenance fluid requirements

In infants and children, fluid requirements (Table 3.6) are usually based on the method of Holliday and Segar. This, however, is not suitable for infants <4 weeks of age as they have very wide range of requirements, depending on:
- ambient conditions, e.g. incubator or Babytherm®
- clinical condition, e.g. phototherapy, pyrexia, burns, or other insensible losses may increase requirements, whereas PDA or chronic lung disease decrease requirements.

In addition, especially in preterm infants, fluid administration should also allow for the physiological weight loss over the first 5–10 days of life (up to a maximum of 10% of birth weight), always maintaining urine output at 1–4 mL/kg/h.

Table 3.6 Normal maintenance fluid requirement

Premature infant	1st day of life	60–150 mL/kg/day
	2nd day of life	70–150 mL/kg/day
	3rd day of life	90–180 mL/kg/day
	>3rd day of life	Up to 200 mL/kg/day
Term infant	1st day of life	60–80 mL/kg/day
	2nd day of life	80–100 mL/kg/day
	3rd day of life	100–140 mL/kg/day
	>3rd day of life	Up to 160 mL/kg/day
Child > 4 weeks of age, ≤ 10 kg		100 mL/kg/day
Child from 10–20 kg		1000 mL + 50 mL/kg/day for each kg over 10
Child >20 kg		1500 mL + 20 mL/kg/day for each kg over 20

Fluids administered

Newborn
- 10% dextrose solution
- Sodium supplementation is not usually required in the first 24 h (low urine output); after that time 2–4 mmol/kg/day (adjusted primarily on serum sodium values and changes in weight)
- Potassium 1–3 mmol/kg/day (not usually required in the first 24 h)
- Calcium 1 mmol/kg/day (only in the first 2 days of life or if required)

Infancy and childhood
A variety of intravenous solutions can be used (Table 3.7). To maintain normal physiological concentrations, 1–3 mEq/kg/day of potassium and 2–4 mEq/kg/d of sodium are typically required.

Table 3.7 Common intravenous fluids

Intravenous fluid	Glucose (g/100mL)	Na⁺ (mEq/L)	K⁺ (mEq/l)	Cl⁻ (mEq/L)	Osmolality (mOsmol/L)
5% dextrose	5	–	–	–	252
10% dextrose	10	–	–	–	505
Normal saline (0.9% NaCl)	–	154	–	154	308
½ Normal saline (0.45% NaCl)	–	77	–	77	154
5% dextrose with ½ N saline	5	77	–	77	406
5% dextrose with ¼ N saline	5	34	–	34	329
Lactated Ringer's	0	130	4	109	273
Hartmann's	0	131	5	111	278

Post-surgical fluid administration

In the first 24–48 h post-surgery, patients usually require a fluid restriction to 50–75% of full maintenance calculated as above. However, this varies depending on:
- the quantity of fluids received in theatre
- clinical condition
- losses from drains, nasogastric tubes or stoma, which should be replaced with normal saline (with or without added K⁺).

During the first 24 h after surgery, patients can develop a hyponatraemia, due to haemodilution and/or SIADH (syndrome of inappropriate antidiuretic hormone secretion), which is associated with neurosurgery, head injury, pain and stress. It is therefore strongly recommended to measure serum electrolytes within 24 h of surgery for all children on IV fluids for more than 12 h.

Route of administration

IV fluids can be administered via peripherally or centrally placed catheters. In newborn infants, or other conditions where dextrose is administered at >10%, peripheral administration is not recommended because of complications due to hyperosmolar solutions.

Monitoring

- Serum electrolytes should be measured before surgery, within the first 24 h after surgery, and daily thereafter whilst on IV fluids (or more frequently during correction of previous fluid or electrolyte disturbances). In stable patients remaining on IV fluids, three times per week is adequate.
- Children should be weighed daily (if the clinical condition allows).
- Urine output, and other fluid losses, should be compared with fluid administration (including drugs) at least every 24 h, or more frequently depending on clinical condition (e.g. abnormalities in heart rate, blood pressure and capillary refill time).

Common fluid and electrolyte disturbances and their treatment

Dehydration/oedema

- If a patient presents with some of the signs of dehydration (hypotension, tachycardia, long capillary refill time, dry mucosa, low urine output, slow responses), fluid infusion rates should be checked. Haemodynamic instability should be treated with initial resuscitation (starting at 20 mL/kg of isotonic solution such as Ringer lactate or normal saline), the cause investigated and intensive care support sought.
- Mild oedema, as an inflammatory response, is not uncommon in the first 48 h after surgery. In the presence of oedema it is still important to check fluid infusion rates and measure urine output.

Sodium (normal value: 135–145 mmol/L)

Hyponatraemia

- Is common after surgery (as described above).
- It is important to exclude spurious hyponatraemia due to hyperglycaemia.
- Treatment depends on the fluid status of the patient.
- If hypo- or hypervolaemic, fluid status should be gradually corrected first with isotonic solution.

If normovolaemic, serum sodium should be corrected with NaCl infusion using the formula:

$$Na_{required} = [(Na_{desired} - Na_{actual}) \times 0.6 \times body\ weight]$$
(safe rate of correction < 25 mEq/L over 48 h, not exceeding 0.5mEq/L/h)

Hypernatraemia

- Usually due to haemoconcentration/excessive fluid losses.
- Other causes of hypernatraemia are renal or respiratory insufficiency, or can be related to drug administration.
- Treatment is via gradual correction of fluid status and of plasma osmolality (not exceeding 0.5 mEq/L/h change in plasma sodium), with appropriate electrolyte-containing solutions.

Potassium (normal value: 3.5 - 5 mmol/L)

Hypokalaemia

- Is commonly iatrogenic or due to renal or gastrointestinal problems (e.g. vomiting, pyloric stenosis, ileus, ileostomy loss).
- Treatment is with KCl infusion (1–3 meq/kg/d).

Hyperkalaemia

- Can be iatrogenic or due to renal problems but can also be caused by cell lysis syndrome (e.g. trauma) or malignant hyperthermia.
- It is important to exclude false hyperkalaemia due to haemolysis of the blood sample.
- Treatment is to stop all sources of additional K^+ and to promote movement of K^+ from the extracellular fluid into the cells, using insulin (plus glucose to avoid hypoglycaemia) or with inhaled or nebulized or IV beta-agonists (salbutamol). If other therapies fail, dialysis may be necessary.

Acidosis (pH <7.35) and alkalosis (pH >7.45)

- Respiratory – $PaCO_2$ is >45 mmHg (acidosis) or <35 mmHg (alkalosis). Treatment is via appropriate respiratory support.
- Metabolic – bicarbonate <21 mmol/l (acidosis) or >26mmol/l (alkalosis). In metabolic acidosis it is useful to check the anion gap [= $Na^+ - (Cl^- + HCO_3^-)$, which is normally 12 ± 2 mEq/L] to understand the underlying cause and correct the existing deficits. It is also important, before treatment with sodium bicarbonate bolus, to check the volaemic status because this condition can be due to tissue hypo-perfusion.

Further reading

Modi N. Fluid and electrolyte balance. In: Rennie JM (ed). *Roberton's Textbook of Neonatology.* Churchill Livingstone, 2005, pp335–54.

Robertson J, Shilkofski N (eds). *Harriet Lane Handbook* (17th edn). Phildelphia: Elsevier Mosby, 2005 (useful detailed reference tables).

Extracorporeal membrane oxygenation (ECMO)

This is a form of extracorporeal life support that utilizes the principles of cardiopulmonary bypass to provide prolonged support for infants, children and adults with severe cardiac or respiratory failure who are failing conventional intensive care therapies (Box 3.1).

Box 3.1 History of EMCO

During the 1960s, Theodore Kolobow developed a successful silicone membrane oxygenator, leading to the first case of prolonged extracorporeal support in 1972. Robert Bartlett, the father of ECMO, commenced the first clinical ECMO programme in the late 1970s.

Epidemiology

By 2008, the Extracorporeal Life Support Organization (ELSO) had registered >36,400 cases overall. Most were for respiratory failure – 21,900 in neonates, >3600 in children and >1400 in adults; others were for cardiac support (> 8000 – 40% neonatal, 50% paediatric age and 10% adults). ECMO was used as a form of resuscitation in ~1000 cases.

Types of ECMO

Blood is drained from the venous circulation, typically through a cannula placed via the right internal jugular vein (RIJV) into the right atrium, and continuously passed through a modified cardiopulmonary bypass (CPB) circuit where it is oxygenated and cleansed of CO_2 before being delivered back to the patient at a controlled temperature. Unlike CPB, not all the circulating volume is diverted into the circuit, maintaining some pulmonary blood flow. This, and the absence of a large blood reservoir, ensures continuous flow of blood allowing a lower level of anticoagulation compared to CPB. A pump (usually roller, sometimes centrifugal) ensures continuous flow of blood through the circuit and back to the patient.

There are two methods of delivering ECMO support:

Veno-arterial (VA) delivery

Oxygenated blood from the circuit is returned (usually via the right common carotid artery (RCCA)), into the ascending aorta and the systemic arterial circulation. This results in a degree of circulatory support in addition to respiratory support and is the method of choice for patients with isolated cardiac failure or combined cardiac and respiratory failure. The blood draining into the ECMO circuit is 'true venous' blood and, if some cardiac output is maintained, the reduced proportion of deoxygenated blood not drained through the circuit continues to flow through the pulmonary circulation. Blood ejected from the left ventricle into the aortic arch will mix with the richly oxygenated blood from the ECMO circuit. Excellent oxygenation can be achieved with this modality. Potential disadvantages reflect the method of cannulation and the direct return of blood into the aorta and, in turn, the cerebral circulation and the risk of embolic episodes.

Veno-venous (VV) delivery

The oxygenated blood from the circuit is returned into the venous circulation, either directly into the right atrium or via the femoral vein. Adequate native cardiac output is necessary for this method of support although, in patients where myocardial contractility is reduced secondary to hypoxia, the improved oxygenation can result in improved cardiac function and a reduction in inotrope requirements. As the oxygenated blood re-enters the venous circulation, all blood is directed through the pulmonary circulation and the pulmonary arterial system is exposed to well-saturated blood, facilitating resolution of pulmonary hypertension. Venous blood drained into the ECMO circuit will inevitably be mixed with some returned oxygenated blood, leading to a degree of 'recirculation' of oxygenated blood in the venous cannula. This method avoids the need for arterial cannulation and (in the absence of an ASD or VSD), is not associated with cerebral emboli.

Physiology

The balance between oxygen delivery and tissue consumption is reflected in the oxygen content of venous blood after tissue extraction. As blood drains into the circuit, continuous in-line venous saturation measurements (SvO_2) are used as a guide to adequacy of oxygen delivery.

Oxygen delivery

This is managed by optimizing the Hb concentration and increasing ECMO blood flow. The rate of blood flow through the circuit is calculated as a percentage of the patient's cardiac output, and initial flows are typically set at around 50% of predicted cardiac output. Early oxygenators used a silicone rubber membrane. Recent advances in hollow fibre technology using polymethylpentene (Medos®) have resulted in greater oxygenator efficiency and reduced circuit prime volume. Oxygenators have a maximum rated blood flow beyond which the efficiency is compromised so the choice of oxygenator is determined by the patient's weight.

Carbon dioxide extraction

The countercurrent gas flow in the oxygenator results in extremely efficient CO_2 transfer (x6 that of oxygen), and occasionally CO_2 is added to the gas mix to prevent the physiological effects of hypocarbia. The CO_2 content of the post-oxygenator blood is determined by the rate of flow and the air/O_2/CO_2 ratio of the gas mix, with improved clearance achieved by increasing the rate of gas flow or reducing the CO_2 content of the gas mix. Typically patients with respiratory failure have high $PaCO_2$ when ECMO is commenced. Close monitoring is required in the early stages to ensure a controlled, gradual reduction towards normocarbia.

Heat exchange

Before blood is returned to the patient, normothermia is usually restored by a countercurrent heat-exchanger. This can also be used to induce hypothermia in appropriate cases.

Various ports are available for the administration of medications or fluids and the circuit is a ready site for extracorporeal renal (or hepatic) support.

Cannulation techniques

A double-lumen catheter is used in infants for VV ECMO. Venous blood is drained into the circuit as for VA ECMO but the oxygenated blood is returned through a separate lumen with side holes (only) and the cannula is positioned, using echocardiography, to direct the 'arterial' jet towards the tricuspid valve. Only 12 Fr, 15 Fr and 18 Fr cannulae are presently available, restricting use to patients between 2.5 and 12 kg. Catheters can be placed in the RIJV using a Seldinger technique or by an open surgical approach. In older age groups, VV ECMO is carried out through two percutaneously placed cannulae with the RIJV cannula typically utilized for venous drainage and a femoral venous catheter inserted for return of the oxygenated blood.

The commonest vessels for cannulation in VA ECMO are the RIJV and the RCCA. Following completion, both vessels are usually ligated though some advocate repair of the artery where possible. Alternatively, both arterial and venous cannulae can be placed percutaneously and can be removed safely without sequelae. Post cardiac surgery, intra-operative CBD cannulae may be left in place where appropriate.

Management of ECMO

- 'Rest' ventilator settings (i.e. reduced inspiratory pressures and rate but relatively high PEEP and inspiratory time – to maintain some lung distension, and avoid barotrauma)
- $FiO_2 = 0.3$–0.4
- Regular chest physiotherapy (particularly in meconium aspiration syndrome)
- Anticoagulation (continuous heparin infusion) – monitored using the activated clotting time (ACT). Keep levels at 180–210 s

If VA ECMO is used for low cardiac output state, normal ventilatory settings should be used to maintain normal pulmonary venous oxygen levels and preserve adequate coronary oxygen delivery.

Direct circulatory support is offered in VA ECMO, although the effects on left ventricular ejection need to be considered. Although the return flow from the ECMO circuit is non-pulsatile, if left ventricular function is maintained, ejection against the return flow just results in reduced pulsatility. However, if left ventricular dysfunction exists, the increased afterload can exacerbate left ventricular failure, leading to ventricular dilatation, pulmonary oedema, and reduced myocardial perfusion. In practice, this rarely happens in the neonate, and in the older child ventricular dilatation is managed by reducing arterial resistance with systemic vasodilators, and by increasing ECMO flows to adequately drain the right side and reduce pulmonary venous return. Occasionally, venting the left side (e.g. by transseptal atriotomy) is required.

Table 3.8 Neonatal respiratory outcome by indication (ELSO international data January 2008)

Indication	Survival (%)
Meconium aspiration	94
PPHN	78
Diaphragmatic hernia	51
Sepsis	75
Pneumonia	58
RDS	84
Air leak syndrome	74

Over the past 15 years, novel therapies such as high-frequency ventilation, surfactant replacement and inhaled nitric oxide have reduced the numbers of patients referred for ECMO.

ELSO reports a paediatric respiratory survived of 64% for the ECMO run and 56% were successfully transferred or discharged. Commonest reasons for support were viral or bacterial pneumonia.

The overall reported survival for adult respiratory cases was 59% for the run and 51% to discharge or transfer. Results of ECMO in adult respiratory failure are steadily improving, and a recent randomized controlled trial of ECMO versus conventional intensive care for adult respiratory failure (CESAR Trial) showed a significantly better 6 month outcome for those randomized to receive ECMO support.

Neonates who received ECMO support for cardiac problems had a successful run in 58%, and 37% survived to transfer or discharge. Older infants who were supported for cardiac reasons had a 44% survival to discharge and 46% of paediatric cardiac cases over 1 year old survived to discharge. Adults who received ECMO support for cardiac problems survived the run in 46% and 33% survived to transfer or discharge.

Complications (Table 3.8)

Complications can be mechanical (circuit) or patient in origin. Appropriate training and tremendous attention to detail are required to minimize circuit problems during (often) long ECMO runs. Most ECMO patient complications relate to heparinization and the resulting increased bleeding risk.

Further reading

Anonymous. UK collaborative randomised trial of neonatal extracorporeal membrane oxygenation. UK Collaborative ECMO Trail Group. *Lancet* 1996;**348**(9020):75–82.

Bartlett R 2005. Physiology of ECLS. In Van Meurs KP, Lally KP, Peek G, Zwischenberger JB (eds). *Extracorporeal Cardiopulmonary Support in Critical Care*. Ann Arbor, Michigan: Extracorporeal Life Support Organization, 2005, pp5–28.

Walker GM, Coutts JA, Skeoch C, Davis CF. 2003. Paediatricians' perception of the use of extracorporeal membrane oxygenation to treat meconium aspiration syndrome. *Arch Dis Child (Fetal & Neonatal)* 2003;**88**:F70–F71.

Infant milk

While many surgeons leave this area to neonatologists and dieticians, a working knowledge aids discussion and direction.

Breast milk

42% of infants are breast-fed at 6 weeks
21% of infants are breast-fed at 6 months
(UK 2000 statistic)

Initial breast milk, is termed colostrum and is rich in electrolytes and antibodies, which changes after about 3–4 days. Mature breast milk contains carbohydrate (principally lactose i.e. glucose-galactose), fat (triacyl glycerols, long-chain polyunsaturated fatty acids, phospholipids), protein (e.g casein (40%), and the 'whey' proteins (60%) – β-lactoglobulin, α-lactalbumin, lactoferrin, albumin etc), peptides (e.g. epidermal growth factor, somatomedin), water, immunologically active compounds (e.g. IgA, leucocytes), and antibacterial substances (e.g. lysozyme, lactoperoxidase). Table 3.9 Stool bacteriology varies according to the nature of milk feeding. Thus bifidobacteria are predominant in breast-fed infants (80%) versus formula-fed (30%, with rising *E. coli* and *bacterioides* spp)

Table 3.9 Composition of breast and formula milk

	Breast milk (g/L)	Typical formula (e.g. SMA Gold®) (g/L)
Carbohydrate	13	15
Fat	41	36
Protein	13	15

Calorie content ~750 kcal/L (≈3000 kJ/L).

Infant formulas

Formula milks are predominantly demineralized, modified cow's or soy milk based. Actual cow's ('doorstep') milk is inappropriate in first 12 months because of its high sodium, phosphate, and protein content and may cause hypocalcaemia, anaemia and milk curd obstruction.

Preterm formulas for use in hospitals (e.g. Nutriprem LBW®)

These have a higher calorie concentration with increased mineral and vitamin supplementation.

Term formulas (e.g C&G 'Premium'®, SMA 'Gold'®)

Humanized milk suitable for most situations where breast feeding is contraindicated or not sustained.

Term formula – follow on (e.g. C&G 'Step Up'®, SMA 'Progress'®)

For use beyond ~6 months, these tend to be casein dominant in terms of protein (e.g. ~80%) and have a higher mineral content.

Soya-based formulas (e.g Infasoy®, SMA Wysoy®, Isomil®)

Designed for lactose intolerance and cow's milk allergy, ~~~~ mended for preterm infants because of the decreased bioa.. calcium and phosphorus.

Hydrolysed casein-based formulas (e.g. Nutramigen®, Pregestamil®)

Theses are indicated for protein intolerance and are lactose-free.

Hydrolysed whey-based formulas (e.g. Pepti-junior®, Pepdite® and MCT Pepdite®)

These are formulas based on a more hypoallergenic protein source consisting of amino acids and small peptides. They perhaps may be useful when there has been GI tract damage or complication (e.g. NEC). They also contain about half their fat as MCT (medium chain triglycerides – bypasses normal fat digestion process). They are lactose-free.

Caprilon®, because of high (75%) MCT composition is used where there is more of a functional pancreatic or biliary deficit.

Amino acid-based formulas (e.g. Neocate®)

Extensively modified, with free amino-acids, various oils (not MCT) and glucose; indicated in severe protein intolerance and short bowel syndrome.

How much ?

Clearly it is difficult to be prescriptive, but ~150 mL/kg/day is a reasonable guideline.

Fluid ounces (fl oz): In the UK (and US), parents work with 'imperial' units; 1 fluid ounce ≈ 30 mL.

Formulas are reconstituted usually as 1 fl oz water plus 1 scoop of powder.

So, 3 fl oz of water plus 3 scoops is ~ 90 mL.

How much?

Generally, 2.5 oz/lb weight, i.e. an 8 lb baby will require 20 oz of formula. NB 2.2 lb ≈ 1 kg

(The above sum works out as ~550 mL (metric) versus 600 mL (imperial))

Weaning

Weaning is generally advised from 6 months of age (no earlier than 4 months certainly) and usually involves simple bland pureed foodstuffs (e.g. baby rice). 'Finger-food' can be taken from ~9 months. Although there is no rigid time to stop breast/infant milk feeding, one year is probably more than enough.

Further reading

Lucas A, Fewtrell M. Infant feeding In: Rennie J (ed). *Roberton's Textbook of Neonatology*. Churchil Livingstone, 2005, pp281–324.

Neonatal antibiotics

In general, antibiotics in neonatal practice tend to be well-established and conservative (Table 3.10).

Table 3.10 Neonatal antibiotics. Data from Rennie JM (ed). *Roberton's Textbook of Neonatology* (4th edn), 2005

	Dose (mg/kg)	By week of life	Frequency
Penicillin	30	0–1	bd
		1–3	tds
		4+	qds
Amoxicillin, flucloxacillin	50	0–1	bd
		1–3	tds
		4+	qds
Ceftazidime	25	0–4	bd
		4+	tds
Gentamicin	5	Aim for trough level of ≤1 mg/L (after 4th dose)	od
Metronidazole	7.5	0–3	bd
		4+	tds

Neonatal surgery

Assessment of the surgical neonate

Maternal history
- Age
- Blood group, transfusion history, haemoglobinopathy or coagulopathy
- Past medical history (e.g. diabetes, hypertension, thyroid disease, renal disease, and cardiac disease).
- Past obstetric history (e.g. assisted pregnancies, obstetric outcomes)
- Screening tests (e.g. syphilis, herpes, HIV, hepatitis, high vaginal swabs)
- Drug history, including substance abuse
- Family history

Current pregnancy and delivery
- Prenatal ultrasound (liquor volume, end-diastolic flow, growth)
- Labour (e.g. presentation, onset of labour, duration of rupture of membranes, pyrexia)
- Fetal monitoring
- Nature of amniotic fluid and placenta
- Mode of delivery
- Apgar scores, resuscitation required?
- Gestational age and birth weight
- Administration of vitamin K (route and dose)

Examination
Fully undress the child but keep warm under radiant heater or with a blanket. Examine systems in the following order to minimize disturbance and to take advantage of the initially settled child.

General
- Evidence of birth trauma (e.g. cephalhaematomas, cuts, bruises)
- Skin (e.g. jaundice, erythema toxicum, Mongolian spots, milia, hamartomatous lesions)
- Head circumference (normal term neonate 33–38 cm)
- Fontanelle pressure, suture line mobility and moulding
- Ears (e.g. accessory tags, shape, position, pre-auricular pits or sinus)
- Neck masses, lymph nodes and symmetry
- Mouth (e.g. sucking reflex, intact palate)

Cardiorespiratory
- Colour (feet and hands may have a bluish hue but torso should be pink)
- Respiratory rate (40–60 breaths/min), periodic breathing normal
- Abnormal apnoea (breath-holding with cyanosis, grunting, nasal flaring, subcostal recession)
- Heart rate (120–160 beats/min)
- Heart sounds (murmurs common – confirm findings with echocardiogram)
- Femoral pulses (if weak, check upper and lower limb pressures to exclude coarctation of the aorta)

Abdomen

- Asymmetry, masses
- Liver (normal 2 cm below costal margin). Spleen (normally impal...
- Genitalia (male – check for hypospadias, descended testes, hydrocele, inguinal hernia; female – check labia, mucosal vaginal tag (normal), urethral meatus and separate vagina)
- Anus (size, position and patency)

Extremities, spine, joints

- Hands (digits, syndactyly, posture, e.g. Erb's palsy)
- Feet (e.g. talipes equino/calcaneo and varus/valgus)
- Hips (e.g. skin crease symmetry, developmental dysplasia of the hip
- Back (symmetry, alignment, midline swellings, sacral anomalies, sacral pits)

Resuscitation

- Minimize heat loss, dry thoroughly, wrap in blanket, place under radiant heater
- Maintain airway. Suction gently – overstimulus may provoke apnoea/bradycardia

Traditional assessment of the infant's condition at birth involve calculation of the Apgar score (Table 4.1).

Table 4.1 Apgar score (Dr Virginia Apgar, American paediatrician, 1909–1974)

Score	Heart rate	Respiration	Colour	Muscle tone	Irritability
0	Absent	Absent	Blue/pale	Limp	No response
1	<100	Irregular, slow	Pink torso, blue extremities	Mild flexion	Grimace
2	≥100	Crying, active	Pink	Active	Sneeze

Total score 0–10: check at 1, 5 and 10 min post-partum

- Apgar 5–7:
  - stimulate breathing by rubbing chest. Facial mass oxygen as required
- Apgar 4–5:
  - as above. If no response, five breaths with bag and mask
- Apgar 1–3:
  - as above. If no response, commence external chest compressions, 1 breath:3 compressions

Resuscitation drugs (Table 4.2)

Table 4.2 Resuscitation drugs

Drug	Indication	Dose
Adrenaline (epinephrine)*, 1 in 10,000 (IV) [1 in 1000 (IT or diluted)]	Asystole, bradycardia	0.1–0.3 mL/kg (IV), (i.e. 0.01–0.03 mg/kg); repeat *after* 5 min (if no response)
Naloxone (1 mg/mL)	Opioid antagonism	0.1 mL/kg stat (and repeat)
NaHCO₃ (0.5 mEq/mL)	Acidosis	1–2 mEq/kg (slow IV)
Glucose (10%)	Hypoglycaemia	2 mL/kg
Saline (0.9%)	Volume depletion	10 mL/kg (over 10 min)

*Little used in practice in neonates.

Vomiting

Definition

The expulsion of stomach contents through the mouth.

Many normal babies regurgitate (posset) small amounts of milk in the first months of life. This may cause parental concerns but can be ignored if it is not compromising growth or causing other complications. Vomiting is a common symptom in infants and can be associated with virtually any pathology including intestinal obstruction, sepsis, raised intracranial pressure and metabolic abnormalities. Trying to determine the cause of vomiting in an infant may therefore be very challenging.

History and examination

When assessing the patient with vomiting, taking a detailed history is vital. In particular all causes of sepsis must be considered. The age of the patient and the timing and nature of the vomiting may help the differential diagnoses.

Assessment about the nature of the vomiting should include:

- colour – green (bile), yellow (bile), red (blood), brown (old blood)
- force – pyloric stenosis characteristically results in forceful (projectile) vomiting, often some time after completion of the feed. Regurgitation associated with gastro-oesophageal reflux is usually effortless and occurs during or shortly after feeding
- timing – in relation to feeds
- frequency – infrequent vomiting is less likely to result in rapid dehydration
- onset – acute or chronic. Acute vomiting may be a sign of acute illness and immediate investigation may be indicated.

The major complication of vomiting is fluid and electrolyte imbalance and dehydration. This must be corrected by appropriate intravenous fluid replacement (Table 4.3). The severity of dehydration is usually classified by percentage of **body weight loss**.

Table 4.3 Clinical assessment of dehydration

% Dehydration	Clinical features	Volume replacement required (mL/kg)
5	Dry mucus membranes	50
10	Sunken fontanelle, reduced urine output, reduced skin turgor	100
15	Tachycardia, hypotension, depressed conscious level	150

Specific electrolyte disturbances may give important clues to the cause of vomiting (e.g. metabolic alkalosis in pyloric stenosis, hyperkalaemia and hyponatraemia in congenital adrenal hyperplasia).

Non-bilious vomiting

Bilious vomiting suggests intestinal obstruction distal to the insertion of the bile duct in the second part of the duodenum. If the vomiting is non-bilious, intestinal obstruction is unlikely. However, obstruction may still be present above this level and examples are listed below.

Obstructive causes of non-bilious vomiting in infants

- Oesophagus:
  - stricture – peptic, congenital, anastomotic after oesophageal atresia repair
  - foreign body impaction
- Stomach:
  - gastric volvulus
  - antral diaphragm
  - pylorus
  - pyloric stenosis
- Duodenum
  - pre-ampullary atresia
  - malrotation (most have bilious vomiting)

Non-obstructive vomiting

- Gastro-oesophageal reflux (GOR):
  - over 50% of infants at 4 months of age and 5% at 1 year have regurgitation secondary to GOR
  - reflux in infancy does not usually require intervention unless it is causing clinical problems (gastro-oesophageal reflux disease – GORD). These may include faltering growth, aspiration pneumonia, apnoea, and oesophagitis (haematemesis and/or pain). Most clinicians will initially treat GORD in infants with feed thickeners (e.g. Gaviscon®) but will not progress to more intensive treatment (acid suppressants and prokinetic agents) without investigation (e.g. pH probe, upper GI contrast imaging etc)
- Sepsis:
  - vomiting associated with sepsis should resolve spontaneously with effective management of infection
- Raised intracranial pressure
- Metabolic disorders:
  - e.g. congenital adrenal hyperplasia (CAH). In girls this condition causes masculinization and presentation will be at birth because of ambiguous genitalia. In boys, however, the genitalia will look normal and clinical presentation will be delayed with vomiting, dehydration and electrolyte disturbance (hyperkalaemia and hyponatraemia due to lack of aldosterone) (Addisonian crisis)

Bilious vomiting

Bile is produced by the liver and stored in the gall bladder. When it is released via the sphincter of Oddi into the second part of the duodenum it is golden yellow in colour and turns green after contact with gastric acid. Bile does not normally appear in vomitus unless the intestine is obstructed distal to this point; however, it may be present after repeated vomiting.

Green vomiting should always be assumed to be due to obstruction.

Whatever may be causing the lumen of the intestine to be obstructed may also be causing obstruction to the intestinal blood supply, and although luminal obstruction may be managed conservatively vascular obstruction may not. Without blood supply, affected loops of gut will be dead within 6 h, with resulting perforation, peritonitis, and potentially death.

All infants with bilious vomiting should be discussed with surgeons.

Vascular compromise will usually induce a local peritoneal reaction resulting in abdominal tenderness or peritonism. If these features are present, immediate laparotomy is indicated.

In addition to fluid resuscitation, an appropriately sized nasogastric tube should be passed, regularly aspirated and left on free drainage. This decompresses the gut and minimizes the risk of aspiration of gastrointestinal contents.

Intestinal obstruction

Intestinal obstruction at any age is characterized by bile-stained vomiting, abdominal distension and absolute constipation (failure to pass stool or flatus).

If intestinal obstruction is suspected, the following action should be taken:

Clinical assessment
- The abdomen must be assessed for any signs of intestinal ischaemia (tenderness, palpable mass, peritonism) as this will indicate that immediate laparotomy is required.
- Intravenous access must be established and resuscitation and maintenance fluids given.
- A nasogastric tube should be passed, left on free drainage and aspirated regularly.
- Serum electrolytes must be measured and corrected as required and nasogastric losses replaced with appropriate intravenous fluids.
- An abdominal x-ray should be performed.

Surgical referral
Assessment of the cause of intestinal obstruction in the term neonate may follow this sequence:
- inspect the anus for patency (the absence of an anal opening will be obvious in most anorectal anomalies)
- check for inguinal hernia
- digital or instrumental (e.g. Hegar dilator) rectal examination (the anus is narrowed in anal stenosis, decompression may occur in Hirschsprung's disease)
- abdominal x-ray (this is usually diagnostic in duodenal and high small bowel atresia and may be suggestive in malrotation)
- contrast radiology (upper or lower GI contrast study may be required depending on the features on plain x-ray)
- laparotomy.

Functional intestinal obstruction in neonates
This may be multifactorial and differentiation from mechanical causes may be difficult. Causes include:
• sepsis
• maternal factors (e.g. diabetes, medications, narcotics)
• medications (e.g. opiates)
• metabolic disorders (e.g. hypermagnesaemia, hypokalaemia, hypercalcaemia)
• hypothyroidism
• prematurity
• congenital anomalies (e.g. gastroschisis).

Postoperative obstruction
Postoperative ileus will result in bilious gastric contents for some days. Some infants will have persistent bilious aspirates and even vomits in the absence of obstruction because of an incompetent pylorus (e.g. duodenal atresia) or prolonged distal dysfunction (e.g. gastroschisis).

Gastrointestinal bleeding

Bleeding from the gastrointestinal tract is uncommon in this age group; nonetheless certain key causes can be identified.

Aetiology

It is important to exclude a coagulopathy (e.g. vitamin K deficiency) or systematic cause (e.g. thrombocytopaenia) before embarking on a series of specific GI investigations. Similarly, regurgitation of swallowed maternal blood needs exclusion in the newly born by an Apt's test (alkali (NaOH) denatures adult but not fetal haemoglobin – causing a colour difference).

Upper GI bleeding, i.e. haematemesis
* Oesophagitis, gastritis, Mallory–Weiss tear
* Gastroduodenal ulceration
* Cow's milk allergy
* Pyloric stenosis
* Gastric and mid-gut volvulus
* Fore-gut duplication cyst
* vascular malformation
* NG tube trauma

Lower GI bleeding, i.e. melaena (black stool), haematochezia (red- or maroon-coloured stools) or simply fresh, red blood
Depending on the severity, all of the above can also manifest with melaena etc. Other causes may grouped into predominantly:
* infective, e.g. enteric pathogens (*Campylobacter jejuni, Clostridium difficle* etc), also indirectly – hemolytic-uraemic syndrome via *E. coli* O157:HZ)
* structural, e.g. duplication cyst, vascular malformation, Meckel's diverticulum
* inflammatory, e.g. NEC, Hirshsprung's disease (enterocolitis), cow's milk allergy
* ischaemic e.g. intussusception, midgut volvulus,
* anal fissure

Investigations

The investigation of GI bleeding in neonates must be individualized to the specific scenario and based on clinical features. Suspicion of a mid-gut volvulus (gasless abdominal plain film, peritonitic abdominal examination etc) needs rapid progression to a laparotomy rather than a leisurely series of investigations more appropriate for cow's milk allergy for instance.

Within this spectrum of possibilities consider blood profile (FBC including WBC differential for eosinophils, coagulation tests), plain and contrast abdominal radiography (upper and lower), Meckel (Tc^{99m}) scintiscan, faecal microscopy (for eosinophils, ova, cysts, and parasites), and culture; and allergy tests (serum total and specific IgE, skin-prick tests, food challenge or exclusion diets). Upper and lower GI endoscopy is technically difficult in neonates, but persistent bleeding may warrant it. Angiography remains the preserve of specialist institutions, and is chiefly used where a congenital vascular malformation is suspected.

Management

Again, the specific management depends on the specific cause. Resuscitation always takes precedence. Consider passage of a NG tube in upper GI bleeds with saline lavage to determine the degree of ongoing bleeding. 'Blind', or rather presumptive therapy with H_2 receptor antagonists (e.g. ranitidine) or PPIs (e.g. omeprazole) may be appropriate in the NICU setting with sick infants. Cow's milk protein intolerance is largely treated by conversion to a casein-hydrolysate formula (e.g. Pregestimil®).

Further reading

Arvola T, Ruuska T, Keranen J et al. Rectal bleeding in infancy: clinical, allergological and microbiological examination. *Pediatrics* 2006;**117**:e760–8.

Lazzaroni M, Petrillo M, Tornaghi R et al. Upper GI bleeding in healthy full-term infants: a case-control study. *Am J Gastroenterol* 2002;**97**:89–94.

Maayan-Metzger A, Ghanem N, Mazkereth R, Kuint J. Characteristics of neonates with isolated rectal bleeding. *Arch Dis Child (Fetal and Neonatal)* 2004;**89**:F68–F70.

Ohtsuka Y, Shimizu T, Shoji H et al. Neonatal transient eosinophilic colitis causes lower gastrointestinal bleeding in early infancy. *J Pediatr Gastroenterol Nutr* 2007;**44**:501–5.

Failure to pass meconium

The word 'meconium' derives from *meconium-arion*, meaning 'opium-like', in reference either to its tarry appearance or to Aristotle's belief that it induced sleep in the fetus (Wikipedia).

Meconium is the sticky, viscous, black or dark-green first-passed product of the newborn intestine. It contains swallowed amniotic fluid, lanugo, bile, intestinal secretions, epithelial debris, and mucus. In itself it causes problems if passed *in utero* (as meconium-stained liquor) indicating fetal distress, and if is inhaled where it sets up a marked pulmonary inflammatory pnumonitis (meconium aspiration syndrome).

Normal term neonates should pass meconium within 48 h. Failure to pass stool together with abdominal distension suggests distal gastrointestinal obstruction.

Only about one-third of normal preterm neonates pass meconium in The first 24 h, and one-third will still not have done so by 48 h.

Surgical causes
- Anorectal malformation
- Hirschsprung's disease
- Meconium ileus
- Meconium plug syndrome
- Ileal or colonic atresia
- Small left colon syndrome (offspring of diabetic mothers)

Management
After resuscitation, assess the degree of abdominal distension – is it compromising respiratory effort? Are there any masses? Perform a careful perineal exam: is the anus normally sited? (The anus is normally sited more than one-third of the distance between the fourchette (girls)/crotum (boys) and the coccyx.) Is it patent? Gently pass a lubricated probe to assess. Casual examination may embarrassingly miss an imperforate anus as there is often a blind-ending pit.

Investigation
Plain abdominal radiograph is often diagnostic; contrast enemas can be useful in diagnosis and treatment; suction rectal biopsy if Hirschsprung's disease suspected; gene probe/sweat test for cystic fibrosis if there is meconium ileus.

Further reading
Weaver LT, Lucas A. Development of bowel habit in preterm infants. *Arch Dis Child* 1993; **68**:317–20.

Jaundice

Jaundice is the clinical sign of a raised bilirubin (usually detectable at >50 micromol/L) and is named from the Old French for yellow (jaunice).

Normal values

Bilirubin (3–20 micromol/L), conjugated (<5 micromol/L)

Bilirubin metabolism

Bilirubin is an open chain tetrapyrrole with eight side chains (molecular weight = 585) and a metabolic by-product of red cell breakdown (largely in the spleen). Haem is converted (enzyme: haem oxygenase via biliverdin) to bilirubin, which is transported (on albumin) to the liver in an unconjugated fat-soluble form. Hepatocyte uptake occurs with (enzyme: UDPGT) conversion to the water-soluble form by conjugation with glucuronic acid. This is then excreted into the biliary canaliculus.

Further metabolism occurs in the ileum (to urobilinogen – absorbed and re-excreted in urine) and colon (stercobilinogen – excreted) although the process is poorly developed in infancy.

Causes of unconjugated (indirect) jaundice

Physiological (2–10 days)

Caused by immaturity of neonatal liver enzymes and increased perinatal red cell breakdown. Exacerbated by prematurity, IUGR, breast feeding, cephalohaematoma etc. Treatment depends on postnatal age and total serum bilirubin level. Kernicterus (encephalopathy) is caused by unconjugated bilirubin crossing an immature blood/brain barrier and localizing in the basal ganglia (rare).

ABO and Rhesus incompatibility

(If severe may present as fetus with hydrops or <24 h)
● ABO: group O mother with group A or B infant
● Rhesus: Rh −ve mother (with previous pregnancies) and Rh +ve infant
Direct Coombs' test – evidence of preformed antibodies on red cells.

Breast milk jaundice

Mechanism unknown

Congenital enzyme defects

● e.g. Gilbert syndrome (5% of population, benign), Crigler–Najjar syndrome (types 1 and 2, autosomal recessive, potentially lethal)

Treatment of unconjugated jaundice

Phototherapy, or in severe cases exchange transfusion.

Causes of conjugated (direct) jaundice

Medical
- Alpha-1-antitrypsin deficiency (1 in 2000 births, mutations in SERPINA1 gene on Ch14)
- Giant cell hepatitis
- Cytomegalovirus hepatitis
- Alagille's syndrome (biliary hypoplasia, abnormal vertebrae, pulmonary stenosis, odd facies, probable JAGGED1 mutational abnormality)
- Cystic fibrosis (inspissated bile)
- Galactosaemia (1 in 47,000 defect in enzyme converting galactose into glucose – galactose-1-phosphate uridyl transferase) multifactorial.
- Parenteral nutrition – common on surgical wards

Surgical
- Biliary atresia
- Obstructed cystic choledochal malformation
- Spontaneous perforation of the bile duct
- Inspissated bile syndrome

Investigation of conjugated jaundice in infants (Fig. 4.1)
- Exclude alpha-1-antitrypsin deficiency (serum levels (>30 micromol/L) and phenotype – three possible alleles (M, S, Z))
- Ultrasound – no characteristic signs in biliary atresia but may detect intrahepatic biliary dilatation or choledochal dilatation (normal CBD ~1 mm)
- Percutaneous liver biopsy (suggestive of biliary atresia if cholestatic with ductular proliferation and bile plugging)
- Radio-isotope scan – occasionally used in the absence of biopsy in some centres
- Cholangiogram (laparotomy or laparoscopy) or ERCP (specialist centres only)

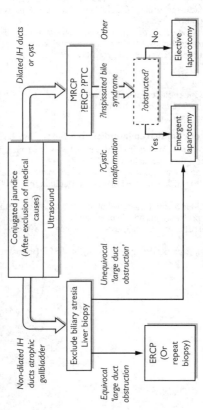

Fig. 4.1 Suggested algorithm for the investigation of conjugated jaundice in the infant.

Parenchymal lung anomalies

There are three main developmental anomalies which may necessitate surgical removal. Although often considered in isolation, it is probably more correct to regard these as a spectrum of disease as there is a great deal of pathological and clinical overlap.

- Congenital cystic adenomatoid malformation
- Lung sequestration
- Congenitial lobar empysema

Congenital cystic adenomatoid malformation

Definition

Harmatous multicystic mass of pulmonary tissue.

Aetiology

Unknown. Characterized by an increase in terminal respiratory structures, forming interconnecting cysts of various sizes.

Classification

See Table 4.4.

Table 4.4 Stocker's classification of congenital cystic adenomatoid malformation

Type	Description
I	Large cysts >2 cm in diameter, with mucus-producing cells
II	Medium cysts <1 cm in diameter, lined with ciliated columnar epithelium
III	Microcystic appearing as a solid mass. Often affects entire lobe or lung. Mainly in stillborn infants

Since its introduction the classification has been expanded to include a Type O and a Type IV.

Incidence

- Not known with precision
- ?1 in 10,000–25,000 pregnancies

Associated anomalies:

May occur in up to 20% of cases (usually type II) and include diaphragmatic hernia, renal, cardiac, and intestinal abnormalities.

Presentation

- Antenatal (80%) – on screening USS. Polyhydramnios or hydrops fetalis (poor prognosis) occurs in 30%
- Neonatal (10%) – progressive respiratory distress due to air trapping within the cysts and pulmonary hypoplasia of the contralateral lung
- Childhood (10%) – recurrent pneumonia or pneumothorax
- Death – ~5% are stillborn
- A high proportion of those detected antenatally will be asymptomatic at birth and for a long time thereafter

Diagnosis
- Antenatal:
  - cyst size, i.e. >5 mm macrocystic versus <5 mm microcystic (Adzick classification)
  - Progression, i.e. serial US can show an increase, decrease or resolution
- Postnatal:
  - CXR– sharply outlined, irregularly shaped, radiolucent areas of variable sizes; air-fluid levels; mass, or mediastinal shift
  - Doppler USS (may show anomalous systemic blood supply)
  - CT with IV contrast

Differential diagnosis
Congenital diaphragmatic hernia, pulmonary sequestration, or congenital lobar emphysema.

Management
Antenatal (see also pages 58–59)
Serial monitoring with USS. Fetuses with hydrops and macrocystic disease may need thoraco-amniotic shunting. Fetal surgical resection is controversial but possible.

Symptomatic
Excision of affected lobes

Asymptomatic
Controversial. CCAM can spontaneously regress and therefore some maintain observation is the treatment of choice. However, there is a significant risk of infection, plus rare cases of malignancies developing e.g. bronchioalveolar carcinoma, rhabdomyosarcoma, and squamous cell carcinoma; supporting prophylactic excision.

Surgery
Postero-lateral thoracotomy. Single or multiple lobectomies. Segmental resection is possible for localized disease or bilateral involvement. Thoracoscopic excision is possible but can be technically difficult due to failure of the affected lung to collapse.

Specific complications
- Incomplete excision, resulting in recurrence of symptoms, prolonged air leak, or development of malignancies
- Postoperative mediastinal shift

Pulmonary sequestration

Definition
Congenital non-functioning lung tissue with no tracheo-bronchial communication. This has a characteristic yet anomalous systemic arterial supply. Two types may be seen (Table 4.5):
- intralobar sequestration (ILS) – sequestered lung within the normal lung. Some authors have suggested these are an acquired anomaly following chest infection
- extralobar sequestration (ELS) – separate from the normal lung and outside the visceral pleura.

Although the majority are found within thoracic cavity, some ELS may be found below the diaphragm.

Table 4.5

	Intralobar	Extralobar
Gender (M:F)	1:1	4:1
Anatomy	Lower lobe (~95%), left-sided	Basal intrathoracic and upper abdominal, left-sided
Frequency	75%	25%
Blood supply	Abdominal aorta (75%)	Thoracic/abdominal aorta (80%)
Venous drainage	Pulmonary vein (98%)	Systemic vein (75%)
Association	Oesophagobronchial fistula (rate)	Diaphragmatic hernia, bronchogenic cyst, CCAM

Incidence
~6% of all congenital lung malformations.

Aetiology
Thought to be due to an accessory lung bud developing from the primitive foregut. Development prior to pleural formation results in ILS, while later development causes ELS.

Clinical features
ILS tends to present later with chronic cough and recurrent pneumonias in the same anatomic location, or poor exercise tolerance, or congestive cardiac failure if there is a large systemic arterio-venous shunt.

Most (60%) ELS present earlier as an antenatally-detected anomaly (±polyhydramnios, fetal hydrops, or pleural effusion), as a coincidental anomaly (e.g. CDH) or postnatally with respiratory distress, chronic cough, or recurrent chest infections. Some have feeding difficulties, vomiting, abdominal pain if there is a communication with the GI tract.

The key feature to show is the characteristic systemic arterial blood supply. CXR is of limited use but Doppler ultrasound is non-invasive and may show this feature. CT, MRI, MRA are all useful and have generally supplanted angiography.

Management
Some authors simply adopt a conservative strategy if asymptomatic but this will need long-term follow-up.

Surgery
Excision is usually recommended to prevent infection, hemorrhage or arterio-venous shunting. This may involve a formal lobectomy or segmentectomy where the lesion is discrete. ELS should be easy to resect without the loss of normal lung tissue.

Thoractomy is a traditional approach but thoracoscopic excision is possible.

The anomalous blood supply is often out of proportion for the tissue supplied and needs to be precisely defined to prevent untoward haemorrhage.

Pre-operative embolization of the arterial supply has been reported both as an aid to later surgery or occasionally as the only intervention.

Congenital lobar emphysema

This is probably caused by a defect in bronchial developmental resulting in 'valve-like' function allowing air in but not out. Thus the lobe becomes over-distended and compresses adjacent normal lung tissue.

Distribution
- Left upper lobe (50%)
- Right middle lobe (20%)
- Right upper lobe (20%)

Clinical features

Presents with respiratory distress in first few days of life. There may be signs of mediastinal shift, hyper-resonance, and transillumination (clear differential is with pneumothorax) may be seen. The CXR shows hyper-lucency in the upper lobes, typically. If symptoms allow then a CT scan should resolve diagnostic problems.

Surgery

Once diagnosed, consider urgent thoracotomy and lobectomy. Selective bronchial intubation has been suggested as a temporizing measure.

Box 4.1 Scimitar syndrome

This is a congenital anomaly in which an anomalous pulmonary vein drains into the IVC or its junction at the right atrium. An association exists with hypoplasia of the right lung, hypoplasia of the right pulmonary artery, and an anomalous systemic vascular supply to the lung.

Further reading

Congenital cystic adenomatoid malformation

Burge D, Babu S. Structural anomalies of the airways and lungs. In: Burge DM, Griffiths DM Steinbrecher HA *et al* (eds). *Paediatric Surgery* (2nd edn) 2005.

Davenport M, Warne SA, Cacciaguerra S *et al*. Current outcome of antenatally diagnosed cystic lung disease. *J Pediatr Surg* 2004;**39**:549–56.

Stocker JT, Madewell JE, Drake RM. Congenital cystic adenomatoid malformation of the lung. *Hum Pathol* 1977;**8**:155–71.

Sundararajan L, Parikh DH. Evolving experience with video-assisted thoracic surgery in congenital cystic lung lesions in a British pediatric center. *J Pediatr Surg* 2007;**42**:1243–50.

Pulmonary sequestration

Corbett HJ, Humphrey G. Pulmonary Sequestration. *Paediatr Respir Rev* 2004;**5**:59–68.

de Lorimier A. Respiratory problems related to the airway and lung. In: O'Neil JA, Rowe M, Grosfeld JL St Louis, MO *et al* (eds). *Pediatric Surgery* (5th edn). Mosby-Year Book Inc, 1998 873–97.

Foregut duplication cyst

This encompasses a spectrum of abnormalities arising from the primitive embryonic foregut (mouth to mid-duodenum). Most common are bronchogenic cysts and enteric duplication cysts.

Bronchogenic cysts

Abnormal budding of the tracheal diverticulum from the primitive foregut may cause cyst formation. The level of the abnormal budding accounts for the variety of positions that bronchogenic cysts etc are found.

Majority surround the carina, but other locations include peri-hilar, within the lung, para-oesophageal, in the neck/tongue, or subdiaphragmatic.

Histopathology

Thin-walled cystic structure, lined with respiratory epithelium and filled with viscid mucus.

Incidence

Rare (<5% of mediastinal masses). Slight male preponderance.

Clinical features

The majority are usually diagnosed in adulthood. Some present with recurrent pneumonia or atelectasis secondary to compression effects or due to the connection with the bronchial tree. Compression of the bronchi/trachea as a neonate can result in respiratory distress. This could also cause congenital lobar emphysema, which can often cause confusion in the diagnosis. Uncommonly they may be a source of haemorrhage or haemoptysis.

Incidental finding on CXR or antenatal ultrasound.

Diagnosis

Chest x-ray and CT or MRI.

Differential diagnosis

* Tumours, e.g. lymphoma, neuroblastoma and teratoma
* Foreign body
* Lobar emphysema

Surgery

Complete surgical excision recommended due to eventual development of symptoms and the reported risk of malignant transformation. Can be performed open or thoroscopically, depending upon cyst location.

Further reading

Philippart A. Benign mediastinal cysts and tumors. In: O'Neil JA, Rowe M, Grosfeld JL et al (eds). *Pediatric Surgery* St Louis, MO (5th edn). Mosby-Year Book Inc, 1998.

Ribet ME, Copin MC, Gosselin B. Bronchogenic cysts of the mediastinum. *J Thorac Cardiovasc Surg* 1995;**109**:1003–10.

Oesophageal atresia

Embryology

The foregut divides lengthways by the appearance of lateral mesodermal ridges, becoming complete around the 26th day of gestation. Incomplete fusion seems to explain TOF, if not OA.

Types

- OA and distal TOF (80%)
- OA alone (10%)
- OA and proximal TOF (<5%)
- OA and proximal and distal TOF (<5%)
- TOF alone (4%)

Incidence

1 in 3000; slight male predominance, no racial variation

Associations

Multiple but the ones of note are:
- other atresias (duodenal and ano-rectal)
- cardiac anomalies
- VATER (vertebral, anorectal, tracheo-esophageal, renal (radial)
  VACTERL is the same association (with cardiac) but misspelled! Need 3+ features to be so named
- CHARGE (coloboma, heart, atresia choanal, retarded growth, genital hypoplasia, ear defects). Autosomal dominant. Usually mutation in CHD7 gene
- chromosome (e.g. trisomy 21, 18).

Clinical features

OA and failure to swallow amniotic fluid and saliva cause most clinical features. Thus, polyhydramnios (seen in ~30%) and absence of stomach bubble on US may allow a prenatal diagnosis. Frothing or being excessively mucosy should be obvious on the day of birth. Difficulty with feeding means you should change the midwife! The diagnostic procedure should be an attempt to pass a 'proper' naso-gastric tube (8 Fg and beyond), with a CXR. This should show the uncurled tip at the level of T3–5, and no further. Distal intestinal gas means there is an additional TOF. More subtle signs on the CXR may include, vertebral body anomalies, a right-sided aortic arch, signs of aspiration, and the large distended stomach of an associated duodenal atresia.

Management

If you can manage the saliva and potential for aspiration then these infants are perfectly safe for weeks. A Replogle tube is ideal and allows continual suction with avoidance of end-hole occlusion. Most will come to surgery early, but a different strategy should be adopted for those deemed as long-gap OA. All need appropriate work-up (including echocardiography) and there is really only one scenario where urgent surgery is contemplated (see later).

Surgery – primary repair OA and TOF (Fig. 4.2)
- ?Preliminary bronchoscopy (identify any proximal TOF)
- 3rd/4th/5th left postero-lateral thoracotomy (level depending on size/ position of upper pouch)
- Extrapleural approach – divide intercostal muscles and strip pleura off posterior structures
- Identify azygous vein (ligate or respect)
- Identify (proximity to vagus), sling and oversew TOF
- Identify/mobilize upper pouch – facilitated by manipulation from above
- Oesophageal anastomosis – now typically single-layer monofilament (5/0, 6/0). A trans-anastomotic tube allows early feeding

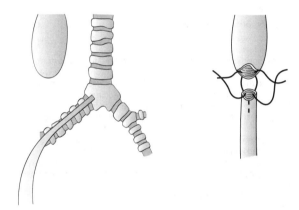

Fig. 4.2 Oesophageal atresia with distal TOF. Ligation of TOF and primary end-to-end anastomosis.

All of this can of course be accomplished thoracoscopically – although its true role in the real world has yet to emerge. It has been compared to operating in a matchbox!

Box 4.2 TOF and RDS

Dangerous combination of a ventilated preterm infant (stiff, low com- pliant, RDS lungs) with a TOF which is prone to gas escape via the TOF into a distended stomach. Associated with rupture. Surgical solution is to ligate urgently the TOF (leaving the anastomosis potentially for another day). Medical solution is high-frequency oscillation (to reduce mean airway pressure). Endoscopic occlusion is possible using embolec- tomy balloon etc.

Complications
- Anastomotic leak (<10%) – early major leak (consider re-exploration and revise) versus later, minor leak (should close spontaneously)
- Stricture (20–30%) – consequence of leak usually. Assess with contrast. Balloon or rigid dilatation. If multiple, then consider revision or occasionally replacement
- Reflux (>40%) – predisposed and may contribute to stricture development. Early fundoplication should be considered for symptoms
- Fistula recurrence (<5%) – now not common
- Tracheomalacia – becomes problematic after some weeks typically, with 'death' or 'drop' episodes. Improves with tracheal growth. Interventions include tracheopexy, aortopexy, and endolumenal stenting

Long-gap oesophageal atresia
Suspected because of absence of distal gas. There are many options and none are ideal:
- delayed primary anastomosis – needs an initial open gastrostomy (to feed) and promote expansion of the small stomach. An EUA will evaluate the gap (in vertebral bodies) using contrast, or sound in the distal part. The ends tend to come closer (requires 6–8 weeks though). When ends are apparently overlapping then aim for elective thoracotomy and anastomosis. Some authors believe that a flap created from the upper pouch can facilitate this often-difficult anastomosis
- Foker technique – in contrast to above, an early thoracotomy is performed and multiple tension sutures are placed on the distal oesophagus, with ends left outside the chest wall. These are progressively tightened causing lengthening and facilitating later anastomosis (1–2 weeks)
- oesophageal replacement – if delayed typically requires cervical oesophagostomy and gastrostomy.

The outcome in term infants with only OA is excellent with a corresponding reduction in outcome for those who have low birth weight or associate (particularly cardiac anomalies) (Table 4.6)

Table 4.6 Spitz prognostic classification (1994) (successor to Waterston)

Group		Survival (predicted) (%)
I	>1.5 kg, no anomalies	>98
II	<1.5 kg *or* major cardiac anomalies	~60
III	<1.5 kg *and* major cardiac anomalies	~20

Further reading

Holcomb GW, Rothenberg SS, Bax KMA *et al.* Thoracoscopic repair of esophageal atresia and tracheoesophageal fistula: a multiinstintutional experience. *Ann Surg* 2005;**242**:422–30.

Nasr A, Ein S, Gerstle JT. Infants with repaired esophageal atresia and distal tracheoesophageal fistula with respiratory distress: is it tracheomalacia, reflux or both? *J Pediatr Surg* 2005;40 1612–15:

Quan L, Smith DW. The VATER association. Vertebral defects, Anal atresia, T-E fistula with esophageal atresia, Radial and Renal dysplasia: a spectrum of associated defects. *J Pediatr* 1973;**82**:104–107.

Spitz L. Lessons I have learned in a 40 year experience. *J Pediatr Surg* 2006;**41**:1635–40.

Spitz J, Kiely EM, Morecroft JA, Drake DP. Oesophageal atresia: at risk groups for the 1990s. *J Pediatr Surg* 1994;**29**:723–75.

Congenital diaphragmatic hernia

Incidence
1 in 2500 live births – a new case is encountered every 24–36 h in the UK.

Types
- Posterolateral diaphragmatic hernia (of Bochdalek):
  - left – 85%
  - right – 12%
  - bilateral – 2%
  - agenesis – 1%
- Anterior hernia (of Morgagni) – seen usually in later infancy and childhood (better prognosis).

Associated anomalies
These are seen in up to 40% of those antenatally diagnosed and have a grave prognosis and a dismal survival of <10%:
- central nervous system
- cardiac
- chromosomal disorders.

Familial associations are rare (< 2%).

The 'hidden mortality' are *in utero* deaths, and terminations recorded from population-based studies and malformation registries and provide the best indicator of true survival.

Lung hypoplasia and pulmonary hypertension account for the high mortality in isolated CDH.

Management
The antenatal diagnosis of CDH is usually made by maternal ultrasound in 70–80% of cases in the UK. Amniocentesis is recommended to karyotype the fetus and exclude chromosomal anomalies (almost invariably lethal). Referral for prenatal counselling should be coordinated by a multidisciplinary team (obstetrician, neonatologist, and paediatric surgeon).

Some centres offer prenatal intervention for isolated CDH, using biometric measurement of the fetal lung–head ratio (LHR) to guide prognosis. An LHR ≤1.0 and a liver-up position have been considered as markers of such poor outcome to warrant intervention (e.g. FETO balloon). Nonetheless, an American randomized trial comparing fetal intervention versus standard postnatal care failed to identify significant survival benefit using hysterotomy-applied tracheal occlusion. Further trials refining LHR entry criteria for fetal intervention are anticipated (European FETO task group). Other modalities to assess lung maturation in the fetus such as MRI lung-volumetry continue to be explored but require validation.

Elective delivery of the fetus with CDH should be planned near term (≥37 weeks) and coordinated in a tertiary specialist unit. Better outcomes for 'live born' cases are now reported in 'high volume' centres (>80% survival).

Resuscitation

Prompt elective intubation, nasogastric decompression, and vascular access to permit pre- and postductal gas monitoring. Inotrope support (e.g. dobutamine) may be required.

Permissive hypercapnea ('gentle ventilation') strategies

In previous times, much of the lung damage appeared to be related to barotrauma and the effects of sustained high-pressure, high-frequency ventilation. Recent improvements in survival have been attributed to strategies designed to limit this damage and protect the vulnerable hypoplastic lung.

Other elements might include:

- HFOV (high-frequency oscillatory ventilation)
- management of pulmonary hypertension should be guided by serial bedside echocardiography and include the use of iNO and, more recently, sildenafil
- ECMO (available since the early 1980s, in USA, and early 1990s in the UK) to treat resistant pulmonary hypertension and provide a period of 'lung rest'. There is wide variation in institutional success rates across Europe and North America, with different entry criteria. The UK ECMO randomized trial did not show a survival advantage in the CDH subgroup (albeit with small numbers)
- liquid ventilation (perfluorocarbons) is subject to experimental study.

Surgery – repair of diaphragmatic hernia (Fig. 4.3)

Surgical repair is scheduled as a semi-elective procedure after stabilization of labile physiology. Aim for $FiO_2 \leq 0.3$.

- Subcostal (appropriate to side) incision. Visualize defect and reduce herniated viscera. On right, division of hepatic ligaments, and rotating liver helps its reduction
- ?Hernial sac (~10%) – requires excision
- Dissect posterior rim – although this may be sparse. A subcostal slide can be created in the anterior diaphragm rim
- Aim for primary closure (possible ~70%), preferably using non-absorbable (e.g. Ethibond®) sutures.

A prosthetic (Gore-Tex®) or bioprosthetic (Surgisis®) patch can be used to repair larger defects (~30%). Other innovative options include use of rotated muscle flaps, e.g. latissimus dorsi, although these are probably best suited to recurrent hernias.

Abdominal compartment syndrome is possible with too-tight wound closure, and consideration should be given to a prosthetic patch closure in these circumstances.

Most surgeons have abandoned the routine use of a chest tube.

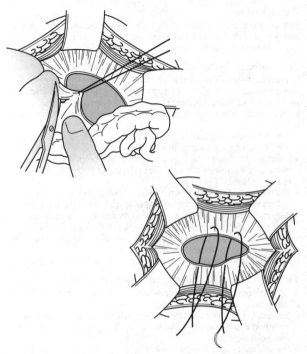

Fig. 4.3 Operative repair of Left CDH – the posterior rim of the diaphragm is mobilized after reducing the hernia contents to aid primary closure. Non-absorbable sutures are used to close the defect. Reprinted with permission from Congenital diaphragmatic hernia. (In: *Paediatric Surgery* (2nd edn). London: Hodder Arnold)

Postoperative course and complications

Infants are returned to intensive care. Surgery rarely improves their cardiorespiratory status immediately, and typically several more days of weaning will be required.

- Pleural effusion – invariable, but intervention (e.g. needle thoracentesis) only required if there is evidence of mediastinal shift and clinical deterioration
- Chylous effusion – presumed to be due to division of lymphatic trunks in posterior dissection. Recognized by milky nature if feeding, or high lymphocyte count if not. Total parenteral nutrition ± octreotide is usually effective for persistent effusions
- Gastro-oesophageal reflux and feeding problems – increased incidence and presumed to be due to anatomical (crural) disruption and perhaps chronic lung disease. Initially treated with medical therapy but may require fundoplication ± gastrostomy

- Chronic cardiorespiratory disease – as a consequence of pulmonary hypoplasia/hypertension and iatrogenic lung injury following barotrauma
- Skeletal and chest wall deformity (pectus excavatum, scoliosis).
- Neurocognitive deficits – secondary to neonatal hypoxia and use of ECMO
- Prosthetic patch revision and re-herniation reported in ~ 50% of long-term survivors

Box 4.3 Minimally invasive repair of CDH

This has been performed successfully in infants and older children with good respiratory function. The easiest approach appears to be from above (i.e. thoracoscopically). Care should be exercised in 'high-risk' newborns with physiological instability given invariable hypercarbia associated with insufflation. In the short term, outcomes appears comparable to the traditional open operation.

Further reading

Ba'ath ME, Jesudason EC, Losty PD. How useful is the lung-to-head ratio in predicting outcome in the fetus with congenital diaphragmatic hernia ? A systematic review and meta-analysis. *Ultrasound Obstet Gynecol* 2007;**30**:897–906.

Conforti AF, Losty PD. Perinatal management of congenital diaphragmatic hernia. *Early Hum Dev* 2006;**82**:283–287.

Gucciardo L, Deprest J, Done E *et al.* Prediction of outcome in isolated congenital diaphragmatic hernia and its consequences for fetal therapy. *Best Pract Res Clin Obstet Gynaecol* 2008;**22**:123–38.

Harrison MR, Keller RL, Hawgood SB *et al.* A randomised trial of fetal endoscopic tracheal occlusion for severe fetal congenital diaphragmatic hernia. *N Engl J Med* 2003;**349**:1916–24.

Diaphragm eventration

This may be:
- congenital – pulmonary development may also be impaired *in utero*
- acquired – due to phrenic (C 3, 4, 5) nerve injury secondary to birth trauma; cardiac surgery (typically PDA ligation) or resection of mediastinal tumours.

Clinical features

Paradoxical diaphragm movement may adversely affect respiratory function leading to need for ventilation or difficulty with weaning. CXR shows an elevated hemidiaphragm (usually left-sided) while real-time US/fluoroscopy shows the abnormal movement. Bilateral eventration is also possible.

Echocardiography is recommended in babies with congenital eventration, to rule out cardiac malformations. Intestinal malrotation should be excluded in those with feeding problems.

Although conservative treatment and spontaneous restoration of function is possible in a few, indications for surgery include ventilator dependency, persistent feeding problems, and failure to thrive with recurrent respiratory infections.

Surgery – diaphragmatic plication

The diaphragm may be approached via a subcostal or thoracic incision. Place a radially aligned series of non-absorbable sutures (e.g. Ethibond®) with care to avoid branches of the phrenic nerve. These should be tied to achieve a bunched, low, flat diaphragm.

In severe cases the paralysed segment resembles the membranous sac seen in a CDH. If so, then excision of this attenuated membrane may be performed with primary suture of the defect.

Minimally invasive thoracoscopic repair is also feasible.

Further reading

Yazici M, Karaca I, Arikan A et al. Congenital eventration of the diaphragm in children: 25 years' experience in three pediatric surgery centres. *Eur J Pediatr Surg* 2003;**13**:298–301.

Pyloric stenosis

Incidence

1 in 500 live births (Caucasian); 1 in 1000 (Asian and African)

Epidemiology

Male predominance (4:1), siblings (10% risk), possible association with Hirschsprung's disease.

Aetiology

Unknown, although clear genetic component because of familial cases.

Clinical features

Projectile, non-bilious vomiting between 3 and 6 weeks of age. Typically, the baby is unsettled and hungry with a history of failure to thrive. Dehydration usually obvious if history >3 days.

- Look for – visible peristalsis.
- Feel for – an olive-sized 'tumour' in the right hypochondrium or midline.
- Test feed (milk, water or even air (via nasogatric tube)) may facilitate above features.

Investigations

- US (sensitivity >95%), used if the examination is equivocal and history is suggestive. Normal wall thickness (≤3 mm), diameter (≤10 mm), length (≤18mm) – in term infants.
- The differential diagnosis might include other causes of non-bilious vomiting such as possetting, overfeeding, GORD, sepsis, cow's milk protein intolerance, and lactose intolerance.

Management

The classical electrolyte imbalance is due to loss of Na^+, Cl^-, K^+, H^+, and water in the acid vomiting. Infants are therefore dehydrated with a hypokalaemic, hyponatraemic, metabolic alkalosis (high pH, raised $[HCO_3^-]$). The urine pH may be alkaline or, paradoxically, acid.

Fluid replacement

Calculation of (i) resuscitation, (ii) maintainence, and (iii) replacement of ongoing losses. Contemplate surgery only when all abnormality is corrected.

The typical stock IV fluid is 0.45% saline with 4% or 5% dextrose (10% dextrose in the neonate) with 10 mmol of potassium per 500 mL used as maintenance fluid.

Surgery – pyloromyotomy (Figs 4.4 and 4.5)

This was first described in 1907, by Conrad von Ramstedt (1867–1963).

Although mostly performed as an open procedure it may also be performed using a laparoscopic technique. A recent RCT demonstrated some benefits from the latter approach.

Open procedure
- Incision (right upper quadrant muscle-cutting or supra-umbilical incision with delivery of the pylorus into the wound)
- Pyloromyotomy (longitudinal split using blade and mosquito clip to allow the underlying mucosa to bulge. Caution with fornix of duodenum in distal part of split)

(i)   (ii)

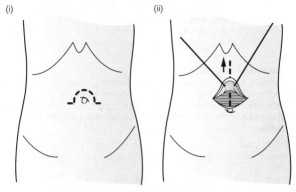

Fig. 4.4 Pyloromyotomy – (i) circumumbilical incision, (ii) skin hooks providing traction to expose epigastrium. Divide linea alba in midline, as near to xiphisternum as possible.

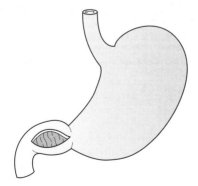

Fig. 4.5 Pyloromyotomy incision.

Laparoscopic procedure
- Supine position CO_2 working pressure ~8 mmHg
- Three ports (open Hasson technique):
  - 5 mm laparoscope – umbilical insertion
  - 3 mm working port (x2) – RUQ andLUQ
- Immobilize proximal duodenum using an atraumatic grasper. The pyloric incision can be then be made using the back of a hook diathermy or an arthroscopic cold-knife. The muscle is then spread using an atraumatic grasper, or a Tan spreader

NB mucosal integrity and absence of perforation should always be confirmed at the end of whatever technique is chosen by insufflation of air into the stomach via the nasogastric tube.

Postoperative management
At present, there is no consensus, nor compelling evidence, for a standardized as opposed to an *ad libitum* postoperative feeding regimen. The parents need to be made aware that most infants can have further vomiting after the procedure. Feeding is occasionally delayed by the surgeon if complicated by a mucosal perforation.

Complications
- Serosal laceration (treat conservatively unless there is significant bleeding)
- Mucosal perforation (operative closure when recognized)
- Wound infection (higher if umbilical wound (5%), use prophlactic antibiotic on induction)
- Incomplete pyloromyotomy (<2%)

Further reading

Najmaldin A, Tan HL. Early experience with laparoscopic pyloromyotomy for infantile hypertrophic pyloric stenosis. *J Pediatr Surg* 1995;**30**:37–8.

St Peter SD, Holcomb GW 3rd, Calkins CM *et al.* Open versus laparoscopic pyloromyotomy for pyloric stenosis: a prospective, randomized trial. *Ann Surg* 2006;**244**:363–70.

Tan KC, Bianchi A: Circumumbilical incision for pyloromyotomy. *Br J Surg* 1986;**73**:399.

Malrotation and volvulus

Malrotation refers to abnormal rotation and fixation of the embryonic mid-gut.

Embryology

Mid-gut rotation based on changing positions of two component loops, (duodeno-jejunal and the caeco-colic) as they go into and out of physiological hernia.
- Stage 1 (5th–10th week) – rotation of DJ flexure, anticlockwise *behind* the SMA to lie in LUQ
- Stage 2 (10th week) – 270° rotation of caeco-colic loop from LLQ to lie in front of DJ flexure
- Stage 3 (11th week onwards) – continuation of anticlockwise rotation of caeco-colic pole to RLQ and fixation

The commonest malrotation (Fig. 4.6) is failure of final 90° caeco-colic rotation from RUQ to RLQ and fixation. This results in proximity of DJ flexure and ileocaecum and hence a narrow-based, short mesentery. This predisposes to a volvulus.

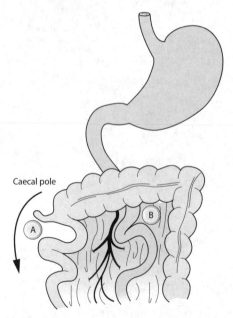

Caecal pole

Fig. 4.6 Commonest type of malrotation with failure of descent of caecal pole – untoward proximity of base of mesentery (A and B) make volvulus likely.

Incidence
- 0.5–1% of the population (from post-mortem studies)
- 1 in 6000 live births become symptomatic (50–75% within first month of life and 90% within a year)

Associations
- Congenital diaphragmatic hernia
- Abdominal wall defects (exomphalos and gastroschisis)
- Cardiac heterotaxia syndromes
- Duodenal web/stenosis (~10%)

Clinical features
Malrotation can be entirely asymptomatic, but may be a cause of upper intestinal obstruction either by extrinsic compression from abnormal peritoneal bands (Ladd's bands), or because a volvulus has occurred.

Bile vomiting is the usual presenting feature (~70% in those <2 years, and ~50% in those >2 years, but others include abdominal pain, diarrhoea, anorexia, irritability, failure to thrive, altered blood in stools and fever).

The examination may vary dramatically, depending on the presence or absence of volvulus and if there is mid-gut necrosis. If the latter, then infants are shocked with a tender distended abdomen. In the absence of volvulus, the signs may be minimal with perhaps dehydration if vomiting has been prolonged and a scaphoid abdomen. It is rarely diagnosed on asymptomatic children who undergo an upper GI contrast.

Investigations
- Abdominal x-ray may show a distended stomach with paucity of gas distally.
- Upper GI contrast study is now regarded as the key investigation showing the DJ junction on the right of the midline. So-called 'corkscrew' sign of proximal jejunum implies the twisting nature of the volvulus.
- Lower GI contrast study – looking for caecal position.
- US (or CT scan), looking for relative position of SMA and SMV – normally SMA is to the left of SMV. 'Whirlpool sign' is US equivalent of corkscrew!

Differential diagnosis
Lies between congenital causes of upper GI obstruction (e.g. duodenal atresia/tenosis) and features of bowel ischaemic seen in NEC.

Management
Resuscitation (including NG aspiration, IV fluids and antibiotic therapy).

Surgery – Ladd's procedure (Box 4.4, Fig. 4.7)
- RUQ muscle-cutting (occasionally periumbilical)
- Recognition (and immediate correction) of volvulus. Further steps are dictated by whether mid-gut is viable or not
- For uncomplicated malrotation, the aims are then to correct extrinsic duodenal compression and prevent a volvulus in the future. Thus, division of Ladd's bands and confirmation that there isn't an underlying

bowel stenosis or atresia fulfills the former, while widening the mesentery and separating the two ends of the mid-gut, the latter. Practically, this means replicating the original state of 'non-rotation', where the proximal loops are entirely right-sided and the caecal pole and colon are entirely left-sided

- ?Appendicectomy – excision or inversion

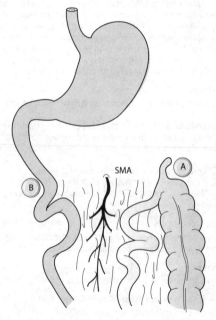

Fig. 4.7 Ladd's procedure with reversion to non-rotated position – note reversed positions of A and B.

Mid-gut volvulus

Unequivocal necrosis mandates intestinal excision, but sometimes this can be difficult to be absolutely sure about, in which case if there is doubt it is reasonable to leave the decision for a different time – a second-look laparotomy (24–36 h), preferably performed by a senior surgeon. The alternatives to consider for complete mid-gut necrosis depend on what is sensible and available, but might range from surgical nihilism (i.e. nothing) and withdrawal of treatment to primary jejunocolic anastomosis and treating the consequences of short bowel syndrome (particularly if small bowel transplantation is a realistic possibility).

Complications
- Short gut syndrome (see page 260)
- Ischaemia–reperfusion syndrome following detorsion – multiple experimental possibilities – few practical suggestions
- Recurrence of volvulus (2–5%)
- Adhesional small bowel obstruction (up to 10%)
- Sometimes malrotation is the first sign of an intestinal dysmotility syndrome

Further reading

Godgole P, Stringer MD. Bilious vomiting in the newborn. How often is it pathologic? *J Pediatr Surg* 2002;**37**:909–11.

Moore KL, Persaud TVN. *The Developing Human. Clinically Oriented Embryology* (7th edn). Philadelphia Saunders, 2003.

Intestinal atresia

Embryology

There are two conflicting hypotheses which have been suggested as appropriate for different parts of the intestine. These are (i) failure of recanalization for duodenal and true rectal atresia, and (ii) intrauterine ischaemic intestinal reabsorption for the remainder of jejuno-ileocolic atresias.

Failure of recanalization (after Tandler – 1900)

This implies that there is a 'solid-stage' in duodenal development (possibly at 5th week gestation), which is by no means certain.

Vascular accident/ischaemia

Based on experimental observations in fetal puppies by Janie Lowe and Christian Barnard in 1950s, who could reproduce all types of atresia by *in utero* mesenteric vascular ligation.

Bland–Sutton classification (modified, Fig. 4.8)

- Type 1 – membranous diaphragm, mural continuity
- Type 2 – cord joining two ends.
- Type 3 – complete separation ± 'v'-shaped mesenteric gap
- Type 4 – multiple (see later)

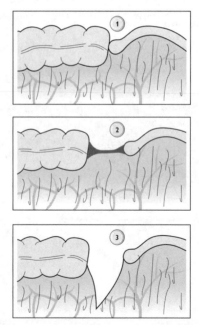

Fig. 4.8 Bland–Sutton classification

Pyloric atresia

Least-common site for atresia – and therefore consider underlying disorder, e.g. epidemolysis bullosa (known as Carmi syndrome), hereditary multiple intestinal atresia.

Duodenal atresia, stenosis, and web

Incidence

1 in 5000 live births (higher in Finland at ~1 in 3000); M=F

Associations

- Trisomy 21 (~25%, if unselected)
- ?Hirschsrpung's disease
- VATER constellation – careful with OA/TOF as gastric perforation likely, look for vertebral and rib anomalies (20%), check for cardiac and renal anomalies (20%)
- Annular pancreas (Box 4.5)

Clinical features

In UK, about 50% of these will now be detected on antenatal US screening (see page 66). In remainder, the classical presentation will be with day 1 bile-stained vomiting if it is infra-ampullary (60%), or simply vomiting if supra-ampullary (40%). Most have a scaphoid abdomen, due to collapsed distal intestine. The only investigation should be a straightforward AXR, with air as the contrast medium and show the classical 'double-bubble'. This picture, but with some distal air, may also suggest duodenal stenosis or malrotation.

Box 4.5 Annular pancreas

- Derived from ventral and dorsal pancreatic precursors. Although can be asymptomatic, associated with underlying duodenal stenosis/atresia
- Aim to perform duodenoduodenostomy over pancreatic bridge – avoid actually dividing ring
- Association with pancreatitis later on in life

Surgery – duodenoduodenostomy

- RUQ muscle-cutting – although laparoscopic repair is certainly possible it is not common.
- Examine all parts of the duodenum and small bowel. Exclude associated malrotation and be careful not to miss 'wind-sock'-type of duodenal membrane.
- Look at gall bladder – ?contains bile.
- Mobilize (Kocherize) duodenal ends and retract hepatic flexure of colon inferiorly.
- Most common anastomosis is probably Kimura 'diamond' (Fig. 4.9), which is simply two incisions orientated at 90° to achieve a self-opening appearance when joined.
- Occasionally with gross proximal dilatation, consideration should be given to excisional or tapering duodenoplasty.
- Transanastomotic tubes (TAT) have been largely abandoned given the availability of parenteral nutrition.

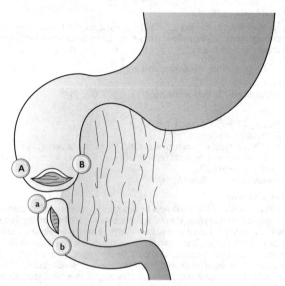

Fig. 4.9 'Diamond' duodenoduodenostomy. Initial enterotomies (AB and ab) are at 90° to each other. Sutured so that 'a' is midpoint of back wall and 'b' midpoint of front wall.

Complications
- Anastomotic leak
- Poor gastric emptying – makes you wish you'd put a TAT in!
- Biliary damage – persistent conjugated jaundice & white stool

Jejunoileal atresia and stenosis

Epidemiology
- 1 in 5,000 with no gender predilection
- Higher incidence in twins and black and Asian (versus white) infants
- No real associations, other than as complication of abdominal wall defects
- Jejunal : ileal 2:1

Clinical features
Perhaps the majority in the UK will present with abnormal antenatal imaging, but the classical postnatal features are bile vomiting, distension, and failure to pass meconium. These are usually isolated anomalies and therefore infants are normal term and otherwise healthy.

An AXR will show distended, centrally placed small bowel loops. The fewer the loops, the more proximal the atresia. Fluid levels may be apparent – if not ?meconium ileus. Intralumenal calcification may suggest a particular type of familial intestinal atresia.

Surgery – jejunal atresia

- Supraumbilical – muscle-cutting
- Proximal bowel will be distended and hypertrophied, down to the level of the atresia. Thereafter, anything could have happened. Ideally the remainder of the mid-gut will be intact, albeit disused. Sometimes there has been a greater degree of distal intestinal deletion evident perhaps as an 'apple-peel' ileum, or there are multiple atretic segments ('string of sausages') Box 4.6 and 4.7
- Primary jejunal (or ileal) anastomosis is the ideal. The problem is size disparity and this needs to be carefully considered before planning the anastomosis. Sometimes, judicious suturing (taking more of the larger part) will allow a safe functioning 'funnel-shaped' anastomosis or opening the distal end along the anti-mesenteric aspect and achieving an 'end-to-back' anastomosis. If no problems with bowel length then consider resection of the dilated part, back to a more normal calibre
- Anti-mesenteric tapering of the hypertrophied side may be considered to match better the distal opening. Either way, single-layer fine (5/0, 6/0) monofilament sutures should be used
- Stomas – should be considered if unstable infant and truly precarious distal bowel. Always leave access to distal bowel so that intestinal content can be re-fed. This will allow growth and marked improvement in distal bowel quality, essential for when it is rejoined later

The main prognostic observation which should be documented and detailed is the length of residual viable bowel, in order to assess the likelihood of short bowel syndrome (see page 260).

Small bowel length

Normal bowel length in neonates
Stretched and anti-mesenteric:
• Term ~ 300 cm
• Preterm ~200 cm
(After Touloukian *et al. J Pediatr Surg* 1983;18:720–3 and Delriviere *et al. Transplantation* 2000;69:1392–6.)

- >100 cm – long-term problems unlikely but short-term PN might be required
- 100–50 cm – long-term problems probable, TPN essential. Consider reconstruction (if anatomically possible) if no early progress
- 50–20 cm – long-term TPN, aim for early intestinal reconstruction (if anatomically possible)
- <20 cm – aim for long-term TPN with small bowel transplantation

> **Box 4.6 Hereditary multiple intestinal atresia – a genetic defect**
>
> Typically spontaneous (despite name). Has multiple (>15) membranous-type atresias within small and large bowel (beware the pyloric atresia). Intraluminal content has putty-like consistency. Most have underlying immunological deficit and outcome is appalling. Only survivors have had SB and bone marrow transplants.

> **Box 4.7 Apple-peel atresia (aka Christmas tree, maypole etc)**
>
> Caused by distal superior mesenteric arterial loss, with retrograde blood supply from marginal colonic vessels (always tenuous). The residual ileum spirals around its vascular axis.

Colon atresia

Unusual site for atresia – may be associated with gastroschisis where the colon (and usually jejunum) is 'pinched-off' by closing defect. If isolated, then commonest site is the watershed between mid- and hind-gut (i.e. the distal transverse colon). In common with atresia, the proximal colon is hugely distended (resembling a banana) and more so if the ileo-caecal valve is intact and competent, The AXAR should show a distended right-sided loop with a single fluid-level.

Surgical management should aim for proximal resection of the most grossly dilated part and colo- (or ileo-) colic anastomosis.

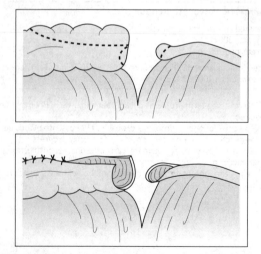

Fig. 4.10 Tapering enteroplasty. For gross disparity, excise antimesenteric aspect and reconstruct to achieve a smaller proximal diameter.

Further reading

Dalla Vecchia LK, Grosfeld JL, West KW et al. Intestinal atresia and stenosis: a 25 year experience with 277 cases. *Arch Surg* 1998;**133**:490–6.

Davenport M, Bianchi A, Doig CM et al. Colonic atresia: current results of treatment. *J R Coll Surg Edinb* 1990;**35**:25–8.

Kimura K, Mukohara N, Nishijima E et al. Diamond-shaped anastomosis for duodenal atresia: an experience with 44 patients over 15 years. *J Pediatr Surg* 1990;**25**:977–9.

Spitz L, Ali M, Brereton RJ. Combined esophageal and duodenal atresia: experience of 18 patients. *J Pediatr Surg* 1981;**16**:4–7.

Meconium ileus, peritonitis, and plug

Meconium ileus

This is due to inspissated meconium plugs becoming impacted within the distal ileum. The proximal small bowel is dilated and filled with tenaciously adherent dark-green meconium. This is termed simple meconium ileus. This may become complicated by segmental bowel volvulus, atresia, perforation and peritonitis.

Epidemiology
- 10% of infants with CF will present with MI
- 90% of infants with MI will have CF (Box 4.8)

Clinical features
Antenatal US in the second and third trimester may detect dilated or echogenic bowel loops. Complicated MI may be indicated by development of an abdominal pseudocyst and mural calcification.

After birth, there will be bile vomiting and abdominal distension. The meconium-filled loops may be appreciated especially in the right lower quadrant. Rectal examination should show mucus plugs only.

Plain AXR usually shows air-filled bowel loops, which may have a 'soap-bubble' appearance due to the admixture of swallowed air with meconium (Neuhauser's sign). US shows a similar appearance of thick-walled bowel loops filled with echogenic material. Contrast enema should show a micro-colon, perhaps with some reflux beyond the IC valve.

> **Box 4.8 Diagnosis of cystic fibrosis**
>
> - Genetic analysis – up to 20 of commonest mutational variants (e.g. ΔF508) can be identified
> - Immunoreactive trypsin on dried blood spot – raised in CF, but can be non-specific
> - Sweat test – demonstrating raised [Cl⁻] >80 mmol/L. Needs sufficient sweat and often only successful after a few weeks

Management
As usual, infants require NG decompression, IV fluids, and broad-spectrum antibiotics as initial management. For those without radiological evidence of complication then this is followed by Gastrografin® enema (Box 4.9).

> **Box 4.9 Gastrografin® enema**
>
> (meglumine diatrizoate and polysorbate 80 as a wetting agent – osmolality ~1600 mosmol/L)
> This is instilled by a rectal catheter under screening. The hyperosmolar solution should mix, soften and break up impacted meconium, allowing onward transit over the next 6–8 h. Perforation (10%) is possible leading to surgery. Monitor fluid status carefully because of the potential to 3rd space. Quoted success rate varies up to 50%.

Surgery

A number of options are available depending on nature of complicaton, infant stability, and operator experience.

Manual clearance

If uncomplicated MI is found, then a catheter passed via an enterotomy in the proximal small bowel can aid Gastrografin® (1/2 strength) irrigation and manual break-up of meconium. It is essential to confirm that the contrast passes into and through the micro-colon prior to finishing. Unresolved obstruction will inevitably lead to grief.

Enterostomy

If adequate bowel decompression is not achieved, then a distal ileostomy is fashioned. The best option is probably a simple loop or double-barrel stoma, although in the past more complicated arrangements were constructed. For instance, a Bishop–Koop stoma was an end-to-side anastomosis leaving a spout brought to the surface as a stoma. The advantage was that in the absence of distal obstruction then there was intestinal continuity.

Formal ileostomy closure can be performed after 6–8 weeks following a distal contrast study to confirm patency. Refeeding of the distal limb in the interim will improve bowel quality and improve the microcolon calibre.

Meconium peritonitis

This is an aseptic peritonitis due to intrauterine intestinal perforation resulting in spillage of meconium. A peritoneal chemical reaction occurs with formation of foreign body granuloma and calcifications. Usually, the site of perforation may be sealed by the resulting pseudocyst. This can occupy up to two-thirds of the abdominal cavity. Most are due to underlying MI, but not all, and any *in utero* perforation will cause it.

Clinical features

Most have signs of obvious intestinal obstruction, but occasionally the perforation and distal obstruction clears *in utero*. Usually the intestine is intact, although atresias may be found. If the processus vaginalis is patent at the time the perforation occurs, calcification or hernias may involve the scrotum. Ascites may also be present.

AXR may show the characteristic calcifications (amorphous and irregular or curvilinear suggesting cystic loculation or coating of the peritoneum). Ascites may give a 'ground-glass' appearance, and rarely pneumoperitoneum may be seen if the perforation is still present. Rarely, fluid and meconium can pass into the chest, presumably through congenital communications, resulting in meconium thorax.

Management

Those infants with obstruction or perforation are candidates for surgery. Again there are a number of possibilities including bowel resection and primary anastomosis and enterostomy.

Meconium plug and small left colon syndrome

Some authorities regard these as essentially the same pathology, perhaps due to varying degrees of intrauterine colon dysmotility. Notwithstanding this, meconium plug syndrome is a distal colon obstruction due to an impacted mucus plug(s). This may be recognized following digital or instru-mental examination of the rectum, or at the time of contrast enema. Once cleared, then normal bowel function should rapidly return.

Small left colon syndrome, associated particularly with infants of diabetic mothers (>50%), has a characteristic radiological contrast appearance with a transition zone at splenic flexure. Various histological abnormali-ties have been described. Again, contrast enema should be performed and be therapeutic.

In both conditions, Hirschsprung's disease is a differential diagnosis and suction rectal biopsy should be performed to actively exclude it. CF is much less likely as an underlying diagnosis.

Further reading

Boix-Ochoa J, Lloret J. Meconium peritonitis. In: Puri P (ed). *Newborn Surgery*. London: Edward Arnold, 2003, pp471–7.

Kiely E. Meconium ileus. In: Puri P (ed). *Newborn Surgery*. London: Edward Arnold, 2003, pp465–70.

Rangecroft L. Neonatal small left colon syndrome. *Arch Dis Child* 1979;**54**(8):635–7.

Rescorla FJ, Grosfeld JL. Contemporary management of meconium ileus. *World J Surg* 1993;**17**:318–25.

Necrotizing enterocolitis

Necrotizing enterocolitis (NEC) is the most common surgical emergency in the newborn, yet still its aetiology remains obscure.

Incidence
- 1.7% of all infants admitted to NICU in UK
- 15% of <1500 g infants
- ~10% are term infants

Pathogenesis
The precise mechanism remains elusive, but low birth weight (<1500 g), prematurity, early enteral feeding, and sepsis are among known risk factors. Breast milk confers some protection. It is likely that a combination of compromised gut mucosa, pathogenic bacteria, and luminal substrate results in impaired gut barrier function, activating an inflammatory cascade and causing bowel injury in susceptible individuals.

Clinical features
Predominantly gastrointestinal and includes abdominal distension, feed intolerance, bile vomiting, and blood in the stool. May be accompanied by features such as lethargy, temperature instability, recurrent apnoea, bradycardia, and blood glucose instability. Examination may show erythema and oedema of the abdominal wall, tenderness, palpable bowel loops, or a mass. Look for systemic signs of sepsis, DIC, and haemodynamic instability as evidence of progression (e.g. blood gases, platelet count, coagulation studies and lactate level).

Investigation
The earliest finding on abdominal radiograph is multiple gas-filled loops. Pneumatosis intestinalis (intramural gas) is diagnostic of NEC. This may be cystic (bubbly appearance) or linear (Wriggler's sign). Persistent dilated loops, intraperitoneal fluid, portal vein gas and free air can be seen (Fig. 4.11).

Bell classification (1978)
See Table 4.7.

Table 4.7 Bell classification of necrotizing enterocolitis.

Stage I	Suspected	Non-specific small bowel distension
Stage II	Definite	pneumatosis intestinalis, portal vein gas
Stage III	Advanced	pneumoperitoneum

After Bell MJ et al. Ann Surg 1978;187:1–7.

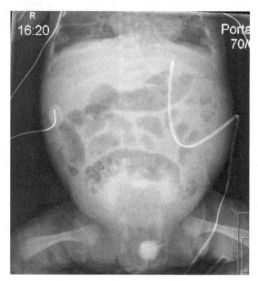

Fig. 4.11 AXR of infant with definite NEC showing widespread pneumatosis.

Management

Supportive measures include gut rest (NBM, NG tube, and TPN), and broad-spectrum antibiotics (standard regimen 10 days). Indications for surgical intervention are debatable but include perforation, intestinal obstruction and 'failure' of medical management. Serial AXR will give the best indication of deterioration.

Surgery

The principle aims of intervention include removal of necrotic gut, peritoneal lavage, and restoration/diversion of GI tract. A spectrum of options is available, dependent on infant stability under GA:
- proximal ileostomy (± resection)
- resection and primary anastomosis
- 'patch, drain and wait'
- 'clip and drop' – technique for multifocal NEC, to avoid immediate reconstruction or stoma, implies second-look laparotomy in 24–48 h.

Peritoneal drainage

This has been advocated; however in two recent trials no benefit has been demonstrated, by PD alone. One trial has shown that 74% of infants treated by PD required a delayed 'rescue' laparotomy.

Aim for stoma closure once acute episode has resolved. Distal contrast studies are mandatory to exclude stricture and ensure distal bowel patency.

Complications
- Mass/abscess formation
- Fistula (interloop, enterocutaneous)
- Stenosis
- Short-bowel syndrome.
- Recurrence (~5%)

Outcome

Mortality remains at 20–30%, and is related to extent of NEC, complications together with gestational age, birth weight, and co-morbidities. Survivors are significantly more likely than gestation-matched controls to be neurodevelopmentally impaired.

Further reading

Bell MJ Kosloske AM, Benton C et al. Neonatal necrotising enterocolitis. Theraputic decisions based upon clinical staging. Ann Surg 1978;**187**:1–7.

Hall NJ, Curry J, Drake DP et al. Resection and primary anastomosis is a valid surgical option for infants with necrotizing enterocolitis who weigh less than 1000 g. Arch Surg 2005;**140**:1149–51.

Rees CM, Hall NJ, Eaton S, Pierro A. Surgical strategies for necrotising enterocolitis: a survey of practice in the United Kingdom. Arch Dis Child Fetal Neonatal Ed 2005;**90**:F152–F155.

Hirschsprung's disease

History

Named after a Danish paediatrician, Harald Hirschprung (1830–1916), who presented typical cases at a congress in Berlin in 1886. Tittel in 1901, first observed the characteristic lack of ganglion cells, but this was only confirmed some years later. Orvar Swenson (1909–present), an American surgeon, performed the first pull-though operation in June 1947.

Incidence

- 1 in 4500 births (in UK)
- M:F 4:1 (ratio reversed in long-segment variant)

Associated anomalies

- Trisomy 21 (~15% of all cases)
- Waardenburg syndrome (WS4) – white forelock, deafness
- Hypoventilation syndrome
- Kaufman–McKusick syndrome (hydrometrocolpos, polydactyl)

Aetiology

There is failure of migration of neural crest cells resulting in absence of ganglion cells (should reach colon by 12th week gestation). Thus HD will always involve the rectum but have a variable proximal extent. Most, termed short-segment disease, extend to mid-sigmoid, while total colon involvement seen in 3–12% of cases. Although aganglionic segment is contiguous, there are rare reports of skip lesions.

Although the precise mechanism is unknown, mutations in the RET proto-oncogene on Ch10 have been found to be present in most familial cases and RET 'knockout' mice can be used as a model of aganglionosis. Others include endothelin B receptor (EDNRB), endothelin 3 (EDN3), GDNF, ECE1 and SOX10.

Clinical features

Cardinal feature is failure to pass meconium within the first 48 h of life, and this can be accompanied by signs of intestinal obstruction (e.g. distension, bilious vomiting, and poor feeding). A smaller proportion will present later in life with chronic constipation. On examination, it is important to exclude subtle anorectal malformations which may present in a similar way. A digital rectal examination will often result in temporary relief of the obstruction, and a gush of meconium may follow.

Initial failure to pass meconium can be seen in meconium plug syndrome, small left colon syndrome, meconium ileus, and anorectal malformation.

Investigation is directed at excluding other causes of distal intestinal obstruction and confirmation of HD. Abdominal x-ray is relatively non-specific; a distal contrast study may show a 'transistion zone' of relatively normal bowel, going into proximally distended bowel.

Rectal suction biopsy

This is a key test (may have to be open biopsy in older childre
for aganglionosis in myenteric and submucosal plexi, +ve acet)
rase,

Management

The aim is to resect the aganglionic segment and recreate a functional
ano-rectal reservoir (pull-through operation). This is usually delayed by 3–
6 months, with daily rectal washouts (typically with saline) by the parents
in the interim – to ensure intestinal decompression. It is crucial to ensure
this occurs, and if it doesn't – because of poor technique, parental dis-
quiet, or because is pathologically unsuitable (e.g. long segment disease),
then a loop colostomy should be performed.

Surgery – the pull-through operation (Fig. 4.12)

There are a number of variants, having the same principle of resection
of ganglionic bowel and restoration of GI continuity. The transistion zone
must be defined either prior to (e.g. at time of a colostomy) or during
definitive surgery by frozen section.

The dissection of the recto-sigmoid segment proceeds along the wall of
the bowel, with ligation/coagulation or the mesenteric vessels. The bowel
that is pulled through needs to be mobilized to lie within pelvis without
tension.

Swenson operation

Distal resection of all affected bowel down to anus, with restoration colo-
anal anastomosis. Risk of injury to anterior structures in boys (e.g. prostate, vas deferens).

Duhamel operation

This leaves the distal rectum *in situ*, with most of the dissection posteri-
orely to create a retro-rectal tunnel. The normal bowel is brought down
and a long side-to-side anastomosis (stapled) is created between this and
the anterior (aganglionic) rectum.

Soave (endorectal) operation

A plane is developed within the rectum between the mucosal and the
muscle layers. The mucosa is removed down to the anus, leaving a sleeve
of rectal muscle, through which normal bowel is pulled through and anastomosed to the anus.

Most of the above abdominal dissection and preparation can be accomplished laparoscopically, which minimizes the postoperative recovery
period. Further, a transanal approach has been described, avoiding the
abdominal part completely.

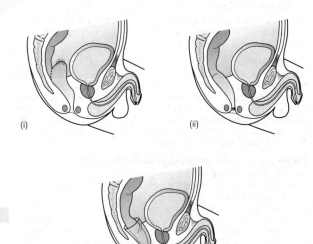

Fig. 4.12 Pull-through operations. (i) Duhamel, retrorectal tunnel and long side-side anastomosis; (ii) Swenson, coloanal anastomosis; and (iii) Soave, endorectal muscle sheath with colo-anal anastomosis.

Complications

Late complications can be divided into incontinence, constipation, and enterocolitis. The incidence of incontinence has fallen significantly with improved understanding of the position of the neorectal anastomosis (above the level of the internal sphincter). However, constipation is still a problem for a significant number of children (~30%), and it may be necessary to repeat rectal biopsies to exclude a pulled-through transition zone.

Enterocolitis affects 15–30% of children, and may occur before and after pull-through surgery. Its aetiology is unknown, but it is responsible for significant morbidity and even mortality in these patients. Diagnosis is made on clinical criteria of abdominal distension, explosive (bloody) diarrhoea, fever, and general malaise. Treatment involves antibiotics (e.g. metronidazole, oral vancomycin). Recurrence is possible, but it may respond to sodium cromoglicate.

Further reading

Dasgupta R, Langer JC. Evaluation and management of persistent problems after surgery for Hirschsprung disease in a child. *J Pediatr Gastroenterol Nutr* 2008;**46**:13–19.

Pierro A, Fasoli L, Kiely EM, Drake D, Spitz L. Staged pull-through for rectosigmoid Hirschsprung's disease is not safer than primary pull-through. *J Pediatr Surg* 1997;**32**:505–509.

Shankar KR, Losty PD, Lamont GL et al. Transanal endorectal coloanal surgery for Hirschsprung's disease: experience in two centers. *J Pediatr Surg* 2000;**35**:1209–13.

Anorectal malformation

Embryology

The hindgut initially extends into the body stalk, as the allantois, but then develops as a pouch towards its caudal end – the entodermal cloaca (latin – sewer). The cloacal membrane extends from the umbilicus towards the tail bone. There is ingrowth of mesoderm toward the midline to form symphysis, pubis, and lower anterior abdominal wall (5th to 6th week), leaving the now posteriorly placed ectodermal cloacal membrane. Coincident with this is a lateral mesodermal ingrowth which separates the cloaca into an anterior urogenital sinus (with its attached Müllerian and Wolffian ducts) and a posterior anorectum. Breakdown of the ano-rectal membrane occurs and allows fetal defaecation from about 15 weeks.

Introduction

Anorectal malformations (ARMs) are a wide spectrum of anomalies in which the distal end of the hindgut fails to develop a normally patent opening in the anatomically correct position, i.e. in the centre of the anal sphincter complex. In most cases the anus is imperforate and the intestine terminates in an abnormal fistulous connection to the perineum, urethra, or bladder in males, or to the perineum or vestibule in females. ARMs range from isolated minor displacements of the distal rectum, which have an excellent functional prognosis, to complex anatomical variants with deficient pelvic musculature and associated genito-urinary, neurological and spinal anomalies, which carry a poor functional prognosis.

Incidence

- 1 in 5000 live births
- ~2% have +ve family history

Aetiology

- Unknown but likely to be multifactorial with a genetic component

Associated anomalies (50–60%)

- Genitourinary, e.g. vesicoureteric reflux, renal dysplasia, cryptorchidism
- Spinal, e.g. hemivertebrae, hemisacrum, tethered cord, myelomeningocele
- Cardiac, e.g. atrial septal defect, PDA, tetralogy of Fallot
- Gastrointestinal, e.g. TOF, intestinal atresias, malrotation
- Gynaecological, e.g. hydrocolpos, bicornate uterus, vaginal septum
- Genetic, e.g. trisomy 21

Assessement

- Management of life-threatening associated anomalies, NG tube, IV fluids with clinical assessment for any cardiac anomaly (± echocardiography)
- Renal US, AP and lateral x-rays of the lumbar spine and sacrum
- Definitive assessment of the ARM should be deferred until 24 h or so, to allow normal prograde passage of meconium and gas to the limit of the ARM. The presence of perineal meconium suggests fistula and low anomaly in male. If a colostomy is already present, a high-pressure distal loop stomogram can be performed prior to surgery

Classification

Formerly classified as **low, intermediate, or high,** depending on the relationship to sphincter complex, However, the following system in Table 4.8, initially proposed by Alberto Peña (1938–present), and adopted at an international conference in 2005 provides a more practical description.

Table 4.8 Krickenbeck classification (2005)

Major clinical group	Rare/regional variants
Perineal (cutaneous) fistula	Pouch colon
Recto-urethral fistula (i) prostatic or (ii) bulbar	Rectal atresia/stenosis
Recto-vesical	Recto-vaginal fistula
Vestibular fistula	'H' fistula
Cloaca (i) < 3cm or (ii) > 3cm common channel	

Need for colostomy?

Low lesions in boys (e.g. recto-perineal fistula) can be treated without covering stoma. In girls, the need for a stoma in managing a recto-vestibular fistula is arguable. Higher anomalies or more-complex arrangements (e.g. recto-vesical fistula in boys or cloacal anomaly in females) should undergo a delayed staged repair with an initial stoma.

Posterior sagittal anorectoplasty (PSARP)

Indicated for most ARMs without perineal fistulas:
- midline incision – extending from the mid-sacrum to the perineal body, dividing anal sphincter complex in saggital plane
- identification of rectum – dissected from urethra, or bladder neck in boys and from the vagina in girls. Closure of fistula – NB common wall
- mobilization of rectum – allow enough to bring through anal sphincter complex (identified by electrostimulation) and suture to perineal skin
- high or complex lesions may require an additional abdominal approach, either by laparotomy or laparoscopy, to separate the fistula and rectum.

Persistent cloaca

These are complex anomalies in which the urethra, vagina and rectum all terminate in a single common channel with a single perineal opening. Complex reconstructive procedures may be necessary and so these are usually managed in specialist centres. The prognosis for urinary, bowel, and sexual function is better if the common channel is less than 3 cm in length.

Complications

- Anastomotic leak
- Anal stricture
- Recurrent fistula
- Damage to the urethra, ureters, vas deferens, or seminal vesicles
- Constipation – more obvious in low anomalies (20–40%)
- Soiling

> **Box 4.11 Bowel control**
>
> Bowel control is the ability to detect, retain, and evacuate flatus, liquid stool, or solid stool at appropriate times. This requires:
> - normal sphincter function
> - normal anorectal sensation
> - normal colonic and recto-sigmoid motility.

Outcome

In general, the higher the lesion the poorer the prognosis.

Over 80% of patients with a perineal fistula will be continent, but in patients with a bladder neck fistula or with cloaca (common channel >3 cm), then <10% will be continent. Bowel management may be required to treat constipation or soiling, which may involve dietary manipulation, laxatives, medications to decrease bowel motility, or bowel irrigation (either by enema or via a Malone appendicostomy).

Further reading

De Vries PA, Peña A. Posterior sagittal anorectoplasty. *J Pediatr Surg* 1982;**17**:638–43.

Peña A, Levitt M: Anorectal malformations. In: Grosfeld JL, O'Neill JA, Fonkalsrud EW, Coran AG (eds). *Pediatric Surgery*. Philadelphia, PA: Mosby, 2006, pp1566–89.

Peña A, Levitt M. Anorectal malformations. In: Spitz L, Coran AG (eds). *Operative Pediatric Surgery*. London: Hodder and Arnold, 2006, pp479–502.

Umbilical anomalies

Embryology

This is a complex junction in embryonic development. There are two key extra-embryonic structures destined to disappear – the allantois (Greek – sausage: ill-defined role in mammals, but excretion and oxygen exchange role in birds), and the yolk sac. The former is a tubular structure connected with the developing bladder (and its hindgut precursor). The latter connects with the developing midgut and has a nutrient role from the second to fourth week. Furthermore, the entire mid-gut loop protrudes through the umbilical ring in order to accommodate the expanding embryonic liver (returns by 12th week).

Urachal remnants and vitello-intestinal duct

Normal urachal involution leaves the median umbilical ligament, which is neighboured by two paired structures radiating from the mature umbilicus – medially the obliterated umbilical arteries and laterally the inferior epigastric arteries arising from external iliac artery and gaining access to the posterior rectus sheath.

Failure of urachal involution leads to either a median urachal cyst or a fistula capable of leaking urine. Congenital bladder outlet obstruction (e.g. posterior urethral valves, prune belly syndrome) may predispose to persisting urachal leakage.

Persistence of the vitello-intestinal duct (VID) may lead to a fistula commincating with the distal ileum, an umbilical sinus, or simply a Meckel's diverticulum. The duct may also be completely obliterated but a fibrous connection persists.

Clinical features

There is a multiplicity of presentations, including an abnormal-looking umbilicus with prolapse, polyp, or persistent discharge (purulent/mucoid/urine/faeces); abdominal pain (secondary to diverticulitis or urachal sepsis); intestinal obstruction (volvulus around fibrous cord or intussusception with Meckel's as lead point); and gastrointestinal haemorrhage (ulceration of Meckel's diverticulum).

Assess discharge if present, and probe the umbilical opening to determine the direction of the tract. Ultrasonography is useful to show cystic variants and to exclude further urological abnormalities and obstruction. A fistulogram should also provide a guide to the anatomy.

The treatment is surgical excision with excision of the urachus or VID, and may include a bowel resection for a Meckel's diverticulum.

Umbilical granuloma

This is much more common than any of the above conditions and occurs where granulation tissue fails to epithelialize following cord separation, leading to persistent discharge, often secondarily infected. It can be treated by cauterization using silver nitrate (75%) sticks, or more formally by surgical excision.

Omphalitis

Umbilical cord sepsis is often polymicrobial but usually caused by *staphylococcal* or *streptococcal* spp. Management includes resuscitation if unwell, swabs for microbiology, and appropriately delivered antibiotics (e.g. flucloxacillin). Late presentation or ineffective treatment may allow progression to necrotizing fasciitis or peritoneal sepsis. A possible longer-term complication is portal vein thrombosis from ascending infection.

Further reading

Ameh E, Nmadu PT. Major complications of omphalitis in neonates and infants. *Pediatr Surg Int* 2002;**18**:413–16.

Nagar H. Umbilical granuloma: a new approach to an old problem. *Pediatr Surg Int* 2001;**17**:513–14.

Pacilli M, Sebire NJ, Maritsi D et al. Umbilical polyp in infants and children. *Eur J Pediatr Surg* 2007;**17**:397–9.

Exomphalos

Exomphalos (aka omphalocele) is a congenital abdominal wall defect arising from a failure of visceral return from its normal extrabdominal location around 10–12 weeks' gestation. Characteristically viscera are covered with a sac (formed from peritoneum, Wharton's jelly and amnion), although this can rupture *in utero* (<5%). The umbilical cord should be an integral part of the sac.

Incidence
1 in 5000 live births (slight male predominance)

Types
- Hernia of umbilical cord – small defect containing single intestinal loop
- Exomphalos minor – defect <5 cm. Typically only containing intestinal loops
- Exomphalos major – defect >5 cm, and typically contains central globular liver

Malrotation or non-rotation is invariable in major exomphalos and may also be identified in minor variants.

Embryology
The genesis of exomphalos is controversial but probably due to embryonic failure of midline fusion of cephalic, lateral, and caudal folds from 3 weeks of gestation.

Associations
- Chromosomal, e.g. trisomies 13 and 18; Pallister–Killian syndrome
- Cardiac anomalies, e.g. tetralogy of Fallot
- Pentalogy of Cantrell – originally upper midline exomphalos, diaphragmatic defect, sternal cleft, ectopia cordis, and intracardiac anomalies
- Lower midline syndrome, e.g. bladder/cloacal extrophy, imperforate anus, colon atresia, etc
- Beckwith–Wiedemann syndrome – macroglossia, macrosomia, islet cell hyperplasia (causing hypoglycaemia), and an increased risk of intra-abdominal tumours such as Wilms' and hepatoblastomas

Management
Non-operative
Allows eschar to form, with slow epithelialization of the amniotic surface and later secondary surgical closure of the ventral hernia. This is preferable in premature infants with other major anomalies. Agents such as silver sulfadiazine or other non-toxic anti-bacterial dressing have been used. Once skin-covered, then an abdominal binder may encourage development of the abdominal cavity. Secondary fascial closure is still a major undertaking.

Surgery
- **Elective primary closure** – for all minor and some major defects. Liver mobilized and separated from normally adherent sac to allow safe abdominal cavity return. Ladd's procedure for malrotation. Fascial closure facilitated with prosthetic patches (e.g. Gore-tex®, Permacol® or Surgisys®)

- **Staged silo repair** – sac excised (occasionally retained) and replaced by prosthetic silo which allows deliberate slow cavity expansion (7–14 days) and visceral return completed by secondary defect closure. Fascial closure is facilitated with prosthetic patches. Skin cover may still be problematic.

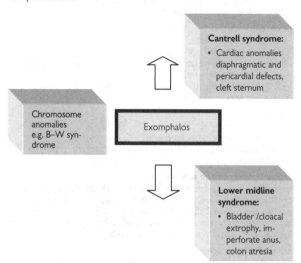

Cantrell syndrome:
- Cardiac anomalies diaphragmatic and pericardial defects, cleft sternum

Chromosome anomalies e.g. B–W syndrome

Exomphalos

Lower midline syndrome:
- Bladder /cloacal extrophy, imperforate anus, colon atresia

Fig. 4.13 Relation of exomphalos with other syndromes.

Further reading

Rijhwani A, Davenport M, Dawrant M et al. Definitive surgical management of antenatally diagnosed exomphalos. *J Pediatr Surg* 2005;**40**:516–22.

Gastroschisis

Embryology

Premature interruption of the right omphalomesenteric artery, results in ischaemic injury to the anterior abdominal wall through which herniation of the intestine occurs (possible mechanism).

Epidemiology

- 4–6 per 10,000 live births
- Sporadic with a small risk of recurrence
- Rising incidence seen in most countries, with some marked regional variation (reason obscure)
- ~25% of infants have other anomalies – usually related to the gastro-schisis (e.g. undescended testes)

Aetiology

Risk factors include:

- low maternal age ×10 risk for mothers <20 years age
- exposure to vasoactive substances, e.g. smokers ×4 risk, class A and B drugs ×4 risk.

Antenatal detection and surveillance

Maternal serum alpha-fetoprotein is raised in 100% of affected fetuses. The 20-week US anomaly scan detects the majority. Further US surveillance is used to assess bowel dilatation and wall thickness. Bowel dilatation may indicate the need for early delivery. Both polyhydramnios and oligohydramnios may indicate associated atresia.

Antenatal intervention

Amnioinfusion or amnioexchange has been used to dilute digestive compounds that may cause bowel injury but remains experimental. Similarly, fetoscopic enlargement of the defect has been performed in some cases.

Obstetric management

Spontaneous vaginal delivery in a surgical centre is recommended. Induction of labour before 38 weeks to reduce risk of late third trimester fetal loss is routine practice in most UK centres. There is no role for preterm delivery less than 36 weeks. Rate of emergency section is ~50%. Amniotic fluid and bowel are typically bile stained.

Postnatal appearance

- Intestine appears normal
- Intestine thickened and matted together ('peel')
- Intestinal atresia (10%) may be seen, occasionally multiple, but rarely with perforation
- Closed gastroschisis (antenatal loss of mid-gut and therefore associated with jejunal atresia and short bowel syndrome)
- Ischaemia of mid-gut due to volvulus or kinking of mesenteric vessels

Postnatal management

Passage of a nasogastric tube and placement of secure cannula for intra-venous fluid replacement of serous fluid losses. Exposed bowel can be wrapped with cling film but ideally placed in a preformed silo as soon as possible. Antibiotics are routine (penicillin and gentamicin).

Surgery – repair of gastroschisis

There are a number of different surgical approaches with the object of visceral reduction and fascial closure. Conventionally the first stage is performed under GA as soon as possible after delivery:

- primary fascial closure (± prosthetic patch)
- ventilation is invariable for several days with a risk of abdominal compartment syndrome
- secondary fascial closure – if there is initial failure to achieve visceral reduction then a silo is placed and a slower reduction achieved over the next 7–14 days, with a return to theatre for completion of fascial closure. This customized silo requires widening of the defect and fashioning of, typically silicone sheeting. An IV infusion bag is a cheaper alternative.
- Alternatively, a number of techniques have been described to achieve the same object without anaesthesia:
- cotside reduction and primary closure – gentle manual reduction at the cotside can be achieved in selected infants, with closure of the defect with a suture or dressing
- preformed silo (Figs 4.14 and 4.15) – a preformed silo can be placed at the cotside in most cases and then managed by serial reduction until the viscera have returned. Closure of the defect is then performed either by using steristrips alone, or by suturing under GA. Close attention should be made to the colour of the bowel, and the defect should be widened if there is concern.

Intestinal surgery

- Resection for perforation, ischaemia, or NEC
- Atresia – immediate or delayed intestinal anastomosis for atresia is performed according to bowel condition. Stomas may be formed
- Intestinal refashioning – longitudinal intestinal lengthening (Bianchi operation), serial transverse enteroplasty (STEP), placation, or tapering for dilated dysmotile segments of bowel can be done at birth or as a delayed procedure

Specific complications

- Early:
  - abdominal compartment syndrome
  - fascial wound dehiscence
  - necrotizing enterocolitis
- Late:
  - Parenteral nutrition-associated cholestasis
  - intestinal failure-associated liver disease (IFALD)
  - intestinal failure resulting from short bowel or dysmotility or both
  - adhesive small bowel obstruction
  - intestinal stricture

Outcomes

Parenteral nutrition is required for ~30 days before full enteral feeding is established. Mortality is less than <10% but mostly relates to IFALD and factors associated with small bowel and or liver transplantation. Most long-term survivors lead normal lives.

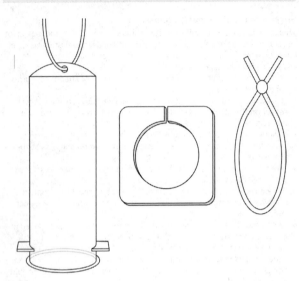

Fig. 4.14 Preformed silo – contruction.

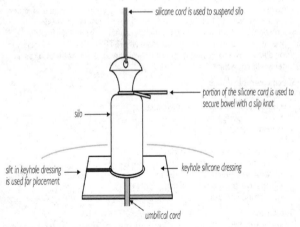

silicone cord is used to suspend silo

portion of the silicone cord is used to
secure bowel with a slip knot

silo

slit in keyhole dressing
is used for placement

keyhole silicone dressing

umbilical cord

Fig. 4.15 Preformed silo application.

Further reading

Bianchi A, Dickson A, Alizai NK. Elective delayed midgut reduction – no anesthesia for gastroschisis: selection and conversion criteria. *J Pediatr Surg* 2002;**37**:1334–6.

Charlesworth P, Njere I, Allotey J et al. Postnatal outcome in gastroschisis: effect of birth weight and gestational age. *J Pediatr Surg* 2007;**42**:815–18.

Owen A, Marven S, Jackson L et al. Experience of bedside preformed silo staged reduction and closure for gastroschisis. *J Pediatr Surg* 2006;**41**:1830–5.

Silo Information – Medicina Ltd, Unit 2, Rivington View Business Park, Station Road, Blackrod, Bolton BL6 5BN; www.medicina.co.uk; email: info@medicina.co.uk.

Biliary atresia *et al*

Biliary atresia

Obliterative process with destruction of bile ducts and most common cause of paediatric liver transplantation in the developed world.

Incidence

1 in 15,000 (UK); 1 in 9,000 (Japan)

Aetiology

Unknown, theories include aberrant early bile duct development, perinatal viral infection, aberrant immune response, abnormalities of bile acids; all postulated but not proven.

Clinical features

Prolonged conjugated jaundice (>2 weeks), pale stools and dark urine (100%). Abnormal antenatal ultrasound due to cystic change in the biliary tree (5%). Other anomalies, e.g. the cardiac anomalies associated with BASM (biliary atresia splenic malformation syndrome; Box 4.12) (5%). Vitamin K-dependent coagulopathy (3%).

Box 4.12 Biliary atresia splenic malformation (BASM) syndrome (10%)

Consists of polysplenia or asplenia, and cardiac anomalies, situs inversus, malrotation, preduodenal portal vein, absent vena cava.

It has a worse prognosis despite being diagnosed earlier. Possibly due to defect or derangement in early bile duct development as the other associated anomalies also occur in the first trimester.

Cystic biliary atresia (5%)

A form of developmental biliary atresia with a better prognosis, discriminated from choledochal malformation by cholangiogram showing disordered intrahepatic ducts.

Classification (according to most proximal level of obstruction)

- **Type 1** (~5%) – common bile duct (gall bladder contains bile)
- **Type 2** (~3%) – common hepatic duct
- **Type 3** (>90%) – where there is no visible bile-containing proximal lumen and the obstruction is within the porta hepatis

Surgery – the Kasai portoenterostomy (Fig 4.16)

The aim of surgery is to excise all extrahepatic biliary remnants and anastomose the transected portal plate to a jejunal Roux loop (~40 cm in length).

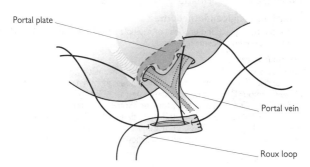

Fig. 4.16 Schematic illustration of Kasai portoenterostomy.

Outcomes
- Clearance of jaundice (to normal in ~50%)
- Preservation of native liver at 5 years (~50%)

Complications
- Ascending cholangitis (~20%)
- Portal hypertension (oesophageal varices and splenomegaly)

Liver transplantation is indicated for persisting jaundice and liver failure, varices resistant to endoscopic therapy, severe failure to thrive, and hepato-pulmonary syndrome.

Inspissated bile syndrome

This is caused by precipitation of insoluble bilirubin in the biliary tree and hence occluding the CBD.

Clinical features

Affected infants are usually premature and have underlying haemolysis, dehydration, or episodes of sepsis. The diagnosis is suggested by dilatation of the bile ducts on ultrasound and visualization of sludge in the ducts and gall bladder.

Treated by percutaneous transhepatic cholangiogram and biliary lavage, although ~50% will come to open surgery.

Spontaneous perforation of the bile duct

Obscure aetiology, with a perforation occurring typically at the junction of the common hepatic duct and cystic duct.

Clinical features

Presents with bile ascites, jaundice, and subcutaneous bile discolouration in the first weeks of life. Diagnosis suggested by US (free intraperitoneal fluid ± mass in RUQ) and confirmed by radio-isotope scan. It is treated by operative placement of a T tube in the CBD, or occasionally by direct closure (if there is no distal obstruction). Good prognosis.

Choledochal malformations (see page 236)

Liver haemangioendothelioma

These can be solitary and unilobar or multiple and bilateral and ~40% will also have cutaneous haemangiomata.

Clinical features

There is a range of presentations from asymptomatic to hepatomegaly and cardiac failure (from futile arteriovenous shunting). Investigated by US with colour-Doppler flow studies, contrast CT scans, and ultimately angiography. Only treat if symptomatic. Some are steroid responsive, others require resection (if unilobar), hepatic arterial ligation/embolization (to reduce blood flow), or (rarely) transplantation. Vincristine has also recently been used for some bilobar lesions.

Further reading

Davenport M, De Ville de Goyet J, Stringer MD *et al.* Seamless management of biliary atresia in England and Wales (1999–2002). *Lancet* 2004;**363**:1354–7.

Davenport M, Tizzard SA, Underhill J *et al.* The biliary atresia splenic malformation syndrome: a 28-year single-center retrospective study. *J Pediatr* 2006;**149**:393–400.

Persistent hyperinsulinaemic hypoglycemia of infancy (PHHI)

Background

PHHI is the most important cause of severe and recurrent hypoglycaemia in neonates and infants. It is characterized by autonomous insulin production requiring concentrated continuous IV dextrose therapy to maintain normal plasma glucose levels.

Incidence

- ~1 in 40,000 live births (Europe)
- More common in consanguineous families

Aetiology

- Unknown
- Associations include Beckwith–Wiedemann, Perlman, Usher type 1c and Soto's syndromes and congenital disorders of glycosylation. Familial forms have been linked to mutations in genes (*ABCC8* and *KCNJ11*) encoding the SUR 1 and Kir 6.2 subunits of the pancreatic β-cell K^+ ATPase channel respectively.

Pathology

There are two distinct pathological subgroups (Fig. 4.17):
- diffuse disease is characterized histologically by abnormal, prominent β-cell nuclei with capacious cytoplasm throughout the pancreas
- focal adenomatous disease is characterized by crowded β-cells with abnormal nuclei and shrunken cytoplasm. The distinction between these two subtypes is critical for successful surgical management of this condition.

Presentation

PHHI may present at any time from birth (in severe cases) to age 18 months (after weaning following increased time between feeds). Clinical features include jitteriness, tremors, convulsions, apnoeas, tachypnoea, and a high-pitched cry. Examination may reveal macrosomia, mild hepatomegaly, and facial dysmorphism, with a high forehead, globular nose, short columella, and thin upper lip.

Diagnostic criteria

- Fasting hypoglycaemia – plasma glucose <3 mmol/L
- Hyperinsulinism – plasma insulin >3 mU/L
- Undetectable or low fatty acids and ketone bodies
- requirement for significant amounts of IV dextrose to maintain plasma glucose above 3 mmol/L – infusion of >10 mg/kg/min
- Response to IM or S/C glucagon – 0.5 mg glucagon increment in blood glucose level >1.5mmol/L

Imaging and investigations

Focal lesions are typically 2.5–7.5mm in diameter, which renders imaging modalities such as ultrasound, CT, and MRI inadequate for the differentiation of diffuse or focal disease. Recently the non-invasive 18F-L-dopa PET scan is becoming the imaging method of choice to differentiate focal from diffuse disease.

Diffuse disease
Abnormalities in beta cells throughout
the pancreas (large nuclei)

Focal disease
A focal lesion with rest of pancreas normal

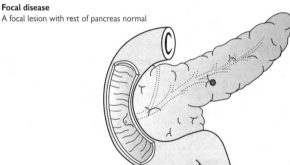

Fig. 4.17 Pathological subgroups of PHHI: a, diffuse disease – abnormalities in beta cells throughout the pancreas (large nuclei; b, focal disease – a focal disease with the rest of the pancreas normal.

Medical management

A central venous catheter is placed to allow access for regular blood glucose management and continuous infusion of IV dextrose ± glucagon. This is given in conjunction with continuous nasogastric feeds. Oral dia-zoxide (5–20 mg/kg/day in three divided doses) and, as a second line, octreotide (5–35 microgram/kg/day in four divided doses) are used to medically inhibit insulin secretion.

Surgery for PHHI

This is indicated in persistent hypoglycemia resistant to medical therapy. The approach depends on whether the disease is focal or diffuse in nature. Near-total pancreatectomy is indicated in diffuse disease not responding to medical treatment, resecting approximately 95% of the pancreas (Fig. 4.18).

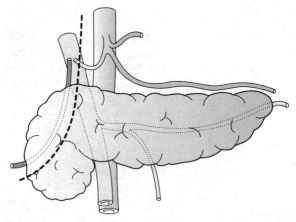

Fig. 4.18 Near-total pancreatectomy.

Open procedure
A supra-umbilical muscle-cutting incision is used and the pancreas exposed. If focal disease is present, the lesion is resected with an appropriate margin. If the disease is diffuse, a near-total pancreatectomy is performed leaving a small portion of pancreas near the common bile duct.

Laparoscopic procedure
In some centers, a limited laparoscopic excision of the pancreas including the focal lesion is perfomed. A near-total pancreatectomy can also be perfomed laparoscopically.

Postoperative management
The patient is initially managed on the high-dependency unit with regular plasma glucose measurements and IV dextrose as required. Occasionally transient rebound hyperglycaemia is seen and the patient may require temporary treatment with insulin.

Specific complications
- Persistent hypoglycaemia (following inadequate resection of diffuse lesions)
- Diabetes mellitus (up to 90% of patients will require regular insulin by the age of 15 years)
- Exocrine insufficiency (may require enzyme supplementation)
- Common bile duct damage

Prognosis
Persistent hypoglycaemia is associated with psychomotor retardation; 10% of patients with intractable hypoglycaemia requiring surgery will continue to be severely neurologically impaired.

Further reading

Aynsley-Green A, Hussain K, Hall J *et al*. Practical management of hyperinsulinism in infancy. *Arch Dis Child (Fetal Neonatal Ed)* 2000;**82**:F98–107.

McAndrew HF, Smith V, Spitz L. Surgical complications of pancreatectomy for persistent hyperinsulinaemic hypoglycaemia of infancy. *J Pediatr Surg* 2003;**38**:13–16.

Sacrococcygeal teratomas

Teratomas (Greek – monster) are defined as 'tumours derived from all three primitive germ cell lines, i.e. endoderm, epiderm and mesoderm'. They are usually congenital in origin (with the notable exception of ovarian teratomas/dermoids in adults) and are claimed to be the commonest solid tumour to be found in infancy. Typically these are midline tumours whose possible site of origin describes a question mark in the sagittal plane (thus anterior mediastinum, craniopharynx, posterior mediastinum, and the sacrococcyx as the dot in this analogy).

Classification

Altman (1974) classification depends on the level of tumour in relation to perineum:

- type 1 – almost completely external
- type 2 – most external, less pelvic
- type 3 – less external, most pelvic
- type 4 – entirely pelvic.

Histological classification

This is accorded importance depending on the degree of tissue maturation and proportion of neural elements, and may have some prognostic importance.

Clinical features

Almost 95% should be detectable on maternal ultrasound and hence delivery can be planned in centres with appropriate obstetric and surgical facilities. Serial US and Doppler studies should evaluate both fetal and maternal wellbeing, looking for signs of fetal cardiac failure (i.e. hydrops), polyhydramnios, the maternal mirror syndrome (i.e. pre-eclampsia, hypertension), and local complications such as hydronephrosis, cyst rupture and bleeding. Antenatal intervention is possible in ~5% of fetuses, and can be regarded as standard (e.g. amniocentesis and cyst drainage) or experimental (alcohol sclerotherapy, laser photocoagulation of feeding vessels, and *in utero* excision).

Obstetric management

Obstructed labour is probable with large tumours subject to vaginal delivery. Formerly this mandated early elective Caesarean section, although prelabour cyst drainage may allow vaginal delivery in selected cases.

Postnatal management

Whatever the mode, the obstetric hand may well resect some of the tumour and some may need urgent resuscitation and operative control of haemorrhage. Most can await elective operative excision after defining proximal extent of tumour and involvement of urinary system (US/MRI). Note that involvement to sacral promontory may warrant a combined laparotomy/pelvic approach. Baseline α-fetoprotein and β-human chorionic gonadotrophin is important (normal in neonate <150,000 kU/L).

Surgery – sacrococcygeal teratoma (Fig 4.19)

- 'Skydiver' position
- Urinary catheter and povidone-iodine-soaked ribbon gauze packed into anorectum
- Appropriate incision now controversial (because of acceptance of cosmesis), but ranges from simple gentle curving transverse, through a 'Mercedes-Benz' (leaving a midline cleft and buttock scar) to 'H-shape'
- Key steps include elevation of skin flaps to expose proximal sacrum and gluteal muscles, ligation of circumferential superficial feeding vessels, gradual separation of solid/cystic mass from soft tissue, laterally to expose the ischial tuberosity and caudally to identify and preserve the ano-rectal muscle complex
- The plane between the rectum and tumour is relatively easy to define and should aid appreciation of the pelvic origin
- Sacrococcygeal junction incised, to expose the median pelvic feeding vessels. Individual ligation and control before tumour (and coccyx) removal
- Drains to posterior rectal space and reconstruction of displaced gluteal muscles to approximate midline

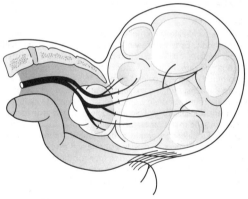

N.B distorted ano-rectal anatomy

Fig. 4.19 Cross-section of type III teratoma showing relationship with coccyx.

Further reading

Altman RP, Randolph JG, Lilly JR. Sacrococcygeal teratoma: American Academy of Pediatrics Surgical Section Survey – 1973. *J Pediatr Surg* 1974;**9**:389–98.

Gabra HO, Jesudason EC, McDowell HP *et al.* Sacrococcygeal teratoma – a 25-year experience in a UK regional center. *J Pediatr Surg* 2006;**41**:1513–16.

Makin EC, Hyett J, Ade-Ajayi *et al.* Outcome of antenatally diagnosed sacrococcygeal teratomas: single-center experience (1993–2004). *J Pediatr Surg* 2006;**41**:388–93.

Limb ischaemia

Pathophysiology

Acute or chronic limb hypoperfusion may result from:
- systemic dysfunction (e.g. severe sepsis – particularly meningococcal septicaemia, birth asphyxia, rhesus incompatibility; and prothrombotic states such as protein S or C deficiency and polycythaemia)
- local arterial insufficiency (e.g. direct iatrogenic trauma from vascular access, adjacent long bone fracture, most commonly displaced supra-condylar fracture of humerus with anterior forearm dislocation).

Pathophysiological mechanisms include direct trauma to arterial wall, arterial spasm, thrombosis, or embolic occlusion and pressure from a hae-matoma. Venous stasis with secondary arterial ischaemia is rare but well described.

Incidence

- ~3% of VLBW and ELBW infants will sustain peripheral vascular injury requiring treatment. Lower limb > upper limb (reflects more common use of femoral arterial cannulation).
- ~5% of older children with supracondylar fracture have vascular compromise and <1% end up with Volkmann's ischaemic contracture.

Clinical features

The limb is cool and pale, with mottling, diminished or absent pulses, and slow capillary refill. Early gangrenenous changes may be reversible, espe-cially in young infants. Full examination of the contralateral limb as well as the hydration and cardiovascular status of the child are important.
- FBC and blood cultures provide a baseline. Where diagnosis is uncertain (no obvious trauma etc), the coagulation profile and a thrombophilia screen (antithrombin protein S and C, plasminogen activity, lupus anticoagulant, and anti-cardiolipin antibodies, *MTHFR* gene mutation, prothrombin gene mutation, factor V Leiden mutation) may contribute.
- Colour-flow Doppler sonography of both limbs is imperative in virtually all cases, being non-invasive, readily available and easily repeatable so that serial imaging can be performed to monitor the effects of treatment.
- Angiography should be used sparingly, particularly in young infants, as arteriotomy and catheter manipulation may result in ischaemia elsewhere.

Interventions

Some conventional management strategies such as elevation and warming of the ipsilateral limb are not recommended as they may potentiate ischaemia.
- Glyceryl trinitrate transdermal patch
- Local papaverine injection around the artery
- Bupivacaine nerve block
- Thrombolysis – tPA is a recombinant protein with thrombolytic activity which works by binding to clot-bound fibrin, producing plasmin and resulting in dissolution

A suggested regimen is shown in Box 4.13.

Box 4.13 Suggested regimen

- Intravenous tPA (0.25–0.5 mg/kg/h) for 6 h
- This is administered with fresh frozen plasma to increase plasminogen available for the action of tPA
- Unfractionated heparin (15–20 U/kg/h) is given concurrently and continued for 24 h to provide low-dose anticoagulation.

This combination is repeated if indicated by incomplete resolution of the occlusion based on clinical and Doppler evaluation.

Surgery

A multidisciplinary approach is recommended with surgery which should be carried out by the most appropriate team member(s) for the individual child (general paediatric, plastic, vascular, orthopaedic). This may involve bony stabilization, arteriotomy, embolectomy, and microvascular reconstruction. Where there is established tissue loss, debridement of soft tissue necrosis and amputation are performed as appropriate.

Further reading

Coombs CJ, Richardson PW, Dowling GJ et al. Brachial artery thrombosis in infants: an algorithm for limb salvage. *Plast Reconstr Surg* 2006;**117**:1481–88.

Gamba P, Tchaprassian Z, Verlato F et al. Iatrogenic vascular lesions in extremely low birth weight and low birth weight neonates. *J Vasc Surg* 1997;**26**:643–6.

Leaker M, Massicotte MP, Brooker LA et al. Thrombolytic therapy in pediatric patients: a comprehensive review of the literature. *Thromb Haemost* 1996;**76**:132–4.

Levy M, Benson LN, Burrows PE et al. Tissue plasminogen activator for the treatment of thromboembolism in infants and children. *J Pediatr* 1991;**118**:467–72.

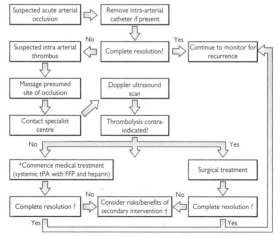

*If not contra-indicated, medical treament may be started prior to transfer to specialist centre,
† i.e. consider surgical intervention if primary treatment was medical and vice-versa

Fig. 4.20 Suggested management for acute arterial thrombosis in infants.

Children's surgery

The acute abdomen

After head injury, abdominal pain is one of the commonest reasons for a child to be admitted to hospital – estimated as 3 in every 1000 children in the UK. Of these, about one-third will have a surgical cause. The rest will have non-specific abdominal pain (NSAP) or other medical causes.

Clinical features

Age

Some conditions are characterized by a peak incidence within certain age groups (e.g. appendicitis – 5 to 15 years; intussusception – 2 months to 4 years; malrotation – the first month of life). Nonetheless be cautious with cases presenting outwith the typical age group (intussusception and malrotation are good examples).

> Pattern recognition is an important element in clinical diagnosis, but atypical presentations must be accommodated.

History

- Consistency of content is important, and inconsistency, particularly in unstable family structures or from carers with dependency problems, needs cautious interpretation. Overcoming communication/language difficulties requires extra care and effort.
- Location of the symptoms requires good definition, e.g. extra-abdominal pathology (pneumonia or oesophageal pathology) may present with epigastric discomfort.
- Duration – persistent abdominal pain of ≥6 h duration warrants hospital admission. In acute appendicitis, 50% of children will have shift of pain.

Examination

Vital signs – temperature pulse and respiratory rate need recording prior to any clinical examination. The following observations are all mandatory:

- **odours** – fetor oris, presence of ketones on the breath
- **inspection –** abdominal wall bruising (in babies less than one year, consider child protection issues and intentional injury), rashes (Henoch-Schönlein purpura, Herpes zoster), abdominal distension, groin lumps, visible intestinal peristalsis
- **palpation** – distraction techniques essential – in the septic irritable baby, allow the infant to become used to touch before palpating
- **auscultation** – of maximal value during an episode of pain
- **percussion –** use to elicit rebound tenderness
- **rectal examination** – for selective use only. Give it the status of an investigation.

Laboratory investigation

- Urine analysis – this is the only routine investigation to be done on children. Leucocytes and nitrates can be detected by strip technology in urinary infection. Positive detection of either or both = midstream sample/SPA for culture and sensitivity.

- White blood cell (WBC) count – if very high (>20 x 10^9 / L), suspect extra-abdominal source for sepsis. If low, consider a viral cause.
- C- reactive protein – commonly used in conjunction with the WBC, with elevation suggestive of bacterial infection. Diagnostic contribution best achieved through serial change rather than an isolated value.
- Biochemistry – general reflection of body systems. Serum amylase – specific indicator of pancreatic inflammation and often overlooked in children.

Radiological investigation

- Abdominal x-ray identifies free extravisceral air, bowel gas distribution, opacities (gall bladder, ureter, bladder, pancreas, faecolith in appendix). Obliteration of psoas shadow may indicate retroperitoneal pathology.
- Ultrasound – free fluid, intra-abdominal collections, calculi, appendicitis, intussusception, malrotation (relative positions of SMA and SMV). FAST (focal abdominal sonography in trauma) identifies intraperitoneal blood.
- CT – visceral injury following trauma (e.g. staging liver and spleen injuries). Routine usage in appendicitis has not resulted in reduction in negative appendicectomy or perforation rates.

Laparoscopy

- Invasive but typical indications would include pelvic inflammatory disease, ovarian pathology, and suspected appendicitis.

Supportive care

Antibiotic usage

Single prophylactic dose where no residual sepsis exists (e.g. non-perforated appendicitis). Therapeutic use determined by clinical response. Increasing awareness of super-infection/resistance indicates the need for restricted spectrum policy

Pain control

Opiate usage will not mask abdominal signs in peritonitis and is a core part of early care.

Fluid management

This should include correction of the calculated fluid and electrolyte deficit, ongoing maintenance requirements, and replacement of continued losses.

Decision making

Computerized decision-making and clinical scores

The use of systems such as the Alvarado scoring system for appendicitis (10-point score based on history, exam findings, and lab values) remain unproven. Supplementation with ultrasound is also of unconfirmed value.

Active observation (i.e. clinical re-evaluation at scheduled intervals – Peter Jones) remains the most reliable diagnostic process in cases of appendicitis, with highest accuracy rates using this management strategy.

Special considerations

Immunocompromised

Typhlitis (caecal inflammation) can mimic appendicitis and is a diagnostic challenge. Ultrasound is particularly useful, remembering the triad of abdominal pain, fever, and neutropenia may not always be present.

Cystic fibrosis

There are many causes for abdominal pain in CF (e.g. appendicitis, mucocele of appendix, distal intestinal obstruction syndrome (formerly meconium ileus equivalent)).

Nephrotic syndrome

Sudden onset of fever and abdominal pain can indicate primary peritonitis. Blood culture should precede laparoscopy/laparotomy. Use antibiotics early to provide cover from *Streptococcus pneumonia* and *E. coli*.

Henoch-Schönlein purpura

Patches of enteritis can cause colicky abdominal pain is well as precipitate small bowel intussusception.

Urinary sepsis

Reflex ileus presenting with abdominal distension along with generalized tenderness may be a manifestation of urinary sepsis (particularly in infants).

Diabetes

Ketoacidosis with severe abdominal pain may be the first presentation; 10% of diabetics have coeliac disease which can present with abdominal pain and low-grade dysmotility resulting in transient small bowel intussusception.

Pneumonia

Abdominal pain, stented breathing and rigid abdomen may give the impression of peritonitis. A high WBC, cough, and abdominal pain requires a chest x-ray.

Further reading

Alvarado A. A practical score for the early diagnosis of acute appendicitis. *Ann Emerg Med* 1986;**15**:557–64.

Douglas CD, Macpherson NE, Davidson PM, Gani JS. Randomised controlled trial of ultrasonography of acute appendicitis incorporating the Alvarado score. *BMJ* 2000;**321**:919–22.

Driver CP, Youngson GG. Acute abdominal pain in children: a 25 year comparison. *Health Bull* 1995;**53**:167–72.

Jones PF. Suspected acute appendicitis: trends in management over 30 years. *Br J Surg* 2001;**88**:1870–7.

Stringer MD, Pledger G, Drake D. Childhood deaths from intussusception in England and Wales (1984 – 89). *BMJ* 1992;**304**: 737–9.

Yanez R, Spitz L. Intestinal malrotational presenting outside the neonatal period. *Arch Dis Child* 1986;**61**:682–5.

Dysphagia

Physiology of swallowing

Swallowing is initiated as a reflex (V, VII, IX, X, XII, via swallowing pattern generator in brainstem) when food/liquid hits the back of tongue and pharynx. There is antero-elevation of the hyoid, depression of the epiglottis, and watertight closure of the larynx so protecting the airway; with relaxation of the cricopharyngeus allowing entry into proximal oesophagus (<1 s). Coordinated peristaltic waves originating in the proximal oesophagus propel the food bolus to the gastroesophageal sphincter (5–6 s). The lower oesophageal sphincter is tonically contracted because of myogenic and neurogenic factors. It relaxes due to vagally mediated inhibition involving nitric oxide as a neurotransmitter.

Dysphagia is uncommon in children, certainly as a *de novo* symptom, and most have pre-existing pathology (e.g. repaired OA etc).

Aetiology

This can be thought of as:
- extrinsic, e.g. cervical rib, pharyngeal pouch, mediastinal mass, duplications cysts, vascular rings
- intrinsic, e.g. oesophagitis, stricture (GOR, post-anastomotic, post-trauma, post-alkali ingestion), web, and achalasia
- intraluminal, e.g. foreign body.

Clinical features

Increasing feeding time or regurgitation of swallowed food are key symptoms, often associated with aspiration manifest as coughing or wheezing. Sometimes this is more obvious at night due to recumbent posture and relaxation. Painful swallowing (odynophagia) is more likely to be secondary to oesophagitis. The grossly distended baggy oesophagus of achalasia is particularly prone to aspiration, or regurgitation of food swallowed some time before. Dehydration, evidence of malnutrition, and halitosis should be actively sought.

Contrast swallow should precede flexible endoscopy. Mostly the cause is all too obvious. Obvious symptoms but no apparent stricture with easy passage into the stomach suggest achalasia. Oesophageal manometry may be available in some centres with an active adult practice but is not essential for most cases.

Vomiting

Physiology

There are two distinct centres within the medulla controlling vomiting (the chemoreceptor trigger zone in the floor of the 4th ventricle and the vomiting centre). Afferent impulses arrive from both the gastrointestinal tract and outside (e.g. middle ear). Efferent impulses are conveyed along sympathetic and cranial nerves VII, IX, and X to initiate increased salivation, reverse peristalsis, and involuntary downward movement of the diaphragm.

Clinical features

- **Bile (green) staining** is important and strongly suggests intestinal obstruction distal to the ampulla of Vater. Such children have surgical pathology until proven otherwise.
- **Non-bilious vomiting** may be due to obstruction at the oesophagus, pylorus, or the proximal duodenum (see other causes below however).
- **Haematemesis** is rare; 'coffee ground' vomiting suggests gastric cause, ingestion of red food and drinks can mimic haematemesis so take a careful history. Forceful 'projectile' vomiting may suggest hypertrophic pyloric stenosis.

Effortless vomiting after feeds in newborns is most commonly 'posseting' – benign common gastro-oesophageal reflux. Take a careful feeding history – what volume of feeds? Breast or bottle? How often? A chubby well-hydrated baby that vomits after feeds is often overfed.

Assessment

Assess hydration status. The degree of abdominal distension should be noted. In obstruction, this is dependent on the level and duration of obstruction. Tenderness/peritonism may be subtle in infants. Remember to have warm hands. This is impossible to assess in the crying child so you may need to reassess later. Carefully palpate for masses – differential diagnoses are given later in this section. Remember to check for incarcerated inguinal hernia.

Surgical causes of vomiting in the newborn

- Oesophageal atresia
- Duodenal atresia (may be bilious if distal to ampulla)
- Malrotation with volvulus*
- Jejuno-ileal atresia*
- Meconium ileus*
- Duplication cyst*
- Incarcerated inguinal hernia*

*Typically bile-stained.

> Only 40% of all infants referred with 'bile-stained vomiting' turned out to have a surgical cause, in one study from a UK regional referral unit.

Management plan

Resuscitate if shocked – this strongly suggests volvulus and may require urgent laparotomy. Place an 8–10 Fr nasogastric tube to prevent vomiting and aspiration and reduce abdominal distension. Leave open on free drainage and flush regularly with air or saline to keep patent. Commence IV fluid replacement. Plain chest/abdominal x-rays are often diagnostic; contrast studies and USS abdomen may be useful.

Causes of vomiting in the older infant /child

- GOR
- Infantile hypertrophic pyloric stenosis
- Gastroenteritis
- Malrotation with volvulus*
- Appendicitis (may be bilious)
- Intussusception*
- Infection (e.g. UTI, acute otitis, pneumonia)
- Head injury (including non-accidental injury)
- Metabolic causes, e.g. renal failure
- Foreign body ingestion
- Postoperative bowel obstruction*

*Typically bile-stained.

Initial management is as for newborns. Further investigations should be guided by the likely diagnoses from history and examination.

Mallory–Weiss syndrome
Violent retching leading to a mucosal tear at the GOJ, causing appearance of blood within vomitus (George Mallory (1900–1986) Soma Weiss (1898–1942)).
Boerhaave's syndrome
Complete rupture of the oesophagus due to forceful vomiting, leading to mediastinitis, pleural effusion etc. First described in 1723 in a grand admiral of the Dutch fleet who died of this after a particularly heavy meal.

Further reading

Bonadion WA, Clarkson T, Naus J. The clinical features of children with malrotation of the intestine. *Pediatr Emerg Care* 1991;**7**:348–9.

Godbole P, Stringer MD. Bilious vomiting in the newborn: how often is it pathologic? *J Pediatr Surg* 2002;**37**:909–11.

Kenny SE. Acute abdominal emergencies in childhood. *Surgery* 2005;**23**:330–2.

Gastrointestinal bleeding

This varies with age, site (upper or lower GI). and duration (acute or chronic bleeding). Traumatic causes (including NAI) should be obvious, and all haematological causes should be excluded by a normal clotting profile (INR, APTR, fibrinogen level) and platelet count.

Upper GI bleeding

Upper GI bleeding presents with true haematemesis (vomiting of fresh or altered blood – typically brown 'coffee-grounds' but no faeculent odour) or melaena (black stool, hence the name). A detailed history including possible ingestion, trauma, family history (e.g. peptic ulcer disease), previous episode of vomiting before haematemesis, or previous surgery (e.g. gastrostomy tube insertion) will guide diagnosis.

Key causes

- Mallory–Weiss tear (history of initial non-blood retching/vomiting)
- Trauma from gastrostomy tube/button – examination often reveals a worn gastrostomy that cannot be turned, implying some erosion into the gastric wall. Treat by replacing gastrostomy, occasionally may either need to resite gastrostomy or do a formal laparotomy to repair wall and resite
- GOR – usually implies a long history of reflux. Endoscopy diagnostic, but assess severity of GOR with pH monitoring/contrast studies. Treat either with proton pump inhibitors or fundoplication (open or laparoscopic)
- Acute gastritis – beware of acid/alkali ingestion. If severe, treat with sodium bicarbonate irrigation and then proton pump inhibitors
- Peptic ulcers – (usually a strong family history or ingestion of NSAIDs. If confirmed treat with medication but also need to rule out *H. pylori* infection (endoscopic biopsy for CLO test/histology or breath tests). If numerous ulcers, ?Zollinger–Ellison syndrome (measure gastrin levels)
- Oesophageal varices – either caused by obvious liver disease (post-Kasai) or first event of unrecognizd portal vein thrombosis. Treatment by sclerotherapy (infants) or banding. For acute control use a Sengstaken–Blakemore tube and call hepatology team.

Investigations

- Check FBC, G&S (also U&E, LFT, clotting as indicated)
- Upper gastrointestinal endoscopy (required if expectant treatment unsuccessful)

Lower GI bleeding

Can be described as fresh (mixed with stool, on surface of stool or on paper when cleaning perineum), altered (usually with stool) or clots. Other useful diagnostic points are associated abdominal pain, passage of mucus and diarrhoea. In the author's personal series of 250 children investigated with colonoscopy for rectal bleeding, one-third were normal, one-third had IBD, and 10% polyps.

Key causes

- Anal fissure – common at any age. History and examination diagnostic. Treat with laxatives. Use of 0.1% glyceryl trinitrate (GTN) or 2% diltiazem ointment is still debatable. Anal stretch is now discouraged. Internal sphincterotomy is surgical treatment of choice but rarely required.
- Inflammatory bowel disease – increasing incidence with increasing age. Usually present with other pain, diarrhoea, mucus and bleeding.
- Infectious – acute enterocolitis, typically with more diarrhoea than blood loss. Multiple possible organisms (e.g. *Campylobacter jejuni, Salmonella* spp., *Shigella* spp., *E. coli, Clostridium difficle, Aeromonas* spp.; rotavirus; *Entamoeba histolytica*). Stool slide/culture imperative.
- Meckel's diverticulum – occurs in 2% of population, usually presents before the age of 2 years, is 2 feet from ileo-caecal valve and 2 inches long. Bleeding usually presents with brisk rectal bleeding but can be altered blood or even melaena.
- Intussusception (see page 252) – typically infants but <10% occur in older children (?underlying cause e.g. polyp).
- Rectal prolapse – mucosal only is commonest if <5 years; in older child can be full thickness. For mucosal prolapse trial of laxatives may suffice. If not, submucosal injection with 5% phenol in almond oil is treatment of choice.
- Solitary rectal ulcer syndrome. Treatment is aimed at desensitization (with either steroids or short-chain fatty acid enema therapy), biofeedback or surgery. Described operations are many and varied but involve either a perineal or abdominal approach.
- Rectal polyps – histologically, usually juvenile polyps with most (80%) in rectum. Often hard to differentiate from prolapse without an EUA (often parents bring a digital photograph of diagnosis!). Treat by EUA, sigmoidoscopy, and excision. If sigmoidoscopy negative should proceed to colonoscopy. If numerous polyps (>5) then ?polyposis diseases (e.g. familial adenomatous polyposis in colon, Peutz–Jehgers syndrome in small bowel). Rectal cancers are incredibly rare in children.
- Cow milk protein intolerance – can present as rectal bleeding at any age, therefore must be considered as it has led to negative laparotomies. Look for eosinophilia (in biopsy and blood).
- Haemorrhoids – do occur in children! Exclude underlying portal hypertension. Treat underlying constipation. Rarely needs surgical intervention.
- Rare – arteriovenous malformations, intestinal duplications, small bowel polyps.

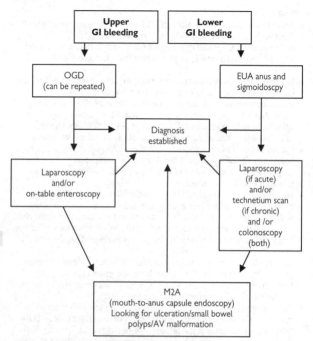

Fig. 5.1 Algorithm – gastrointestinal bleeding in children.

Further reading

De Angelis GL, Fornaroli F, de Angelis N, Magiteri B, Bizzarri B. Wireless capsule endoscopy for pediatric small-bowel diseases. *Am J Gastroenterol* 2007;**102**:1749–57.

Swaniker F, Soldes O, Hirschl RB. The utility of technetium 99m pertechnetate scintigraphy in the evaluation of patients with Meckel's diverticulum. *J Pediatr Surg* 1999;**34**:760–4.

Willets IE, Dalzell M, Puntis JW, Stringer MD. Cow's milk enteropathy: surgical pitfalls. *J Pediatr Surg* 1999;**34**:1486–8.

Foreign bodies

Epidemiology

Peak incidence 6 months to 5 years (older sibling may feed object to younger baby).

Clinical features

You name it, kids will swallow it.

Coins are the most common object. Potentially dangerous objects include button batteries, sharp objects such as toothpicks, open safety pins, razor blades, and multiple magnets that can cause intestinal pressure, necrosis, and perforation.

A history of possible swallowed foreign body *should not be ignored*, as most children will be asymptomatic.

Oropharyngeal foreign bodies

Sixty per cent of foreign bodies are trapped at the level of the cricopharyngeus. Symptoms include discomfort, drooling, airway compromise. Complications are rare but airway obstruction or retropharyngeal abscess can occur.

Oesophageal foreign bodies

Symptoms are subtle but can include a vague sensation of stuck object, gagging, vomiting, dysphagia, neck pain, and occasionally delayed presentation with recurrent chest infections/failure to thrive. Oesophageal perforation presents with symptoms of acute mediastinitis, fever, odynophagia, pneumonitis, and pleural effusion. Cardiac tamponade and acquired tracheo-oesophageal fistulae have also been reported.

Suboesophageal foreign bodies

Reassuringly, over 90% will pass without problem if they get as far as the stomach. Symptoms are rare but children may experience abdominal discomfort/distension, pyrexia, vomiting, rectal bleeding, or signs of gastrointestinal obstruction. Rarely, perforation will result in a child presenting with signs of peritonitis.

Assessment

Carefully assess the airway, oropharynx, respiratory, cardiovascular, and gastrointestinal tract. Plain chest and abdominal x-rays may locate radio-opaque objects. CT scanning is superior but not infallible in detecting foreign bodies and should be considered in difficult cases or where abscess formation is suspected.

Management

In acute airway obstruction the ingested object should be promptly extracted. If this is unsuccessful cricothyroidotomy may be life saving. Asymptomatic oesophageal coins may be safely observed for 12–24 h, as spontaneous passage into the stomach often occurs. Lodged oesophageal foreign bodies will usually require removal by either flexible or rigid endoscopy. Other extraction methods include use of a Foley catheter.

Most objects reaching the stomach can be safely allowed to pass but endoscopy should be performed for button batteries (Box 5.2) or magnets. Large (width >2 cm, length >6 cm) or sharp objects should be followed with serial x-rays: parents should be warned of symptoms requiring re-attendance.

Box 5.2 Disc (button) batteries

- May cause problems related to local current formation and liquifaction necrosis, or rupture and release of toxic chemicals (e.g. alkali, mercury, silver, zinc, cadmium). Fragmentation may occur if lodged in the stomach (because of HCl) but takes >48 h (more common in mercuric oxide cells)
- Need expeditious removal if lodged somewhere (e.g. nose and oesophagus), persists in stomach or there is x-ray evidence of fragmentation.

Further reading

Eisen G, Baron TH, Dominitz JA et al. Guideline for the management of ingested foreign bodies. *Gastrointest Endosc* 2002;**55**:802–806.

Midgett J, Inkster S, Rauchschwalbe R et al. Gastrointestinal injuries from magnet ingestion in children – United States, 2003–2006. *JAMA* 2007;**297**:147–9.

Waltzman M. Management of esophageal coins. *Curr Opin Pediatr* 2006;**18**:571–4.

Abdominal distension and masses

Any organ in the abdomen can cause a mass, and while a 'malignant' mass is always a major concern it is rare and other causes must always be thought of.

Remember that distension is not always caused by a mass. Ascites, free air, or an obstructed viscus is often the cause.

Differential diagnosis

- **Bowel**:
  - adhesions – either primary (e.g. Meckel's band) or, more commonly, post-laparotomy
  - appendix mass – history and examination should give diagnosis, confirmed on USS
  - obstructed inguinal hernia – rarer in children over one year of age, but if you don't examine the inguinal region could be missed
  - constipation – if not thought of then 'missed'. Clues in the history and examination. Either a rectal or plain abdominal x-ray will give the diagnosis. This author has seen diagnosis made on CT on numerous occasions!
  - gastric distension – particular problem post-fundoplication. This is an emergency and should be treated with immediate nasogastric decompression before an x-ray is performed as the patient is at risk of a non-atropine-responsive cardiac asystole
  - inflammatory bowel disease – can present in two ways:
    - acutely tender/distended abdomen with x-ray confirming a toxic megacolon in ulcerative colitis
    - an abdominal mass may develop either at presentation (rare) or as a complication of localized disease in Crohn's disease
  - meconium ileus equivalent – inspissated stool in older child with cystic fibrosis. Treat expectantly with Gastrografin® enema and/or orally
  - intussusception (rare > 2 years). History (e.g. known patient with Peutz–Jegher syndrome) or examination (e.g. leg rash indicative of Henoch-Schönlein purpura) often suggests diagnosis
- **Bladder** (rare):
  - urinary retention – again history and examination should lead to the diagnosis. Causes include phimosis, posterior urethral valves, meatal stenosis, constipation, pelvic masses, or neuropathy
- **Splenomegaly**:
  - neoplastic, e.g. lymphoma or primary tumour or as part of generalized haematological malignancy (e.g. leukaemia)
  - non-neoplastic, e.g. portal hypertension or storage disorders such as Gaucher's disease

- **Hepatomegaly**:
  - neoplastic, e.g. hepatoblastoma in young child, hepatocellular carcinoma in the older child, or benign tumours (focal nodular hyperplasia, haemangioma etc)
  - non-neoplastic, e.g. acute hepatitis, hepatic fibrosis
- **Tumours** (extremely rare in the bowel and bladder but commoner in other organs)
  - ovarian masses – if large enough (> 6 cm), risk of torsion
  - kidneys – e.g. Wilms' tumour. Easier to differentiate from neuroblastoma as child's age increases
  - neuroblastoma
  - lymphoma – lymphomatous deposits presenting with abdominal masses (this could mimic an appendix mass), as a cause of bowel obstruction or lead to urinary retention
  - rhabdomyosarcoma – if prostatic/bladder neck can present with urinary retention
  - lymphangioma, mesenteric and omental cysts
- **Miscellaneous**:
  - Ascites, e.g. urinary, malignant, or chylous
  - free air – perforation
  - haemorrhagic, e.g. post-trauma, pancreatitis
  - pancreatic pseudocyst

Management

- Full history and examination
- Resuscitation as required
- Basic haematological investigations (FBC, U&E, CRP, occasionally amylase)
- If tumour suspected – α-FP, β-HCG, LDH as baseline

Radiological investigations

- Plain abdominal x-rays – often diagnostic
- Ultrasound scan
- CT – advantage is speed of examination, therefore avoiding requirement of general anaesthetic; disadvantage, pictures not as clear, high radiation dose
- MRI – advantage is better anatomical definition, no radiation exposure; disadvantage is GA in younger children, availability

If diagnosis is still uncertain, laparoscopy will allow visual assessment which can proceed to either laparoscopic or open biopsy.

Further reading

Bekiesinska FM, Jurkiewicz E, Iwanowska B et al. Magnetic resonance imaging as a diagnostic tool in case of ovarian masses in girls and young women. *Med Sci Monit* 2007;**13**(Suppl 1):116–20.

Vade A, Azienstein R. Magnetic resonance imaging of abdominal masses in children. *J Pediatr Surg* 1993;**28**:82–8.

Constipation

Definition
Infrequent, painful passage of stools

Aetiology
Diet, parental attitude to toileting

Causes
Mostly idiopathic – typically avoidance of stooling and retention of faeces, which become increasingly firm and bulky making defecation painful, provoking further retentive behaviour and toilet avoidance. Faecal soiling due to paradoxical overflow incontinence is common. Other causes include anal fissures, pelvic mass, neurological – e.g. delayed presentation of lumbosacral spinal pathology such as tethered cord (remember to ask about bladder and lower motor function). Hirschsprung's disease is unlikely if normal stooling in first months of life. Also think of hypercalcaemia or hypothyroidism.

Investigation
Often unnecessary if careful history and exam are performed. Rectal examination is usually unnecessary in the awake infant/child. Consider pelvic ultrasound, serum calcium, and thyroid function tests, rectal biopsy in refractory cases (the minority). Spinal MRI is indicated if a neurological cause is suspected.

Treatment
Thorough explanation of problem and treatment rationale to child and parents in language they understand. Initial evacuation of faecal loading – laxatives/enemas/occasionally manual evacuation. Maintenance treatment comprises diet modification, toileting advice, use of stimulant/osmotic laxatives. (Table 5.1)

The Bristol Stool Chart (Fig. 5.2) is useful for assessment and explanation. Good communication between you and the family is the key!

Further reading

Clayden GS, Keshtgar AS, Carcani-Rathwell I, Abhyankar A. The management of chronic constipation and related faecal incontinence in childhood. *Arch Dis Child Ed Pract* 2005;**90**:58–67.

Lewis SJ, Heaton KW. Stool form scale as a useful guide to intestinal transit time. *Scand J Gastroenterol* 1997;**32**:920–4.

Reisner SH, Sivan Y, Nitzan M et al. Determination of anterior displacement of the anus in newborn infants and children. *Pediatrics* 1984;**73**:216–17.

Bristol Stool Chart		
Type 1	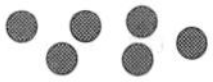	Separate hard lumps, like nuts (hard to pass)
Type 2	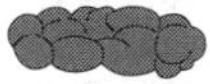	Sausage-shaped but lumpy
Type 3	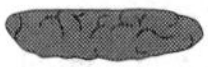	Like a sausage but with cracks on the surface
Type 4	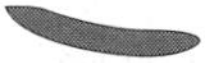	Like a sausage or snake, smooth and soft
Type 5	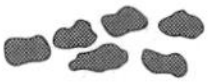	Soft blobs with clear-cut edges (passed easily)
Type 6	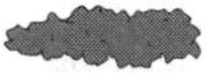	Fluffy pieces with ragged edges, a mushy stool
Type 7	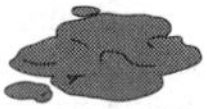	Watery, no solid pieces. **Entirely liquid**

Fig. 5.2 Bristol stool chart. Reproduced by kind permission of Dr K W Heaton, Reader in medicine at the University of Bristol. © 2000 Norgine Ltd.

Table 5.1 Commonly prescribed laxatives

	Mechanism	Dose	Notes
Lactulose	Osmotic	1 mL/kg bd; 5 ml bd (1–5 years); 10 mL bd (5–10 years)	Give with meals, ?dental caries
Macrogols, (e.g. MOVICOL Paediatric Plain® – polyethylene glycol 3350)	Osmotic	1 sachet (6.9 g)/60 mL water – (variable regimens)	
Senna-based (e.g. Senokot®)	Stimulant	Elixir – 7.5 mg/5 mL; 1 mL/kg	Occasional colic
Na picosulfate, (also Picolax®, Laxoberal®)	Stimulant	250 mg/kg for 1 month–4 years, 2.5–5 mg daily for 4–10 years	Occasional colic
Liquid paraffin BP	Lubricant	0.5 mL/kg, contraindicated in children under 3 years	Aspiration pneumonia, anal seepage
Na docusate	Stool softener	Elixir – 12.5 mg/mL, 2.5 mg/kg tds	Bitter taste, avoid combination with senna

Jaundice

Causes

The causes of jaundice in the older child can be divided into:

- prehepatic (typically haemolytic):
  - e.g. hereditary spherocytosis, thalassaemia, sickle cell anaemia, autoimmune haemolysis
  - most are chronic with splenomegaly. Abdominal pain is not usually a feature (aside from sickle cell anaemia, where sickling and splenic sequestration may occur). Urine and stool colour are unaffected
  - Gilbert's syndrome is benign, common, and familial (auto recessive), with transient unconjugated jaundice at times of stress
- Hepatic:
  - infective (e.g. hepatitis A, B, and C (also D and E), infectious mononucleosis, Weil's disease (leptospira), bacterial cholangitis, malaria)
  - metabolic (e.g. Wilson's (Cu), haemochromatosis (Fe))
  - cirrhosis (e.g. post-Kasai biliary atresia)
  - cystic fibrosis
  - tumours (e.g. hepatoblastoma or hepatocellular carcinoma but is rare as should involve both lobes, if jaundiced)
  - distinguish between acute presentation and decompensation of chronic disease. Pyrexia, rigours, tender hepatomegaly suggest former, while signs of chronicity (e.g. spider naevi, clubbing, ascites, splenomegaly) may indentify latter. Pruritus (due to cholestasis) may leave its mark. History of foreign travel, blood transfusion, drug ingestion etc
- post-hepatic (typically surgical)
  - bile duct strictures (including within head of pancreas)
  - choledochal malformations
  - gallstones (typically within CBD, but Mirizzi syndrome is gallstone impacted in neck causing extrinsic compression of common hepatic duct (CHD). Commonest causes either pigmented due to chronic haemolysis, or cholesterol in adolescent, overweight girls
  - tumours (e.g. rhabdomyosarcoma – primary tumour of bile ducts, pancreatic, lymphoma)
  - sclerosing cholangitis (with or without inflammatory bowel disease)
  - usually associated with abdominal pain or discomfort, pruritus, pale stools, and dark urine.

Basic investigation scenarios

Haematological investigation

Anaemia, increased reticulocyte count, and abnormal red cell morphology (e.g. spherocytes, stomatocytes) together with a raised haptoglobin level suggests haemolysis. Osmotic fragility, and red cell enzymes require specialist input.

Laboratory and biochemical investigation
- Split bilirubin distinguishes whether predominatly unconjugated (i.e. probably medical) versus conjugated (possibly surgical). Raised transaminases (e.g. ALT and AST) indicates degree of ongoing hepatocellular damage (grossly elevated in hepatitis). Elevated alkaline phosphatase (NB also bone origin) and γ-glutamyl transpeptidase levels suggest obstructive biliary cause. Low albumin levels suggest chronic liver disease.
- Viral serology.
- Coagulopathy (elevated INR) may be vitamin K-responsive (factors II, VII, IX, X) due to lack of intestinal bile or due to protein production failure of liver failure.
- Percutaneous liver biopsy.

Radiological investigation
Ultrasonography is the key investigation (Box 5.3) in the jaundiced child and dictates investigation strategy. Biliary dilatation and its common surgical causes (e.g. gallstones, choledochal malformations, cysts, tumour) are easily visualized, and Doppler flow studies will give information about portal venous and hepatic arterial flow.

Box 5.3 Approximate normal values

CBD measure ~1 mm in neonates, ~2 mm in infants and <6 mm in adolescents

---

Both CT (contrast-enhanced) and MRI (T_1 weighting is good for anatomical detail, T_2-weighted images which give high signal for tissues with a higher content of free unbound water identify inflammatory or neoplastic tissue) are able to evaluate mass lesions within or outside the liver.

Magnetic resonance cholangiopancreatography (MRCP) defines biliary anatomy (although the common pancreatobiliary junction is a difficult area) and should replace a speculative ERCP.

Radio-isotope studies are useful as a functional evaluation of biliary excretion and to distinguish whether cysts have a biliary connection. Some centres use it in the diagnosis of acute cholecystitis (non-visualization) or post-traumatic bile leaks.

Interventional techniques
There is no lower age limit for either ERCP or percutaneous transhepatic cholangiography (PTC), but because of MRCP they are less commonly performed nowadays. PTC is preferred for hilar obstruction. Therapeutic intervention using wire-guided balloon dilators, Dormia baskets, and indwelling stents can definitively or temporarily treat strictures, remove impacted gallstones and treat traumatic biliary leaks.

Head and neck lesions

Dermoid cysts

These are common and occur along lines of embryological fusion (e.g. lateral corner eyebrow 'external angular', midline of the neck, bridge of the nose, and suprasternal notch). They are non-tender, mobile subcutaneous cysts filled with keratin, hair follicles and sebaceous glands. They slowly enlarge and should be treated by excision.

Thyroglossal cysts (Box 5.4)

Arise as a midline neck swelling just below hyoid bone. This rises with tongue protrusion. Thyroglossal cysts develop from epithelial remnants left after descent of the thyroid from the foramen caecum. Cysts gradually enlarge and eventually become infected (makes excision difficult).

> **Box 5.4 Sistrunk's operation (Walter Ellis Sistrunk – US surgeon 1880–1933)**
>
> Removal of cyst and underlying track down to base of tongue. The central portion of the hyoid bone is also removed. The technique reduces the incidence of recurrence.

Branchial remnants

The branchial apparatus is believed to recapitulate evolution and development, and perhaps is analogous to gill formation in our ancestors. There are five definite clefts.

The most common lesions are derived from the second cleft and include cysts, sinuses or, rarely, a fistula. Branchial cysts are uncommon neck swellings along the anterior border of the sternomastoid. The differential includes cystic hygroma, which is more common. Excision is curative. Branchial sinuses present with small cutaneous openings along the anterior border of the lower third of sternocleidomastoid muscle, which discharge mucous. Occasionally they communicate with the tonsillar fossa (branchial fistula). Treatment is by excision to prevent later infection. Second branchial arch cartilage remnants also may present with skin tags in this region.

First cleft sinuses are rare. They are located at the angle of the mandible and communicate with the external auditory meatus. Third cleft sinuses are very rare. They communicate with the piriform sinus and present with acute thyroiditis and recurrent neck infections.

Cystic hygroma

These are congenital lymphatic malformations and present in early childhood as soft multilocular cystic swellings, often appearing after intercurrent viral infections. They are most often found in the neck and axillae although they can occur anywhere. Large cervical cystic hygromas may present at birth with airway obstruction. Small lesions may require no treatment other than reassurance. Treatment of large lesions is difficult because the cysts tends to infiltrate surrounding tissues making complete surgical excision impossible. Intralesional injection of OK432 (lyophilized product of *Streptococcus pyogenes*) is an alternative to surgery in some cases and appears to work by inducing a vigorous inflammatory response in the cysts which may then regress.

Congenital torticollis

A small lateral swelling in the baby's neck may be noted initially, the so-called sternomastoid 'tumour'. This is an area of fibrosis in the lower part of the muscle, typically transient, resolving after a few months. Sometimes there is a history of dystocia. Shortening of the sternomastoid muscle results in a torticollis with rotation and tilting of the head to the opposite side. Plagiocephaly may also result from untreated cases.

Management is usually conservative with passive exercises to achieve full neck movements. However, unless a full range of movement is restored, hemifacial atrophy and a strabismus may develop. Occasionally it is necessary to divide the shortened muscle surgically but this is no substitute for physiotherapy.

Cervical lymphadenopathy

- Very common cause of neck swelling in children.
- Upper respiratory tract infection is the usual cause. Specific organisms might include (by age) newborn – *Staphylococcus aureus*, GpB *Steptococcus*; pre-school – Gp A *Streptococcus*, *Staphylococcus aureus*, non-tuberculous mycobacterium; school age – Epstein–Barr virus, cytomegalovirus, toxoplasmosis and infectious mononucleosis.
- Differential diagnosis is lymphoma (usually adolescents, ask about 'B' symptoms (e.g. fever, weight loss, night sweats), and biopsy may be necessary.
- Acute suppurative submandibular lymphadenitis occurs in early childhood and is a painful swelling often associated with marked cellulitis. Antibiotics and drainage are required.

Ankyloglossia (tongue tie)

May cause difficulties with breast feeding (baby unable to protrude tongue and latch on) but doesn't impede bottle feeding. The NICE guidelines suggest dividing tongue ties in babies (without anaesthetic) to improve breast feeding. In older children, there is no conclusive evidence that tongue tie division improves speech or feeding problems.

Further reading

NICE. Interventional Procedures Overview – division of ankyloglossia (tongue tie) for breast-feeding. London: NICE, 2005. http://www.nice.org.uk/ip279overview (accessed 11 July 2008).

Ogita S, Tsuto T, Nakamura K *et al*. OK-432 therapy for lymphangioma in children: why and how does it work? *J Pediatr Surg* 1996;**31**:477–80.

Waldhausen JH. Branchial cleft and arch anomalies in children. *Semin Pediatr Surg* 2006;**15**:64–9.

Cervical node infection (uncommon causes)

Certain more exotic infections need to be considered if symptoms/signs are atypical (e.g. prolonged history, poor response to antibiotic, prolonged discharge following I&D).

Non-tuberculous mycobacteria (NTM) (aka atypical mycobacteria)

This category of organisms is clearly distinct from typical pulmonary or intestinal tuberculosis, and includes *M. avium intracellulare*, *M. kansasii*, and *M. chelonei*. These are usually multidrug resistant and typically have a negative Mantoux (PPD) reaction, normal CXR and cause only localized disease.

Clinical features

Prolonged (>4 weeks) indolent nodal infection in children aged 3–6 years is typical. The overlying skin may become reddened and 'brawny', discharging watery, purulent fluid. They are not usually that painful, and have no reaction to conventional antibiotics. Diagnosis is often on clinical grounds as actual culture is slow (8 weeks). Antigens are available for a differential Mantoux test, and in some centres rtPCR can be obtained on excised biopsy material.

Management

The ideal treatment is to excise the infected node(s) and an ellipse of overlying skin. If complete then this has an acceptable risk of fistula formation and is associated with the best cosmesis. However, if there are multiple nodal groups or 'at risk' adjacent nerves (e.g. peri-parotid), then a course of macrolide antibiotic (e.g. azithromycin, clarithromycin) is preferable.

Cervical tuberculosis

The original cause of 'scrofula'. Nowadays it is seen in fairly well-defined scenarios:
- immunosuppressed (e.g. post-transplantation, HIV)
- immigrants
- indigent.

In contrast to NTM, surgery has only a supporting role (drainage of abscess, biopsy) and anti-tuberculous chemotherapy is the mainstay of effective management.

Cat scratch disease

This is under-appreciated, and caused by the pleomorphic Gram-negative organism *Bartonella henselae* (formerly *Rochalimaea henselae*), associated with cats (usually kitten) and their fleas. There is usually a small innoculation papule and regional painful lymphadenopathy some weeks later. Serology and PCR is available. Most disease is self-limiting, but antibiotics (e.g. azithromycin) may be indicated for severe symptoms.

Thyroid surgery

Thyroid surgery in children is uncommon and should be performed only in regional centres after detailed discussion with a multidisciplinary team including a paediatric endocrinologist, an endocrine surgeon with experience in operating on children, a paediatric oncologist, nuclear physician, radiologist, pathologist, and clinical geneticist.

Indications

Benign disease

- Thyrotoxicosis (Graves' disease, toxic adenoma)
- Symptomatic multinodular goitre causing dysphagia, stridor, pain, or discomfort

Malignant disease

- Solitary nodules suspected of being malignant
- Thyroid cancer (papillary, follicular, medullary)
- Prophylactic thyroidectomy for MEN (Table 5.2)

Investigations

Clinical examination of the neck is required to assess the size of the goitre, its retrosternal extension, nodularity and presence of lymphadenopathy. Thyroid function tests (T_3, T_4, TSH) are essential to confirm normal function (with or without thyroxine, antithyroid drugs etc). Serum calcium, thyroglobulin (for well-differentiated thyroid cancer, calcitonin (for medullary carcinoma/hyperplasia), and thyroid antibodies are sometimes required.

Thyroid imaging including neck ultrasound, CXR and sometimes CT and/or MR scans. Ultrasound is invaluable in assessing thyroid nodules and lymph nodes (size, cystic or solid nature, number, blood flow, microcalcifications), and guiding a biopsy needle. Nuclear scans provide information about thyroid function (e.g. radioactive iodine) and expression of specific receptors (e.g. octeotide scan) to stage medullary carcinoma.

Fine needle aspiration cytology is pivotal in assessing potentially malignant thyroid nodules or enlarged lymph nodes. Older children can tolerate it without anaesthesia. Solitary thyroid nodules in children carry a much higher risk of cancer, as compared to the adult population, and negative cytology should not obviate the need for surgical excision and full histological assessment.

Pre-operative laryngoscopy is indicated for all patients who report voice change or who had previous neck surgery.

Surgery

Thyroid surgery is performed through a skin-crease collar incision. At surgery both recurrent and superior laryngeal nerves must be clearly identified and handled gently to prevent their damage. All parathyroid glands should be identified and preserved with their blood supply intact if possible. Devascularized glands should be grafted into adjacent muscle pockets. At the end of surgery, haemostasis is checked and sometimes a small drain is inserted.

The commonest types of thyroid surgery are:

- **lobectomy and isthmusectomy** – performed for solitary thyroid nodules, which are either causing compression symptoms or thyrotoxicosis, or are suspected of being malignant
- **near-total thyroidectomy** – an operation of choice for thyrotoxicosis and large bilateral multinodular goitre
- **total thyroidectomy** – indicated for treating thyroid cancer and as a prophylactic measure in children with MEN2.

Lymph node surgery
- **Central lymphadenectomy** removes lymph nodes adjacent to thyroid and should be performed for tumours >1 cm.
- **Unilateral or bilateral modified neck dissection** with preservation of non lymphatic structures is performed in children with palpable lymph nodes.

Postoperative management

Immediately after surgery, children should be nursed in semi-sitting position with routine observations (blood pressure, pulse, and respiratory rate) checked frequently. Neck swelling or excessive drain discharge must be reported urgently to surgical team.

Dyspnoea or stridor

Potentially life-threatening and may be due to recurrent laryngeal nerve injury or bleeding into the neck (~1%). Immediate intervention at the bedside is required. If there is obvious neck swelling with stridor, the wound should be opened by cutting the skin and deeper stitches, the haematoma should be evacuated and the patient transferred to the operating theatre for further management. Emergency intubation is difficult, and if necessary should be performed by a senior anaesthetist.

Hypocalcaemia

Occurs as a result parathyroid damage. Temporary hypocalcaemia after hemi-thyroidectomy is rare but is common if total thyroidectomy and lymph node surgery is performed. Permanent hypocalcaemia occurs in 1–3% of cases. Serum calcium levels should be checked 12 hourly postoperatively and symptomatic hypocalcaemia (tingling, cramps, tetany – +ve Chvostek +ve Trousseau signs) should be treated urgently with IV 10% calcium gluconate infusion (1.7 mL/kg). Prolonged hypocalcaemia requires treatment with oral calcium and vitamin D_3.

Hypothyroidism

Thyroxine replacement is often necessary. Lobectomy causes hypothyroidism in about 10–20% of children. Maintaining normal thyroid function depends on the volume of remaining thyroid tissue and its functional capacity. The decision to start thyroxine should be based on symptoms and TSH levels during follow-up. After near-total thyroidectomy for benign disease, patients should start thyroxine before discharge from the hospital. The initial dose depends on the patient's age and weight, and should be titrated to achieve a euthyroid state. After total thyroidectomy for cancer, the initial replacement is with short-acting liothyronine (T_3). It reduces the time of withdrawal necessary to render the patient hypothyroid before treatment with radioactive iodine. Once treatment with radioactive iodine is completed liothyronine is replaced with lifelong thyroxine (T_4) with an aim to suppress the TSH to undetectable levels. TSH can stimulate tumour growth, and its suppression is very important.

Voice change

This is caused by injury to the recurrent or superior laryngeal nerves and can be temporary (neuropraxia) or permanent. The risk of injuring a single recurrent laryngeal nerve is ~1% and it causes a hoarse/croaky voice. Injury to both nerves is extremely rare and may require tracheostomy and laryngeal surgery. Injury to the external branch of the superior laryngeal nerve occurs in 2–5% of thyroidectomies and causes voice fatigue and weakness. Patients with an abnormal-sounding voice after surgery should be reassured that these changes are temporary in most cases. They should undergo laryngoscopy if changes persist.

Follow-up and surveillance

After thyroid surgery, especially for thyroid cancer, all children will require lifelong surveillance.

Treatment with radioactive iodine is recommended for most children after total thyroidectomy for papillary and follicular cancer. Radioiodine ablation should be carried about 4 weeks after surgery with a diagnostic scan 6 months later. Regular review should include neck palpation, serum thyroglobulin, and ultrasound with cytology if necessary. Calcitonin is a marker of recurrent disease in medullary cancer.

Table 5.2 Multiple endocrine neoplasia

	Gene	Target organ	Consequence
Type 1 (Wermer)	*MENIN* gene on Ch11 q13	PT, pancreatic islets,	Hyperparathyroidism (hyperplasia), pituitary tumours, rarely gastrinomas
Type 2A (Sipple) (95%)	*RET* mutations	C cells (thyroid), adrenal medulla	Medullary thyroid cancer (invariable), pheochromocytomas
2B (5%)			As above and Marfanoid habitus, mucosal neuromas (thick lips!)

PT – parathyroid.

Further reading

Fleming JB, Lee JE, Bouvet M et al. Surgical strategy for the treatment of medullary thyroid carcinoma. *Ann Surg* 1999;**230**:697–707.

Hegedus L. The thyroid nodule. *N Engl J Med* 2004;**351**:1764–71.

Skinner MA, Moley JA, Dilley WG et al. Prophylactic thyroidectomy in MEN type 2A. *N Engl J Med* 2005;**353**: 1105–113.

Chest wall deformities

Incidence

Pectus excavatum (PE) more common than pectus carinatum (PC) with overall incidence of ~1:300

Epidemiology

Male predominance (4:1). PE often appears in childhood, progressing during adolescence. PC usually appears in adolescence. Family history in 10–15%

Aetiology

- Unknown
- PE associated with:
  - connective tissue disorders e.g. Marfan's syndrome, Ehlers–Danlos syndrome)
  - CDH – particularly after prosthetic patch repair
- PC often associated with asthma

Classification

PE characterized by sternal depression. PC characterized by sternal protrusion. Rare chest wall deformities include:

- sternal clefts
- Poland syndrome (absent pectoralis major/minor muscle, rib anomalies, syndactyly, breast hypoplasia)
- Cantrell's pentalogy (sternal cleft, exomphalos, anterior diaphragmatic defect, absent pericardium with ectopia cordis, cardiac malformations)
- thoracic skeletal dystrophies: e.g. Jeune's syndrome (aka asphyxiating thoracic dystrophy).

Pectus excavatum

Young children are usually asymptomatic. Adolescents may complain of chest pains and fatigue. Other features include scoliosis (5%) and mitral valve prolapse (~20%).

Investigations

- Lung function tests: mild restrictive defects common
- Clinical photographs
- Echocardiogram – if mitral valve prolapse or suspicion of Marfan's syndrome
- Non-contrast CT thorax allows calculation of the pectus index (PI): transverse chest diameter divided anterior–posterior diameter (Fig. 5.3). PI >2.5 significant, >3.2 severe deformity

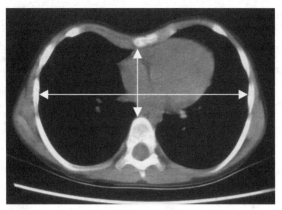

Fig. 5.3 Pectus index – transverse diameter of the thorax divided by the antero–posterior diameter.

Management

Physiotherapy is of no benefit. The Ravitch (Box 5.5) or Nuss (Box 5.6; Fig. 5.4) procedure can be used.

Box 5.5 Ravitch procedure (1949)
Mark M Ravitch, US surgeon (1910–89)

This involves sub-perichondral costal cartilage resection and a transverse osteotomy to correct the sternal depression. Radical, but excellent results are possible. Complications include bleeding and recurrence (usually because of inadequate cartilage resection).

There may be a permanent disturbance of chest wall growth from extensive cartilage resection in young children

Box 5.6 Nuss procedure (1998)
Donald Nuss South African surgeon

A curved metal bar is placed through the thorax behind the sternum to exert continuous pressure on the undersurface of the sternum, correcting deformity. The bar is left in place for 2–4 years to allow skeletal remodelling. It is then removed without recurrence.

Complications include bar displacement (minimized using stabilizing plates), prosthetic infection (bar removal required), injury to intrathoracic structures (minimized by thoracoscopy), pneumothorax (common but rarely significant), and postoperative pain (epidural analgesia mandatory).

See: http://www.nussprocedure.com/

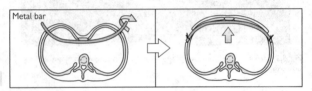

Fig. 5.4 Nuss procedure.

Pectus carinatum

The deformity is often asymmetrical with sternal torsion as well as angulation. The Ravitch procedure is effective. The principle is the same as for PE except that the osteotomy is wedged 'open' with costal cartilage to angle the sternum backwards.

Further reading

Fonkalsrud EW, Dunn JCY, Atkinson JB. Repair of pectus excavatum deformities: 20 years of experience with 375 patients. *Ann Surg* 2000;**231**:443–8.

Haller JA, Kramer SS, Lietman SA. Use of CT scans in selection of patients for pectus excavatum surgery: a preliminary report. *J Pediatr Surg* 1987;**22**:904–906.

Nuss D, Kelly RE, Croitoru DP, Katz ME. A 10-year review of a minimally invasive technique for the correction of pectus excavatum. *J Pediatr Surg* 1998;**33**:545–52.

Shamberger RC, Nuss D, Goretsky MJ. Surgical treatment of chest wall deformities. In: Spitz L, Coran AG (eds). *Operative Pediatric Surgery* (6th edn). London: Hodder Arnold, 2006, pp209–30.

Mediastinal tumours

The mediastinum can be divided conveniently into three compartments: anterior, posterior (paravertebral), and middle (visceral) (Fig. 5.5). Mediastinal tumours are fairly common in children, and approximately 60% are malignant. The commonest tumours are lymphomas (40%) and neurogenic tumours (40%).

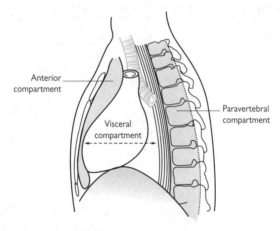

Fig. 5.5 Mediastinal anatomy.

Anterior mediastinum

Lymphoma (Hodgkin's and non-Hodgkin's)

These may present with cough, wheezing, stridor, and 'B' symptoms (i.e. fever, weight loss, night sweats). Mediastinal lymphadenopathy may be seen on CXR and confirmed on CT scan (also assess the trachea for compression because this has anaesthetic implications). Biopsy is essential for diagnosis (fresh tissue).

Treatment

Chemotherapy is the mainstay, and together with steroid administration the tumour may melt away.

Teratomas

These tumours can appear at any age and are often large. Sometimes they are discovered incidentally on CXR (calcified mass) or may cause airway compression. Most are mature benign tumours containing elements of all three germ layers (ectoderm, mesoderm, and endoderm).

Investigations

CXR, CT scan (with contrast), tumour markers (α-fetoprotein, β-HCG)

Treatment

Complete excision via median sternotomy, with adjuvant chemotherapy if malignant

Rare tumours

Thymoma (may be associated with myasthenia), goitre, cystic hygroma

Posterior mediastinum

Neurogenic tumours

- This group includes neuroblastoma (malignant), ganglioneuroblastoma, ganglioneuroma (benign). They enlarge in the paravertebral gutter and may extend into the spinal canal.
- The presentation may include cough, Horner's syndrome (papillary miosis, anhidrosis, ptosis, enopthalmos), paraplegia, and opsoclonus–myoclonus (dancing eyes syndrome).
- Urinary catecholamine metabolites (VMA, HVA) may be elevated; CXR, CT scan, bone marrow biopsy, bone scan should be performed as for investigation of neuroblastoma (see page 306).

Treatment

Excision biopsy (if possible), chemotherapy if malignant

Further paravertebral tumours include neurofibromas, schwanomas, PNETs (primitive neuroectodermal tumour, see page 319), and phaeo-chromocytomas.

Middle mediastinum

Lymphomas and haemangiomas may develop in the visceral compartment.

Bronchogenic cysts

- Congenital airway duplication cysts, lined by respiratory epithelium (ciliated columnar). The majority of these cysts arise adjacent to trachea/bronchi.
- Sometimes cysts can present on the antenatal ultrasound or as an incidental finding on CXR. Respiratory symptoms may include pneumonia, stridor, and chronic cough. The diagnosis is established by CXR and CT scan.

Treatment

Excision

Oesophageal duplication cysts

- Duplication cysts of the oesophagus, which may or may not communicate with the lumen. Some contain ectopic gastric mucosa, which may ulcerate.
- A CXR may show a soft tissue mass and be associated with vertebral anomalies (neuroenteric cyst). Barium swallow may show luminal indentation. CT scan should be definitive.

Treatment

Resection, preserving the oesophagus

Further reading

American Pediatric Surgical Association. http://www.eapsa.org/parents/resources/solid.cfm (accessed 14 July 2008).

Grosfeld JL, Skinner MA, Rescorla FJ et al. Mediastinal tumors in children: experience with 196 cases. Ann Surg Oncol 1994;**1**:121–7.

Okazaki T, Iwatani S, Yanai T et al. Treatment of lymphangioma in children: our experience of 128 cases. J Pediatr Surg 2007;**42**:386–9.

Empyema

Incidence
- 3 per 100,000 (increasing)

Aetiology

The majority follow an acute bacterial pneumonia; occasionally it may be a complication of an oesophageal anastomotic leak or rupture.

Pathogenesis

Empyema progression is divided into three stages:
- **exudative phase** – bacterial infection of pneumonia-associated effusion leads to pus in the pleural space
- **fibropurulent phase** – formation of a loculated pyogenic membrane. Antibiotics penetrate poorly
- **organization phase** – fibrous tissue replaces fibrin. The rind encases the lung preventing re-expansion.

Microbiology
- *Strep. pneumonia* (~75%)
- *Staph. aureus* (10–15%)
- *H. influenzae*, *Strep. pyogenes*, tuberculosis (less common)

Clinical features

Symptoms of pneumonia including cough, breathlessness, fever and malaise. Pleuritic chest pain is common, occasionally with abdominal pain. A child with pneumonia should start to improve after 48 h on IV antibiotics, and lack of improvement suggests an empyema. Pyrexia, tachycardia, tachypnoea, and O_2 saturations <92% in air indicates severe disease. 'Stony' dullness to percussion, reduced breath sounds and scoliosis.

Investigations
- Elevated white blood cell count and CRP
- Blood and pleural fluid for culture
- Mantoux test if tuberculosis suspected

Radiology
- CXR – collapse/consolidation, pleural effusion, scoliosis, mediastinal shift (Fig. 5.6)
- US – effusions easy to identify. Useful to determine whether effusion is loculated
- CT scan with IV contrast – if lung abscess or tumour suspected

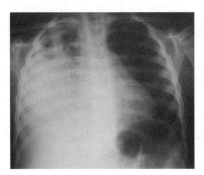

Fig. 5.6 CXR showing empyema.

Management

The cardinal principles are effective antibiotic therapy together with and drainage of the effusion.

Supportive medical therapy
- Oxygen – maintain SaO_2 >95%
- IV fluids if too breathless to drink – watch for hyponatraemia
- Analgesia and antipyretics

Antibiotics
- High-dose cephalosporin or flucloxacillin + amoxicillin IV
- Other antibiotics (e.g. meropenem) may be necessary depending on culture results. Take advice from microbiology.

Intercostal tube drainage and fibrinolytics
Drainage and antibiotics may be successful for early-stage empyemas. There is no evidence that large drains are better than small. Intrapleural fibrinolytics (e.g. urokinase) may improve drainage and may be effective with fine-bore pigtail drains.

Surgery

Early debridement of fibrinous septae and drainage by mini-thoracotomy or video-assisted thoracoscopy (VAT) is highly effective. Decortication is the only effective treatment for an organized empyema. The aim is to free the lung and chest wall from fibrin peel to allow re-expansion. This operation can be difficult and is often associated with significant bleeding and air leak. Blood transfusion is often required.

> The prognosis for empyema is good and lung function generally returns to normal.

Further reading

Balfour-Lynn IM, Abrahamson E, Cohen G et al. British Thoracic Society guidelines for the management of pleural infections in children. *Thorax* 2005;**60**:1–21.

Heffner JE. Multicenter trials of treatment for empyema. *N Engl J Med* 2005;**352**:926–8.

Thomson AH, Hull J, Kumar AR et al. Randomised trial of intrapleural urokinase in the treatment of childhood empyema. *Thorax* 2002;**57**:343–7.

Oesophageal problems (miscellaneous)

Oesophageal stricture

- Congenital (5%) – caused by submucosal fibrosis, ectopic cartilage (tracheobronchial rests), and occasionally a membranous diaphragm. It most commonly affects the lower oesophagus and usually presents in early childhood (after weaning).
- Acquired (95%) – caused by gastro-oesophageal reflux (common), caustic ingestion, or as a complication post-oesophageal atresia repair.

Rare causes

- Epidermolyis bullosa
- Vascular rings – double aortic arch, right-sided aortic arch (aberrant subclavian artery or ligamentum arteriosum). Look for evidence of airway occlusion
- Barrett's oesophagus – lined by gastric mucosa
- Eosinophilic oesophagitis
- Congenital tracheobronchial remnants
- Post-irradiatrion, post-injection sclerotherapy

Symptoms include dysphagia, bolus obstruction, regurgitation, and failure to thrive. The diagnosis is established by contrast swallow and then oesophagoscopy.

Management

Most strictures will undergo some kind of dilatation, although whether a balloon or a rigid (e.g. Savary dilator) method is used depends largely on personal preference.

Further management depends largely on response and underlying aetiology. Thus, peptic strictures are an absolute indication for antireflux surgery after which they will resolve. Congenital strictures also usually require resection.

Resistant stricture?

- Steroids – long history, little evidence
- Mitomycin C – inhibits fibroblasts. Local application (0.1 mg/mL) via endoscope
- Stenting – self–retaining stents, have largely been used post-caustic ingestion
- Oesophageal substitution (see page 232)

Ingested foreign bodies

Accidental foreign body ingestion is common in toddlers and the usual objects are coins and button batteries (see page 201). A CXR should be diagnostic if the object is radio-opaque, and endoscopy if not. Objects tend to lodge in three places: above the cricopharyngeus, adjacent to the aortic arch, and above the OG junction.

Management

Foreign bodies in the lower oesophagus may pass into the stomach so overnight observation may be acceptable; however, others should be removed within a few hours. This involves oesophagoscopy (flexible or rigid) to retrieve the object (or push it into the stomach if harmless). Removal by traction using fluoroscopy and a Foley catheter inflated with contrast is also possible for many objects. If lodged, button batteries must be removed promptly because of the risk of electrolytic corrosion of the oesophagus with ulceration and perforation.

Oesophageal perforation

Spontaneous perforation is rare and is usually traumatic in origin due to iatrogenic (post-dilatation or occasionally nasogastric intubation in neonates), missed foreign body, and caustic ingestion.

Clinical features

Respiratory distress, chest pain, subcutaneous emphysema, drooling, and fever. A CXR may show a pneumothorax (usually left sided), or mediastinal and cervical air. Careful water-soluble contrast swallow will confirm leak and show degree.

Management
- Apply resuscitation principles.
- The development of a hydropneumothorax requires insertion of a chest tube and pleural drainage. The subsequent treatment depends on the nature of injury and the condition of the oesophagus.

Caustic injuries

This may seen as an accidental ingestion in young children, and (rarely) as parasuicide in teenagers.

Alkali causes liquefaction necrosis which destroys the oesophagus. Acid ingestion is less common but causes coagulative necrosis which tends to damage the stomach to a greater degree.

Management

Resuscitation with oxygen, IV fluids, analgesia, and antibiotics. About 95% of children with significant oesophageal injury will have oral burns. Endoscopy should be performed when stable to determine the severity of injury. Contrast swallow may also be performed once the child is able to swallow saliva, to document the extent of injury.

Severe strictures often develop and a feeding gastrostomy is frequently necessary. In the chronic phase, serial dilatations may be necessary. Many children require oesophageal replacement.

Squamous carcinomas can develop in the damaged oesophagus after 20–30 years.

Achalasia

This is an uncommon oesophageal motility disorder in children and adolescents (boys > girls). The aetiology is unknown. The symptoms are characterized by progressive dysphagia, regurgitation, halitosis, weight loss, chest pain, and cough (from recurrent aspiration).

Box 5.7 Chagas' disease

This is a rare South American disease, caused by the protozoa, *Trypanosoma cruzi via* a varity of insect vectors – typically the reduvid or 'kissing' bug, which destroys the oesophageal myenteric plexus, leading to features indistinguishable from achalasia. Similarly autonomic destruction leads to cardiomyopathy.

A contrast swallow shows dilatation of the lower oesophagus, and characteristic 'bird-beak' appearance at the oesophago-gastric junction, which fails to open normally (Fig. 5.7).

Manometry (where available) is diagnostic and shows an abnormally high pressure lower oesophageal sphincter (LOS), which fails to relax on deglutition. Oesophageal peristalsis is reduced or absent.

Treatment

- Endoscopic botulinum toxin (Botox) injection into the LOS causes temporary improvement but is controversial.
- Balloon dilatation of the LOS is effective but has (a) high recurrence rate and (b) risk of oesophageal perforation.
- Heller's cardiomyotomy (extramucosal division of the LOS) is effective (Box 5.8).

Box 5.8 Heller's myotomy

- First performed in 1913, by the German surgeon, Ernest Heller, although he actually used two incisions in the muscle.
- Weakening the sphincter is achieved by longitudinal division of muscle (3–5 cm), as either an open or a laparoscopic approach. Because of the high incidence of GOR, it is often combined with a partial fundoplication (e.g. Toupet). Some surgeons prefer this to a 360° Nissen as peristalsis is invariably impaired.

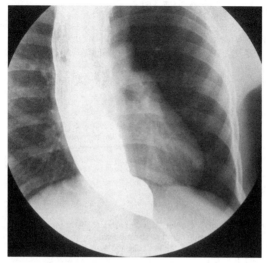

Fig. 5.7 Appearance of achalasia on barium swallow.

Further reading

Oesophageal stricture

Othersen HB, Parker EF, Smith CD. The surgical management of esophageal stricture in children. *Ann Surg* 1988;**207**:590–7.

Rosseneu S, Afzal N, Yerushalmi B et al. Topical application of mitomycin-C in oesophageal strictures. *J Pediatr Gastroenterol Nutr* 2007;**44**:336–41.

Achalasia

Hussain SZ, Thomas R, Tolia V. A review of achlasia in 33 children. *Dig Dis Sci* 2002; **47**: 2538–43.

Oesophageal substitution

While the concept of replacement of a relatively short length of foregut whose only function is to pass solid/liquid from mouth to stomach appears relatively simple, this is beset with surgical complication and problem.

Indications

Permanent oesphageal failure due to 'long-gap' OA, irretrievable stricture (e.g. caustic), neoplasia (e.g. leiomyoma).

Stomach tubes (Fig 5.8)

The greater curve of the stomach can be separated and tubed either iso- or anti-peristalsis (after Gavrilu). It can be limited by length and is probably now the least popular alternative. There are long-term issues related to persistent gastric acid secretion, reflux, and development of proximal pharyngeal Barrett's changes.

Colon transposition

This is probably still the commonest type of substitution performed worldwide.

Three segments of colon can be used (right, transverse and left). Typically the transverse colon can be mobilized on the middle colic artery, or the hepatic flexure on the left colic and marginal artery. Both are anastomosed in isoperistaltic fashion to the cervical oesophagus. Usually the graft is brought through the posterior mediastinum, although it can be transthoracic or retrosternal tunnel. This type of reconstruction has a higher incidence of ischaemic-related complications (e.g. leakage, necrosis) than the others, and long-term issues relate to redundancy and perhaps intrinsic lack of propulsive peristalsis.

Gastric transposition

This is now the most favoured method of substitution following resection of oesophageal malignancy in adult practice, is increasingly popular in children, and can be done laparoscopically.

The stomach is mobilized by dividing the left gastric and the short gastric arteries, maintaining the gastro-epiploic arcade on either side. The distal oesophageal stump is excised and the fundus used for the proximal anastomosis. Further Kockerization of the duodenum and a pyloroplasty achieves enough mobility to reach the cervical oesophageal remnant. A mediastinal tunnel can be created digitally from above and below without thoracotomy, and the stomach pulled up to the neck. Most issues concern the long-term outcome of a large pseudotubular structure in the chest cavity and theoretical problems of aspiration.

Jejunal pedicle graft

Although the standard Roux loop does not reach the upper chest, the same principles can be used to create a graft based on several successive arcades (with some sacrifice of jejunum). This is isoperistaltic and has excellent long-term function.

Free-jejunal grafting and microvascular re-anastomosis in the neck, once advocated, has now been largely abandoned.

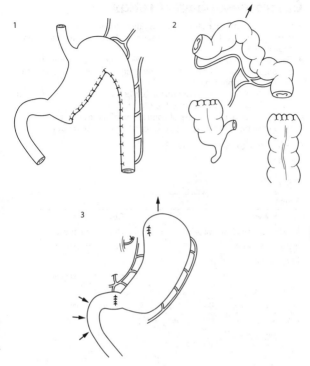

Fig. 5.8 Gastric tube (1), colon (2) and gastric transposition (3).

Further reading

Adamson WT, Tagge EP. Esophageal replacement with colon. In: Spitz L, Coran AG (eds). *Operative Pediatric Surgery* (6th edn). London: Hodder-Arnold, 2006, pp135–44.

Borgnon J, Tounian P, Auber F et al. Esophageal replacement in children by an isoperistaltic gastric tube: a 12 year experience. *Pediatr Surg Int* 2004;**20**:829–33.

Davenport M, Hosie G, Tasker RC et al. Long-term effects of gastric transposition in children: a physiological study. *J Pediatr Surg* 1996;**31**:588–93.

Raffensperger JG, Luck SR, Reynolds M et al. Intestinal bypass of the esophagus. *J Pediatr Surg* 1996;**31**:38–46.

Spitz L. Esophageal atresia. Lessons I have learned in a 40-year experience. *J Pediatr Surg* 2006;**41**:1635–40.

Gastro-oesophageal reflux

- Gastro-oesophageal reflux (GOR) is due to incompetence of the lower oesophageal sphincter mechanism and usually commences in the neonatal period.
- Gastro-oesophageal reflux disease (GORD) refers to the symptoms or complications that may occur when gastric contents reflux into the oesophagus or pharynx.
- Regurgitation of feeds is common in babies and refers to the effortless reflux of gastric contents up to the oro-pharynx.
- Vomiting is an active process of contraction of the diaphragm and abdominal muscles to expel gastric contents from the mouth.

Clinical features of GORD

See Table 5.3.

Table 5.3

Symptoms	Findings
Recurrent vomiting	Oesophagitis
Weight loss or poor weight gain	Oesophageal stricture
Irritability in infants	Barrett's oesophagus
Regurgitation	Laryngitis
Heartburn	Recurrent pneumonia
Haematemesis	Anaemia
Dysphagia	Hypoproteinaemia
Apnoea or acute life-threatening event (ALTE)	
Wheezing or stridor	
Hoarseness	
Recurrent cough	
Arching neck and back (Sandifer syndrome)	

Investigations

Upper GI contrast study

This is useful for detecting anatomical abnormalities (e.g. hiatus hernia – sliding or rolling), but cannot distinguish between physiological and pathological reflux. Other pathology such as pyloric stenosis or malrotation may be shown.

Oesophageal pH study (usually 24 h)

This will detect episodes of acid reflux and is expressed as % of time with pH <4. Upper limit of normality varies with age. Thus:
- 11% – infants
- 5% – 1–9 years
- 6% – >9 years.

Upper GI endoscopy and biopsy

Enables direct visualization and biopsy of mucosa to confirm the presence of oesophagitis. The hiatus can also be inspected and other pathology detected (e.g. primary eosinophilic oesophagitis or candida).

Other investigations

- Gastro-oesophageal scintigraphy – may be useful in diagnosis of pulmonary aspiration and delayed gastric emptying
- Manometry – useful in the diagnosis of motility problems
- US – can be as accurate as contrast swallow in infants and young children.

Management

- Medical:
  - posture/milk thickener (e.g. Nestargel®, Carobel®)
  - antacids (e.g. Gaviscon®)
  - H_2 receptor blockers (e.g. ranitidine 2–4 mg/kg bd)
  - proton pump inhibitor (e.g. omeprazole)
  - pro-kinetics (domperidone/metoclopramide)
- Surgical treatment is reserved for child who:
  - fails medical therapy due to GORD
  - is dependent on aggressive or prolonged medical therapy
  - has persistent asthma or recurrent pneumonia due to GORD
  - has ALTE

Surgery – anti-reflux procedure

Fundoplication – all of these operations elongate the intra-abdominal portion of the oesophagus, buttressed by part of the stomach which is capable of translating variations in intra-luminal pressure directly as a mechanism to shut off the oesophageal lumen:

- complete wrap – Nissen
- anterior – Thal, Dor, Boix–Ochoa
- posterior – Toupet.

While these operations have conventionally been performed as open procedures, laparoscopic fundoplication is increasingly being used.

Other procedures have recently been introduced, although they are not appropriate for use in young children. These include endotherapies:

- endoscopically guided delivery of radiofrequency energy (Stretta)
- endoscopic suturing of the gastro-oesophageal junction (EndoCinch™).

Further reading

Bax KMA, Georgeson K Rothenbergss et al (eds) et al *Endoscopic Surgery in Infants and Children.* Berlin: Springer-Verlag, 2008.

Rowney DA, Aldridge LM. Laparoscopic fundoplication in children: anaesthetic experience of 51 cases. *Paediatr Anaesth* 2000;**10**:133–8.

Rudolph C, Mazur LJ, Liptak GS et al. Evaluation and treatment of gastroesophageal reflux in infants and children: recommendations of the North American Society for Pediatric Gastroenterology and Nutrition. *J Pediatr Gastroenterol Nutr* 2001;**32**:S1–S31.

Choledochal malformations

First recognized by the German anatomist Abraham Vater who described a typical choledochal cyst in 1723; these have a marked geographical variation in incidence (higher in Japan and China) and female predominance (4:1). A proportion will present antenatally on maternal ultrasonography, but most become symptomatic before 4 years of age.

Classification

All choledochal malformations can be divided according to the appearance of extrahepatic dilatation (cystic versus fusiform) and whether the intrahepatic ducts are involved or not. Fig. 5.9 illustrates our current concept.

Common channel

Almost 90% will have an abnormal junction of pancreatic and biliary ducts outside the wall of the duodenum. This allows free intermixing of pancreatic juice and bile, which may cause pancreatitis and (possibly) biliary dilatation and later malignancy.

Caroli's disease

Multiple, saccular dilatations of the intrahepatic bile ducts (may be confined to one lobe). This is different from the other types of CM, having an association with cystic renal pathology (and renal failure) and liver fibrosis (Caroli's syndrome).

Pathogenesis

The cause of most malformations is not known, although the majority are presumed congenital (certainly Type 1c lesions may be diagnosed antenatally). There is a 'reflux hypothesis', stating that the destructive enzyme-rich pancreatic juice causes epithelial damage and mural weakness (and therefore dilatation) in the exposed biliary tree.

Clinical features

The classic triad is jaundice, abdominal pain, and a mass, but is found in about 30%. Abdominal pain may be due to biliary distension, or pancreatitis. Various complications are described including cholangitis, perforation (intra- or retroperitoneal), stone formation, biliary cirrhosis, portal hypertension, and (later) carcinoma.

Investigations

US is the best initial investigation showing the degree of biliary dilatation, stone formation etc. MRCP allows anatomical definition, although visualization of the common channel is still difficult. ERCP is reserved for those with minimal biliary dilation, perhaps with a history of pancreatitis looking for a common channel etc.

Surgery

The aim should be to excise the entire extrahepatic biliary tree (down to the junction of pancreatic duct) with a Roux loop reconstruction, typically at the level of the hepatic duct. Although dilated intrahepatic bile ducts may be left *in situ*, it is important to scope these and correct stenoses and remove stones prior to completion. Cyst excision may be difficult due to preceding infection, and sometimes part of the cyst wall (minus its lining) may be left. Transduodenal sphincterotomy may also be required if the common channel is dilated, especially if filled with debris/stones.

Laparoscopic excision is now possible but in selected (easy) cases.

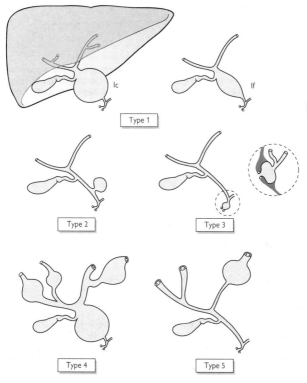

Fig. 5.9 King's College Hospital classification of choledochal malformations.

Gall bladder disease and gallstones

Gallstones are principally of three types: bilirubin pigment (multiple, friable, dark), cholesterol (whitish and often solitary), and mixed. There is some evidence that other types (e.g. pure Ca CO_3) are also specific for children.

There are three usual scenarios:

- post-neonatal – prematurity, TPN, ileal resection. Often asymptomatic, detected by US with underlying cause no longer a problem. Removal debatable
- haemolytic – sickle cell disease (~20% by teenage years), thalassaemia, congenital spherocytosis. Usually teenagers. Prophylactic cholecystectomy is a reasonable option
- Early-onset cholesterol – usually fat and female with family history. Detected because are usually symptomatic. Cholecystectomy indicated.

Clinical features

Abdominal pain, biliary colic, acute and chronic cholecystitis, acute pancreatitis, and obstructive jaundice. US is the most sensitive test and will detect >95% cases. May show thickened wall, sludge, and degree of bile duct dilatation. Suspicion of CBD stones (jaundice, abnormal GGT etc.) requires MRCP for confirmation and then ERCP (including sphincterotomy) for their removal. Follow with deferred cholecystectomy. (Box 5.9)

Acalculous cholecystitis

Associated with sepsis, trauma and some gastrointestinal pathogens (e.g. *Salmonella* spp.). Similar clinical features but obviously without visualization of stones. A non-functioning gall bladder may be demonstrable on radio-isotope imaging. Treated initially conservatively but may need early cholecystectomy, as necrosis and perforation are described.

> ### Box 5.9 Laparoscopic cholecystectomy
>
> First performed in 1987 in France (disputed, but largely by Germans!), but unquestionably is now the standard operation for gall bladder removal.
>   Umbilical camera port (10 mm) and three working ports (5 mm).
> - Requires definition of contents of Calot's triangle (borders – cystic duct, common hepatic duct, and liver – contents cystic artery, cystic lymph node)
> - Division of cystic artery (clips or bipolar coagulation). Division of cystic duct and orthograde removal of gall bladder from bed. Removal via umbilical port.
> - On-table cholangiography is difficult in children due to small size of cystic duct – but may be required in selected cases.

Choledochalithiasis

Stones or debris within the gall bladder can migrate through the cystic duct to the CBD. Sometimes this is symptomless, in others it causes obstruction or, if further distally, pancreatitis.

Clinical features

Stones or debris within CBD may cause abdominal pain and obstructive jaundice, together with pale stools and dark urine. Liver biochemistry will show an obstructive pattern and US and MRCP should define the relevant anatomy. If untreated it may lead to secondary infection (cholangitis) or secondary biliary cirrhosis.

Most examples can now be diagnosed definitively and treated by ERCP and a combination of sphincterotomy and balloon/basket stone extraction.

Portal hypertension

The normal portal venous pressure is ~ 5 mmHg.

Causes

- Idiopathic
- Portal vein occlusion/thrombosis – often congenital, may be related to neonatal sepsis, use of umbilical vein catheter
- Post-biliary atresia surgery
- Congenital liver fibrosis – often related to renal cysts/fibrosis
- Post-pyelephlebitis – portal pyaemia, typically from appendicitis, may heal with liver fibrosis
- Budd–Chiari syndrome – occlusion of hepatic veins (typically by underlying hypercoaguable state) causes hepatomegaly, ascites, and portal hypertension
- Hepatic venopathy – possible complication of anti-cancer chemotherapy

Clinical features

Although presentation with isolated splenomegaly is possible (~20%), most present with GI bleeding (haematemesis and melaena) from oesophageal varices. Known patients may bleed from anorectal varices and haemorrhoids but this is never *de novo*.

Bleeding is often life threatening from the outset. Initial investigations should be guided by the degree of urgency in the mode of presentation, but might include FBC, coagulation tests, liver function tests, abdominal US (and Doppler flow studies of portal vein), and liver biopsy.

Management

Following effective resuscitation with restoration of a normal INR and platelet count (remember hypersplenism), then the key investigation for diagnosis and treatment is an upper GI endoscopy (Box 5.10). Medical therapy to reduce portal pressure may include octreotide (25 µg/hour IV) both in the interim and following.

> **Box 5.10 Endoscopic management of varices**
>
> Two methods: (i) injection sclerotherapy and (ii) banding:
> (i) either intra or para-variceal injection of sclerosing solution (e.g. ethanolamine 5% 1–2 mL to each varix). Repeated every 2 weeks until obliteration
> (ii) using banding attachment (e.g. Saaed Six Shooter®), apply occlusive bands to each varix.
> Currently, (ii) is the better option, but (i) is still used for infants, where there is active bleeding and those where there is pronounced oesophageal scarring.

Surgery – portal pressure reduction

For those where the predominant cause is cirrhosis then liver transplantation is the only definitive surgery possible. Shunt surgery, while effective in reducing portal pressure is associated with an unacceptable incidence of encephalopathy in these cases.

Portosystemic anastomosis effectively reduces portal pressure and usually reduces prograde venous flow. Shunts may be divided into central (e.g. portocaval) or peripheral (lieno-renal), although the distinction is probably semantic. (fig 5.10)

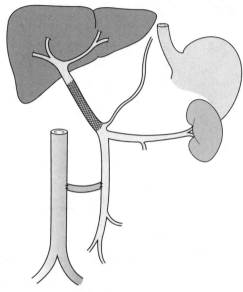

Fig. 5.10 In children, a mesocaval shunt using autologous internal jugular vein is probably the best option, combining a low incidence of thrombosis, retention of splenic function, and reasonable cosmesis, but it requires a patent superior mesenteric vein.

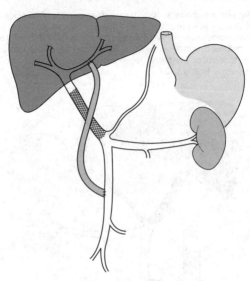

Fig. 5.11 The Meso-Rex shunt is a relatively recent addition and is unique among shunt options because it restores physiological intrahepatic portal venous flow and reduced portal pressure and has no risk of encepaholopathy. The indication is a discrete portal vein occlusion.

Further reading

Howard ER, Stringer MD, Mowat AP. Assessment of injection sclerotherapy in the management of 152 children with oesophageal varices. *Br J Surg* 1988;**75**:404–408.

McKiernan PJ, Beath SV, Davison SM. A prospective study of endoscopic esophageal variceal ligation using a multiband ligator. *J Pediatr Gastroenterol Nutr* 2002;**34**:207–11.

Superina R, Shneider B, Emre S, Sarin S, de Ville de Goyet J. Surgical guidelines for the management of extra-hepatic portal vein obstruction. *Pediatr Transplant* 2006;**10**:908–13.

The pancreas

Acute pancreatitis

Definition

This is an inflammatory disorder of a previously structurally and functionally normal pancreas, characterized by acute inflammation, oedema, and a variable degree of acinar necrosis with an absence of parenchymal fibrosis during the healing phase. There is a spectrum of severity from mild interstitial pancreatitis to severe necrotic pancreatitis (mortality ~20%).

Aetiology

The causes of pancreatitis in childhood include choledochal malformation and pancreatobiliary malunion, enterovirus infection, drugs, severe systemic disease, and trauma (Table 5.4).

While hereditary pancreatitis is rare, the genetic background of the individual (e.g. *CFTR* and *SPINK1* status) may modify an individual's susceptibility to pancreatitis following stimuli such as drugs, infection, and systemic illness.

Table 5.4 Known causes of acute pancreatitis in childhood

Cause	Examples
Systemic illness (15%)	Vasculitis, SLE, haemolytic uraemic syndrome
Gallstones/sludge (10%)	Underlying haemolysis (SCA)
Trauma (20%)	Seat-belt, handlebar, ERCP, non-accidental injury
Common channel and duct anomalies (20%)	Choledochal malformation, pancreas divisum, ampullary stenosis, santorinicele
Infection (10%)	Mumps virus, Coxsackie; HIV; ascariasis
Drugs (12%)	Azathioprine, thiazides, asparaginase, aminosalicylates, sodium valproate, arsenic trioxide, ifosfamide, lamivudine
Metabolic (2%)	Organic acidaemias, mitochondrial disease, hypercalcaemia (hyperparathyroid), hyperlipidaemia (type 1)
Genetic (2%)	*PRSS1* mutations (autosomal dominant) ; *SPINK1* mutations

NB 10–20% will be idiopathic.

Clinical features

The classic presentation of AP is with a triad of abdominal pain, nausea and vomiting which can evolve to an acute abdomen with or without jaundice or circulatory shock. Hyperamylasaemia usually occurs within 2–12 h of the start of an attack, and finding a blood amylase or lipase >3 times the upper limit of normal are simple, relatively sensitive/specific diagnostic tests.

Early imaging with CT or MRI will confirm the diagnosis and allow definition of pancreatic anatomy and perhaps cause (e.g. gallstones, choledochal malformation).

The clinical course in AP is largely determined by events taking place within the first 48 h of the illness. Most children will show signs of spontaneous improvement within this period. Those who deteriorate will have a more complicated clinical course. Although clinical scoring systems exist (e.g. Ransom, Imrie), none are validated in children.

Management
- General supportive care:
  - nil by mouth, IV fluid and NG tube (if vomiting)
  - assess circulation and third space losses (resuscitate with crystalloid, the haematocrit is a good marker)
  - measure and treat hypoxia (nasal prongs, occasionally ventilation)
  - manage hyperglycaemia (insulin)
  - maintain normal electrolytes including ionized calcium and magnesium
  - manage pain (ketamine ideal)
  - reduce gastric acid secretion (e.g. H_2 receptor antagonist)
- Disease-specific treatments (e.g. treatment of vasculitis)
- Non-consensual measures:
  - octreotide (little evidence in favour)
  - prophylactic antibiotics (little evidence in favour)
- Other measures:
  - daily inflammatory markers (e.g. WBC, CRP)
  - Contrast CT scan – looking for severity and ?necrosis
  - ?interval MRI ± secretin stimulation (MRCP) after day 4 to visualize ductal anatomy and pancreatic duct disruption/fluid collection
  - ?ERCP within 72 h if gallstone-related pancreatitis (no consensus)
  - parenteral nutritional support (if illness lasting >7 days)

Role of early surgery
A 'necrosectomy' should be considered if IV-contrast CT scan shows severe necrotizing pancreatitis with a major systemic insult. The aim is to remove inflammatory debris and infarcted tissue.

Acute fluid collection (<4 weeks) and pseudocyst (≤4 weeks)
These are the commonest complications of AP, and are typically retroperitoneal and related to the lesser sac. About one-third will resolve with specific treatment, one-third will require a single needle aspiration, and one-third will require more specific intervention.

Options
- US- or CT-guided needle aspiration of fluid collections/necrotic debris (may be repeated)
- Definitive drainage of pseudocysts (>4 weeks in children to allow capsule to develop). Classically by cyst-gastrostomy (if in lesser sac) or anastomosis of Roux loop to cyst wall. Endoscopic management is now a practical alternative (multiple pigtail catheters across stomach wall) in some centres.

Pancreatic trauma (see also page 387)
Typically caused by innocuous blunt abdominal injury from cycle handlebar in a boy, or from the lap seat-belt in a MVA.

Although most will settle with conservative treatment, those with demonstrable duct injury will invariably cause problems. Early CT/MRCP should be performed to try and predict the need for ERCP.

If the duct can be shown to be leaking (by ERCP) then there are alternative strategies available, from early open surgery and partial pancreatectomy to endoscopic pancreatic duct stenting, which may reduce morbidity.

Chronic pancreatitis

Very much under-recognized in childhood. Should have evidence of:
- Intermittent pain/vomiting
- exocrine impairment (e.g. steatorrhea, low faecal elastase levels (<50 microgram/g)
- Endocrine impairment (overt diabetes is rare, ?abnormal GTT).
- Investigations should include visualization of the pancreatic ducts to exclude an anatomical abnormality, such as pancreas divisum (retention of prenatal duct drainage with dominant dorsal duct draining through accessory pancreatic papilla), common pancreato-biliary channel, and a duct stricture. All these are amenable to surgery with either improvements in duct drainage (orthograde – sphincteroplasty or retrograde – Puestow procedure).

Further reading

Chiu B, Lopoo J, Superina RA. Longitudinal pancreaticojejunostomy and selective biliary diversion for chronic pancreatitis in children. *J Pediatr Surg* 2006;**41**:946–9.

The spleen

Asplenia and polysplenia

The spleen develops in the dorsal mesogastrium and is effectively complete by the 5th week of gestation. Both asplenia and polysplenia can be associated with congenital cardiac anomalies and abnormal visceral situs, and are part of the BASM syndrome (see page 176).

Function

Entirely developed from mesenchyme, the spleen has a multiplicity of roles – immunological (e.g. maturation of B, T, and plasma cells, production of immunologically active agents tuftsin, properidin etc); filtration (e.g. removing encapsulated microorganisms such as *Pneumococcus* spp.); sequestration (e.g. old RBCs and platelets, in order to recycle iron) and in some animals it also has a reservoir function against acute blood loss.

Splenomegaly

In children, the causes of this are legion, but easily palpable spleens are found in infection (e.g. malaria, infectious mononucleosis), portal hypertension (e.g. portal vein thrombosis), and *neoplasia* (e.g. leukaemia, lymphoma). The spleen can be the site for certain infiltrations (e.g. Gaucher's disease), abscess or cyst formation (usually solitary rather than hydatid disease).

Hypersplenism

This is a pathological combination of splenomegaly, anaemia, leucopenia, and thrombocytopenia, and can be secondary (e.g. portal hypertension). A number of haematological abnormalities can cause excessive destruction of one or more cell lines. Thus anaemia may be caused by sickle cell disease, hereditary spherocytosis, or elliptocytosis and platelet destruction caused by idiopathic thrombocytopenic purpura and autoimmune thrombocytopenia.

Surgery – splenectomy

Usually complete, but can be partial for pathology (e.g. ITP, traumatic rupture), as an unexpected adjunct to neighbour surgery (e.g. distal pancreatectomy) (Box 5.11).

> **Box 5.11 Splenectomy – different approaches depending on indication**
>
> Rapid removal for normal-sized spleen – mobilization and division of lieno-renal, lieno-colic ligaments first allowing spleen to rotate into wound allowing control of capsular tears by pressure with control of pedicle (clamp, sling or fingers) before commitment to division.
>
> In giant splenomegaly, access lesser sac first through ligation of gastro-epiploic vessels and early control of pedicle vessels in continuity (artery before veins). Reduces bleeding from pathological adhesions to adjacent viscera.

Complications

Intra-operative
- Neighbour damage (stomach, tail of pancreas, splenic flexure)

Postoperative
- Subphrenic collection
- Haemorrhage (typically from short-gastric vessels)
- Clot propagation from the splenic vein leading to portal vein (1%, higher where haematological anomaly)
- Reactionary thromocythaemia and leukocytosis – appearance of Howell–Jolly bodies
- OPSI (Box 5.12)

Box 5.12 Overwhelming post-splenectomy infection (OPSI)

This was first described by King and Schumaker in 1952, and is due to unrestrained encapsulated bacteria (e.g. *Streptococcus pneumoniae, Haemophilus influenzae, Neisseria meningitides*).
- Incidence: 4% patients without prophylaxis
- Mortality is 50–90%
- Greatest risk is in first 2 years after operation

Post-splenectomy prophylaxis

Vaccinations (ideally before surgery)
- Haemophilus influenzae type B vaccine:
  - immunized, >1 year: 1 additional dose of Hib type B vaccine
  - unimmunized, >1 year: 2 doses of vaccine, 2 months apart
  - <10 years, never immunized: 3 doses, 1 month apart of combined Hib type B vaccine with diphtheria, tetanus, pertussis, and poliomyelitis vaccines
- Pneumococcal polysaccharide conjugate vaccine – at the recommended ages plus:
  - 23-valent pneumococcal polysaccharide >2nd birthday
  - revaccination every 5 years *only* in individuals in whom, after discussion with a haematologist, it is thought that antibody concentration is likely to fall rapidly

- Meningococcal group C vaccine:
  - <1 year: at 2 and 3 months as according to UK immunization schedule
  - unimmunized, >1 year: 2 doses of vaccine, 2 months apart
  - immunized, any age: 1 additional dose
- Annual influenza vaccine
- Prophylactic penicillin (lifelong):
  - oral penicillin V (or erythromycin if allergic) (e.g. 250 mg bd – aged 6–12 years)

Avoid malaria endemic areas, Babesia (tick-borne, Massachusetts islands), *Bartonella bacilliformis* (sandfly, Andes) rigorous precautions advised.

Intussusception

The typical surgical condition of infants, which is still misdiagnosed in paediatric A&E departments throughout the UK.

Definition

Intussusception occurs when one piece of bowel (intussusceptum) invaginates into another (the intussuscipiens). This most commonly (80%) occurs between the terminal ileum and the ascending colon (ileo-colic) but can also occur between the ileum and ileum (ileol-ileal) and the colon and colon (colo-colic), or as a combination (ileo-ileo-colic).

Incidence

Varies between 1.5 and 4 cases per 1000 live births.

Epidemiology

- May occur at any age but 65% occur in the first year of life (peak presentation at 9 months).
- M:F = 3:2 ?seasonal (spring and summer)

Aetiology

Often follows an URTI and is thought to occur as a result of hypertrophy of Peyer's patches within the bowel wall. Recurrent intussusception or intussusception occurring in older age group should raise suspicion of anatomical 'lead-point' (e.g. Meckel's (most common), polyps, appendix, Henoch–Schönlein purpura with haemorrhage, lymphoma, intestinal duplication, or foreign bodies). Intussusception (typically ileo-ileal) can occur post-operatively.

Clinical features

Typically presents with drawing up of legs (pain), vomiting (non- bilious followed by bilious), and pallor. In later stages or if distal bowel involved, blood-stained mucus is passed ('redcurrant jelly stool'). 'Sausage-shaped' mass palpable in right side of abdomen. Anal protrusion of intussusception can occur (late sign).

Plain AXR may show a right-sided soft-tissue mass with small bowel obstruction (~50%). Free air on AXR confirms perforation and urgent surgical intervention is required. Confirm diagnosis with ultrasound (look for pathognomonic sign of 'target lesion' on transverse section, or a 'pseudokidney' sign on longitudinal section.

Management

These infants are often profoundly shocked and may require repeated boluses (20 mL/kg) of resuscitation IV fluid, together with a NG tube and prophylactic antibiotics. Most should then proceed to an attempt at contrast eneva reduction (Box 5.13)

Box 5.13 Hydrostatic/air enema reduction

Similar principle involving sustained intra-colonic pressure to reduce mass and invert bowel. Later technique has superseded former in most centres. Involves catheter, taped securely to buttocks and air application

- Barium – use column 1 m above table, 3 attempts for 3 minutes. Look for 'flooding' into distal ileum
- Air – start at 60 mmHg, max = 120 mmHg – use pressure monitoring device
- Contraindicated – perforation on x-ray. Less likely to be successful if >24 h since onset. If air-enema perforates, decompress abdominal cavity with needle, before surgery

Surgery – reduction of intussusception

- RLQ incision/occasionally transumbilical or RUQ
- Identify mass (this may be on left side of abdomen)
- Squeeze distally (push rather than pull) – this becomes harder as the ileo-caecal junction is reached
- Once reduced – leave alone, return to abdominal cavity, and assess viability in 5 min. If obvious necrosis – resect and primary anastomosis
- ?secondary – this is only really an issue outside of infancy. Look for Meckel's or tumour. Don't be tempted, however, to biopsy thickened bowel or mesenteric nodes in infants.

Complications

- Recurrent intussusception – ~2% of cases but higher if 'lead point' present; most (~60%) occur within 6 months
- Adhesions and small bowel obstruction (1% per year lifetime risk)

Further reading

Guo J, Ma X, Zhou Q. Results of air pressure enema reduction of intussusception: 6396 cases in 13 years. *J Pediatr Surg* 1986;**21**:1201–1203.

Ong N, Beasley SW. The leadpoint in intussusception. *J Pediatr Surg* 1990;**25**:640–3.

Weissberg DL, Scheible W, Leopold GR. Ultrasongraphic appearance of adult intussusception. *Radiology* 1977;**124**:791–792.

Appendicitis

History

Very much a rarity before the 19th century, but increasingly diagnosed from the 1880s. The first successful deliberate removal of an appendix was actually via a scrotal hernia by Claudius Amyand, surgeon at both the Westminster and St George's Hospital, (London) in 1736. The first removal for typical appendicitis is disputed, but Rudolf Kronlein (Germany), Lawson-Tait (UK) and TG Morton (Philadelphia, USA) have all got claims, recognized during the 1880s.

Epidemiology

It is estimated that 7% of the population will have their appendix removed.

Pathology

Early catarrhal inflammation, possibly initiated by luminal obstruction (?lymphoid hypertrophy). There is then increasing luminal pressure, followed by vascular compromise (seen as wet gangrene) and perforation usually at the tip. The timescale is 24–48 h.

Clinical features

Early 'visceral' peri-umbilical, ill-localized abdominal pain, changing and shifting to right iliac fossa (RIF) as increasing involvement of overlying 'parietal' peritoneum. Pain is now sharper, and exacerbated by movement and coughing. Vomiting usual but short-lived. Usually anorexic.

Examination shows local tenderness with degree of reaction elicited in overlying abdominal muscles (ranging from rebound tenderness through guarding to local rigidity). If allowed to progress to perforation, then generalized peritonitis should be all too obvious.

Diagnosis can be 'barn-door' or challenging – often related to the actual position of the appendix. A long history means can mean two things – it is not appendicitis or it is and it has become complicated.

Box 5.14 Pelvic and retrocaecal appendicitis

- Pelvic appendicitis is hidden in the depths of the pelvis and much more midline. There is poor localization and adjacent organ involvement (dysuria/diarrhoea/inability to 'empty' rectum) without RIF tenderness. Consider rectal exam. Look for pelvic mass/collection on US
- Retrocaecal appendicitis is protected by overlying ascending colon, and is extra-peritoneal. Localized signs only on deep palpation. May mimic cholecystitis, pyleonephritis and lumbar pain. Look for right-sided collection on US/CT scan

Investigations (always contentious and no absolutes sadly!)

- Inflammatory markers – white cell count, differential, CRP, ESR
- Urine microscopy, nitrites – and later culture. (NB ~15% will have >10 WBC per high-power field and still have appendicitis)
- US (±graded compression)
- CT – still not perfect, both PPV and NPV ~90%
- MRI – no radiation at least
- Laparoscopy – in adolescent girls this should be strongly considered in preference to blind exploration

Surgery – appendicectomy (open and laparoscopy)

- Incision – original McBurney (Box 5.15) was perpendicular to his line – a Lanz incision (Fig. 5.12) is more transverse within skin crease and is preferred. Centre on point of maximum tenderness
- Muscle splitting – grid-iron refers to split of external oblique, internal oblique and transversus muscles
- Identify appendix, ligate its vessels down to base. Prepare purse-string suture and remove organ. Conventionally the ligated stump is buried in caecal wall
- If not appendicitis, look for evidence of mesenteric lymphadenitis, Meckel's or terminal ileal pathology and examine Fallopian tubes and ovaries in girls

Box 5.15 Charles McBurney (1845–1913) – Professor of Surgery, Roosevelt Hospital, NY

Advocate of early operative intervention. Named maximum point of tenderness as one-third along a line from ASIS to umbilicus.

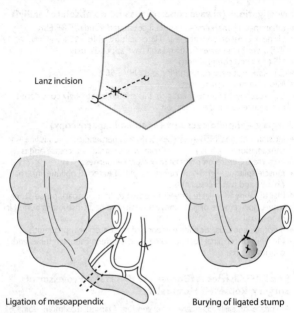

Lanz incision

Ligation of mesoappendix

Burying of ligated stump

Fig. 5.12 (i) Lanz incision is a muscle-splitting incision based on McBurney's point (two-thirds along a line from umbilicus to ASIS). (ii) Ligation of vessels in meso-appendix and ligation of appendix at base, (iii) burying stump using 'purse-string' suture.

Meckel's diverticulum

First described by Johann Meckel in 1809 as a diverticulum on the anti-mesenteric border of the small bowel, derived from the embryological vitello-intestinal duct.

> **Rule of 'twos'**
> - About two inches long and
> - situated about two feet from the ileo-caecal valve
> - Found in 2% of the population
>
> NB – no metric equivalent!

Epidemiology

- Equal sex distribution for asymptomatic Meckel's, but M:F ratio of 3:1 when symptomatic
- Commonly seen in children with oesophageal atresia (12%), ano-rectal malformations (11%), and exomphalos minor (25%)

Clinical features

Approximately 50% of Meckel's are asymptomatic and discovered incidentally, otherwise features are:

- **bleeding** – occurs as a result of ulceration secondary to ectopic gastric mucosa (or pancreatic) within the diverticulum. This may be as altered blood (e.g. melaena-like) or sometimes if massive apparently as a fresh bleed
- **obstruction** – due to it either acting as a lead-point in intussusception or as a volvulus around vitelline remnants attached to the umbilicus. Presents as bile-stained vomiting, abdominal distension, and 'acute abdomen'
- **inflammation** – similar to appendicitis but signs more central. Unlikely to be able to differentiate (unless previous appendicectomy!)
- **miscellaneous** – carcinoid tumours, leiomyomas, leiomyosarcoma, and foreign bodies have all been reported.

A mildly or moderately bleeding Meckel's diverticulum can be diagnosed by a radionuclide 'Meckel's scan' (technetium). Scan is 90% accurate and is dependent on presence of heterotopic gastric mucosa.

Management

Debate continues whether to resect an asymptomatic Meckel's found incidentally, although a recent review demonstrates no advantage in removing it. The chance of it becoming symptomatic during a lifetime is estimated at ~5%. A symptomatic Meckel's diverticulum is resected as a small bowel resection away from its base. This can be accomplished as an open or laparoscopic procedure.

Further reading

Jewett TC Jr, Duszynski DO, Allen JE. The visualisation of Meckel's diverticulum with Tc99m pertechnetate. *Surgery* 1970;**68**:567–70.

Zani A, Eaton S, Rees CM, Pierro A. Incidentally detected Meckel diverticulum: to resect or not to resect? *Ann Surg* 2008;**247**:276–81.

Duplications

These are a rare group of anomalies that can occur anywhere from the mouth to the anus. They are either cystic or tubular in shape and consist of a well-developed layer of smooth muscle, an epithelial lining representing a portion of GI tract, and some attachment to a part of the GI tract (usually paramesenteric).

Embryology

Not fully elucidated, but there are two main theories, derived from either a split notochord (cystic) or as a result of partial twinning (tubular duplications).

Incidence

- ~ 1 in 4500 autopsies
- Male preponderance, with small bowel being commonest site
- Multiple (up to 15%)

Clinical features

- **Cervical** – rarest form of duplication. Majority present at <1 year of age with respiratory distress. Neck mass may be present.
- **Thoracic and thoracoabdominal (see page 126)** – (~25%) Some are classified as neuro-enteric cysts. About one-third of patients have additional cysts below the diaphragm. Most have vertebral abnormalities and the CNS can be involved. Cysts are often found incidentally on chest x-ray or may present with respiratory distress or complications secondary to the gastric mucosa within the cyst.
- **Gastric** – usually cystic and attached to (but not communicating with) the greater curvature. Present with vomiting, poor feeding, or an abdominal mass. Pancreatitis has also been reported.
- **Duodenal** – presents with duodenal obstruction, haemorrhage, jaundice, or pancreatitis.
- **Small intestine** – commonest type of duplication. Can be cystic (majority) or tubular. Clinical presentation varies considerably according to structure and location.
- **Colonic** – cystic colonic duplications may be contained within the abdomen or pelvis, or can communicate with the perineum. These can also communicate with the urological system. Tubular duplications can be associated with duplications of the anus, vagina, and penis. Many of these patients also have vertebral abnormalities.
- **Rectal** – almost half of these are associated with a cutaneous fistulae to the perineum or anus. Presentation may include rectal bleeding, constipation, prolapse, tenesmus, and UTI.

Due to the wide range of different anatomical sites and structural configurations, a considerable number of different investigations are used for diagnosing duplications and also for planning and confirming the feasibility of surgery. These include plain x-rays, CT, MRI, upper and lower GI contrast studies, ultrasound, MCUG, endoscopy, and radionuclide scans (for gastric mucosa).

Management

Surgical removal of any duplication is recommended if that is technically feasible.

One of the main concerns with duplications is the malignant potential of their mucosal lining (particularly with the colorectal duplications). When partial excision is being performed, the entire mucosa still needs to be removed.

Further reading

Ladd WE. Duplications of the alimentary tract. *South Med J* 1937;**30**:363–1.

Orr MM, Edwards AJ. Neoplastic change in duplication of the alimentary tract. *Br J Surg* 1975;**62**:269–74.

Stringer MD, Spitz L, Abel R *et al*. Management of alimentary tract duplication in children. *Br J Surg* 1995;**82**:74.

Short bowel syndrome

This remains difficult to define with respect to anatomy or bowel length but should be thought of as:

- failure to maintain normal nutrition, body weight and internal physiology without external parenteral nutritional support.

- Normal intestinal length in neonates – 200–300 cm
- Normal small bowel length in adults – ~600 cm

Causes

- Intestinal atresia, NEC, midgut volvulus, gastroschisis
- Intestinal dysmotility syndromes – chronic pseudodobstruction
- Microvillus inclusion disease
- Crohn's disease (older children)

Gut adapation is the body's innate response to deficit in the enterocyte mass and may last up to 18–24 months. Controlled by complex network of GI hormones (e.g. growth hormone) and cytokines (GLP-2, EGF, HGF, IL-11). Anticipate improvements in gut function due to increase in surface area (lengthening villi, deepening crypts) and intestinal elongation.

Management

Medical

- Secure, safe vascular access and hence, provision of safe parenteral nutrition
- ?Gut-promoting agents (e.g. glutamine, short-chain triglycerides, pectin)
- Consider gastric hyperacidity and its reduction (e.g. H_2RA, PPI).
- Loperamide (1–2 mg tds, in children)
- Colestyramine – bile salt-binding agent. Interruption of bile salt re-absorption in terminal ileum may exacerbate diarrhoea
- Enteral antibiotics (e.g. cyclical neomycin/metronidazole) to limit bacterial overgrowth
- Octreotide – reduces losses from high-output proximal stomas

Parenteral nutrition-associated cholestasis (PNAC)

Usual cause of mortality in short-bowel syndrome, although actual mechanism obscure. Exacerbated by immature liver, recurrent line sepsis, over-provision of lipid solutions etc.). Often inexorable, once bilirubin starts to rise. Unproven therapies include ursodeoxycholic acid and cholecysto-kinin. Liver transplantation may be needed.

Surgery

The strategy should be to maximize the potential of the native bowel, by provision of an intestinal tube capable of effective prograde peristalsis. Thus:

- restore intestinal continuity – early closure of stomas, or re-feeding intestinal content into distal limb to maintain mucosal integrity and allow further nutrient absorption (by colon and bacterial fermentation of carbohydrate)
- improve native bowel propulsive efficiency (tapering, imbrication, Bianchi lengthening, STEP). The typical indication is a non-propulsive

dilated proximal segment (e.g. jejunal atresia). Thus residual but non-dilated bowel is unlikely to be improved by surgery.

Bianchi longitudinal intestinal lengthening (Fig. 5.13)
Highly original solution, aiming at doubling intestinal length and halving diameter. Improves prograde-peristalsis, by restoring wall apposition.

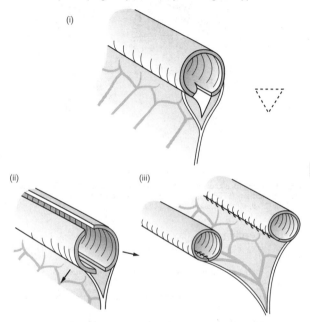

Fig. 5.13 Bianchi bowel lengthening. (i) Separation of mesenteric vessels. The division of vessels between right and left occurs someway short of the actual bowel wall. Develop this 'triangle of dissection'. (ii) Longitudinal division of mesenteric and anti-mesenteric walls. (iii) Isolated, independent hemi-loops.

Serial transverse enteroplasty (STEP) (Fig. 5.14)
Multiple alternate, stapling of dilated bowel, achieves a zig-zag arrangement on untouched mesentery – effectively diminishing bowel diameter and again improving peristalsis and luminal content mixing.

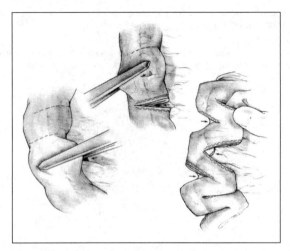

Fig. 5.14 STEP procedure. Taken from Kim HB, Fauza D, Garza J et al. Serial transverse enteroplasty (STEP): a novel bowel lengthening procedure. *J Pediatr Surg* 2003;38:425–9, with permission.

Further reading

Bianchi A. Longitudinal intestinal lengthening and tailoring: results in 20 children. *J R Soc Med* 1997;**90**:429–32.

Javid PJ, Kim HB, Duggan CP, Jaksic T. Serial transverse enteroplasty is associated with successful short-term outcomes in infants with short bowel syndrome. *J Pediatr Surg* 2005;**40**:1019–23.

Sudan D, Thompson J, Botha J et al. Comparison of intestinal lengthening procedures for patients with short bowel syndrome. *Ann Surg* 2007;**246**:593–601.

Kelly DA. Intestinal failure-associated liver disease: what do we know today? *Gastroenterology* 2006;**130**:S70–7.

Inflammatory bowel disease

Epidemiology
- 5.2 cases/100,000 children (<16 years)
- ~60% Crohn's disease, ~40% ulcerative or intermediate colitis
- Commoner in northern latitudes with slight male preponderance

Aetiology

Presumed interaction of genetic and environmental factors leading to dysfunction of immune regulation.

- Numerous candidate genes identified as possible IBD loci though again polygenic inheritance is thought most likely. Loci on chromosome 16 seem more related to Crohn's disease (CD, Box 5.16), though the picture is less specific for ulcerative colitis (UC) where anomalies on chromosomes 2, 6, and 21 have all been implicated.
- Environmental factors studied have included food allergens, ingested substances, gut infections, and most recently MMR vaccination in *Guardian* readers(!).

Box 5.16 Burrill Bernard Crohn (1884–1983) – American gastroenterologist working at Mount Sinai Hospital, NY

His name only appeared first on the paper for alphabetical reasons –much to the chagrin of his more-senior colleagues who were left without lasting fame.

Clinical features

The signs and symptoms vary depending on both the area of gut affected, and the severity and chronicity of the disease process. While many with UC present with an acute history of bloody diarrhoea, and obvious ill-health, in others the presentation may be more subtle and longstanding. Physical signs aside from mild tenderness may be absent except in the rare complication of toxic megacolon.

In CD, the presentation is often more insidious with abdominal pain being the main feature, as well as associated extra-intestinal manifestations such as lethargy and anorexia, and even oral ulceration may be present. Signs may be minimal, but the presence of an abdominal mass and/or peri-anal skin tags and fissures should alert the clinician to the possibility of CD. In addition growth failure, especially accompanied by delay in puberty, may be key diagnostic features.

Investigation

There are no specific blood tests though anaemia may be present and inflammatory markers may be raised. Diagnosis is made on histology with specimens being obtained by gastroduodenoscopy and colonoscopy. Radiology of the small intestine can identify areas of active CD or the presence of complications, e.g. strictures or fistulae.

CD can affect any part of the gastrointestinal tract and may be active in a number of areas simultaneously ('skip lesions'). Pathologically it is a transmural inflammation characterized by the presence of granulomata, whereas UC tends to involve the colon alone and present a picture of acute inflammation confined to the mucosa.

Management

The mainstay of treatment is medical and uses a combination of differing classes of anti-inflammatory medications varying from simple saliciylates (5-ASA compounds), through steroids and to more potent immune-modulators such as azathioprine. More recently the use of ciclosporin and anti-TNF antibodies (e.g. infliximab, adalimumab) has met with some success.

The choice of therapy is dictated by the nature and stage of the disease and is best managed by those with specific experience.

A key treatment in the management of CD has been the use of ele-mental diets, which both maintain nutrition and growth and help control the inflammatory process.

Surgery

Surgery can help manage both the complications of IBD (strictures, fistulae in CD/toxic colitis, or perforation in UC), or reduce disease load to allow possible reduction in the requirement for medication. The timing and type of surgery is again dependent on the stage and severity of disease, and may vary from segmental resection of small bowel, to total colectomy with ileal pouch formation. Correctly applied, surgical intervention can aid the management of IBD.

Outcomes

Both types of IBD run a relapsing and remitting course, and while surgery can 'cure' UC, it cannot do the same for CD. Studies have shown that ~25% of cases with moderate to severe UC will come to colectomy within 5 years of diagnosis, and that surgical outcomes are good. For CD, however, up to 80% have been shown to require some form of surgical intervention within 4 years of diagnosis.

With improvements in medical management and an increasing aware-ness of the need for multidisciplinary management of these cases, including a clearer idea of the place of surgery, then more children will find their management optimized, with consequent improvement in quality of life.

Further reading

Beattie RM, Croft NM, Fell JM et al. Inflammatory bowel disease. Arch Dis Child 2006;**91**:426–32.

Crohn BB, Ginzburg L, Oppenheimer GD. Regional ileitis; a pathologic and clinical entity. JAMA 1932;**99**:1323–9.

Rectal prolapse

Incidence

Rectal prolapse occurs most commonly in children <4 years, with a peak incidence in 2–3 year olds.

Predisposing factors

- Diarrhoeal illness, parasitic worms (developing countries)
- Malnutrition
- Chronic constipation
- Myelomeningocele or bladder exstrophy
- Cystic fibrosis (5%) – occasionally in absence of chest symptoms
- Idiopathic (most) – usually self-limiting.

Clinical features

Straining at stool – ' tenesmus ' and prolonged periods sitting on the toilet may stretch the pelvic musculature and supporting tissues of the rectum leading to prolapse. A 'red rosette' protruding from the anus of the child is often noted by parents. Most commonly the prolapse is incomplete (i.e. mucosal prolapse) with 2–3 cm of swollen rectal tissue appearing from the anus. The differential diagnosis should include rectal polyps, haemorrhoids, intussusception, and proctitis.

Stools should be checked for ova, cysts, and parasites. A sweat test/CF gene probe study should also be considered in the Causcasian population.

Management

As many reduce spontaneously or manually following stooling, an expectant course can be pursued in most children. In the younger (< 4 yrs) with chronic constipation, laxative therapy (e.g. lactulose and Senokot®) is reasonably effective. The older child (>4 years) may prove more resistant. (Fig 5.15)

Surgery

Injection sclerotherapy

- EUA, manual stool evacuation, and proctosigmoidoscopy (to exclude polyps/proctitis)
- Using a proctoscope, sclerosant solution (5% phenol in almond oil, hypertonic 30% saline or 50% glucose) is injected into four quadrants of the rectal submucosa 3–4 cm from the anal verge using a 23-gauge spinal needle. *Be careful anteriorly, given the proximity of the prostate and urethra in boys and vagina in girls.*
- Although repeat injections may be required, some quote ~90% success rate for a single injection.

Thiersch operation

Lithotomy position. Two small radial incisions are made at 12 and 6 o'clock at the anal verge and a PDS suture (0 or 1-0) is threaded from the posterior to the anterior incision deep to the external sphincter muscle. The circumferential suture is tightened with the aid of an assistant's finger or Hegar dilator (10/11 Ch) in the anal canal.

Rectopexy

- Open (including a posterior saggital approach) or laparoscopic.
- The peritoneal reflection is divided and the rectum mobilized. Interrupted 2-0/3-0 non-absorbable sutures are placed between the posterior rectum and fascia over the sacral promontory to provide fixation (70–90% success).

Laxative therapy is required to avoid constipation after all procedures.

Complications

- Perianal abscess may follow sclerosant injection.
- Functional stenosis may can occur if the Thiersch suture is too tight.

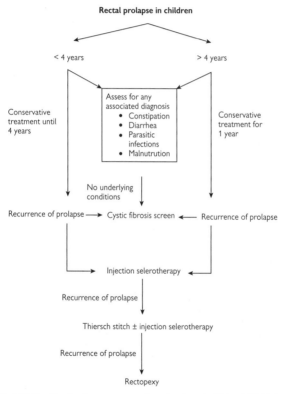

Rectal prolapse in children

< 4 years   > 4 years

Assess for any associated diagnosis
- Constipation
- Diarrhea
- Parasitic infections
- Malnutrution

Conservative treatment until 4 years

Conservative treatment for 1 year

No underlying conditions

Recurrence of prolapse ⟶ Cystic fibrosis screen ⟵ Recurrence of prolapse

Injection selerotherapy

Recurrence of prolapse

Thiersch stitch ± injection selerotherapy

Recurrence of prolapse

Rectopexy

Fig. 5.15 Algorithm for the management of rectal prolapse in children. With kind permission from Springer Science + Business Media: *Dis Colon Rectum* 2005;48: 1620–5. (also with permission of the authors).

Further reading

Antao B, Bradley V, Roberts J et al. Management of rectal prolapse in children. *Dis Colon Rectum* 2005;**48**:1620–5.

Ashcraft KW, Garred JL, Holder TM et al. Rectal prolapse: 17-year experience with the posterior repair and suspension. *J Pediatr Surg* 1990;**25**:992–4.

Koivusalo A, Pakarinen M, Rintala R. Laparoscopic suture rectopexy in the treatment of persisting rectal prolapse in children: a preliminary report. *Surg Endosc* 2006;**20**:960–3.

Bariatric surgery

> *baros* – weight *iatros* – physician (Greek)

Bariatric surgery is the most effective means to achieve durable weight loss with amelioration, if not resolution, of most obesity-related co-morbidities in adolescents.

Definition

body mass index (BMI) = weight (kg) ÷ height^2 (m) (kg/m^2)

Overweight in children = BMI ≥91st centile for age

Obesity in children = BMI ≥98th centile BMI for age

Prevalence of childhood/adolescent obesity

> 14% of 2 to 11 year-olds in England & Wales are obese There will be 1,000,000 obese children in England by 2010.

Epidemiology

- Equally common in males and females
- Increased risk in lower socioeconomic groups, if one or both parents are obese, some ethnic minorities

Aetiology

Chronic positive energy balance.

Presentation

- Co-morbidities – obstructive sleep apnoea, type II diabetes, metabolic syndrome, pseudotumour cerebri, psychosocial dysfunction, hypertension, non-alcoholic steatohepatitis, venous stasis disease, gastro-oesophageal reflux disease, weight-related arthropathies, exacerbation of chronic illnesses, e.g. asthma

Investigation

BMI, waist circumference

Differential diagnosis

Prader–Willi syndrome, hypothyroidism, eating disorder

Surgery

Pre-operative management

Consider for surgery in exceptional circumstances and only as part of a multidisciplinary team (NICE guidelines December 2006). Surgical care and follow-up should be coordinated around the young person and their family's needs and should comply with national core standards as defined in the Children's NSFs for England and Wales. Bariatric surgery is recommended as a treatment option for adolescents with obesity if all of the following criteria are fulfilled:

- BMI $\geq$ 40 kg/m^2 or BMI = >35 kg/m^2 + significant co-morbidity that could be improved if they lost weight
- all appropriate non-surgical measures have been tried but have failed to achieve or maintain adequate, clinically beneficial weight loss for at least 6 months
- the person has been receiving or will receive intensive management in a specialist obesity service
- the person is generally fit for anaesthesia and surgery
- the person commits to the need for long-term follow-up.

Surgery for obesity should be undertaken only by a multidisciplinary team that can provide paediatric expertise in:

- pre-operative assessment, including a risk–benefit analysis that includes preventing complications of obesity, and specialist assessment for eating disorder(s)
- providing information on the different procedures, including potential weight loss and associated risks
- regular postoperative assessment, including specialist dietetic and surgical follow-up
- management of co-morbidities
- psychological support before and after surgery
- providing information on or access to plastic surgery (e.g. panniculectomy) where appropriate access to suitable equipment, including scales, theatre tables, Zimmer frames, commodes, hoists, bed frames, pressure-relieving mattresses, and seating suitable for patients undergoing bariatric surgery.

Bariatric operations

The commonest procedures are the laparoscopic Roux-en-Y gastric bypass (LRYGB, Box 5.17, Fig. 5.16), (restrictive and malabsorptive) and the laparoscopic adjusted gastric band (LAGB, Box 5.18, Fig. 5.17) (restrictive).

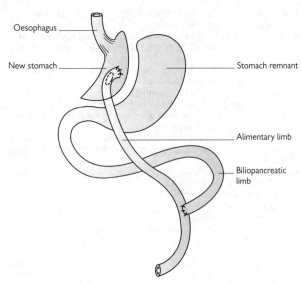

Oesophagus

New stomach

Stomach remnant

Alimentary limb

Biliopancreatic limb

Fig. 5.16

LRYGB typically achieves 75% excess weight loss with ~20% morbidity rate and ~2% mortality.

Box 5.17 Laparoscopic Roux-en-Y gastric bypass

Involves the creation of a small gastric pouch which is drained by a Roux-en-Y jejunal limb. Simple sugars must be limited to avoid the undesirable effects of the dumping syndrome.

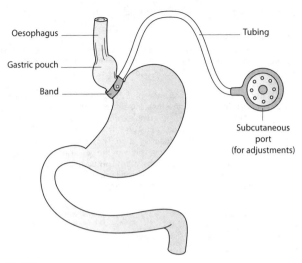

Fig. 5.17

The primary advantage of LAGB is the ease of insertion, with most patients staying in hospital for just one day. It is regarded as safer than LRYGB with a peri-operative complication rate of 1–2%. Late complications are more frequent however, e.g. prolapse of the stomach through the band (15%) and erosion of the band into the stomach (3%). Over 200 adolescents have undergone LAGB without any reported mortality, having a median of 56% excess weight loss at 5-year follow-up.

Box 5.18 Laparoscopic adjusted gastric band

An adjustable band is placed around the stomach to create a 20 mL gastric pouch. A subcutaneous port allows adjustment of the band at subsequent clinic visits.

Further reading

National Institute for Health and Clinical Excellence. *Obesity: guidance on the prevention, identification, assessment and management of overweight and obesity in adults and children.* NICE Clinical Guideline 43; London: NICE, 2006: www.nice.org.uk/CG043 (accessed 14 July 2008).

Reilly JJ. Obesity in childhood and adolescence: evidence based clinical and public health perspectives. *Postgrad Med J* 2006; **82**:429–437.

Abdominal wall hernias

Inguinal hernia

Most problems of the male groin can in some way be attributed to the peculiar need of the testis to flee the abdominal cavity and take residence in an unprotected, but reportedly cooler cul-de-sac of the peritoneal cavity.

Testicular descent is accompanied by a tongue of peritoneum – the processus vaginalis – which envelops and precedes the testis as it slides through the abdominal wall. The complex inguinal 'shutter' mechanism and obliquity of the canal are design features minimizing the possibility of other viscera joining in this scrotal migration. Thus, inguinal hernias arise as a persistence of the processus vaginalis with the deep ring large enough to admit viscera. Persistence, but with a more constrained deep ring, leads to hydrocele formation, and of course varying failure of the whole process – the undescended, ectopic or impalpable testis.

Incidence
- 1–4% (of all children)
- Male predominant (~7:1)
- Most common in children aged <2 years
- ~ 60% right sided, 30% left sided 10% bilateral

Risk factors
- Prematurity (16–25%)
- Previous abdominal wall repair (e.g. exomphalos, exstrophy and gastroschisis)
- Increased intrabdominal fluid (e.g. ascites, VP shunt)
- Chronic cough, cystic fibrosis

Aetiology
- ~98% are indirect resulting from failure of closure of the process vaginalis.

Clinical features
Unilateral or bilateral swelling in the groin, scrotum, or labia which may be intermittent and tends to be most prominent whenever the child cries or strains. It may present as an irreducible swelling associated with bowel obstruction or strangulation.

Commonly the hernia is reduced (Box 5.19) and therefore impalpable at the time of examination. A convincing history (the child's carers should point to the external inguinal ring as the site of the swelling) ± ipsilateral spermatic cord thickening usually justifies surgical exploration.

Consider other possibilities (e.g. hydrocele, hydrocele of the cord, inguinal adenopathy/abscess, torsion of the testis (or appendages), undescended testis, idiopathic scrotal oedema, and, rarely, femoral hernia).

Box 5.19 Reduction of incarcerated hernia – taxis (illegal in adults!)

- Sedation/analgesia/resuscitation
- Maintain gentle but firm pressure back along the line of the canal from the direction of the scrotum. Apply counter-pressure with the other hand to support the anterior cord. Reduction is slow at first then rapid. Success rate should be >90%. If it fails, there is usually an underlying reason – infarcted adherent bowel in sac etc.

Formal surgical repair is recommended within 48 h by open inguinal herniotomy (see page 330) or laparoscopic herniorraphy (see page 343) as preferred.

Hydrocele

Failure of obliteration of the processus may lead to fluid within the cord as a hydrocele of the cord or within the tunica as a scrotal hydrocele. If the processus allows fluid to move both ways according to gravity then this is usually described as a communicating hydrocele.

Incidence

- Common, perhaps as much as 6% of infant males.

Aetiology

While most are congenital, some may be secondary to torsion of the testis or its appendages, infection, trauma, idiopathic scrotal oedema, or, rarely, tumour.

Clinical features

Most are asymptomatic and only rarely are they tense or painful. Communicating hydroceles typically vary in size according to the time of day.

Examination shows a cystic scrotal swelling which you can 'get above' but can't separate from the testis, and which transilluminates. A hydrocele of the cord can occur outside or inside the canal and retains its transilluminability.

Most congenital hydroceles resolve spontaneously by 2 years of age. If a hydrocele persists beyond 2 to 3 years of age or is symptomatic, surgical repair can be recommended. Surgical closure is indicated to improve cosmesis and for symptoms (Box 5.20).

Box 5.20 Operation – ligation of the processus vaginalis

- Skin-crease groin incison
- The PPV is approached, at the level of the superficial ring. Split the cremaster muscle fibres and separate from vas and vessels
- Divide and ligate (e.g. Vicryl®4/0) as high as practical. Retain the distal end and trace it till it opens into the tunica. Open this widely to allow complete drainage.

Complications

- Scrotal haematoma
- Recurrence (~2%) – although possibly due to a missed PPV; consider tunica obliteration such as a Jaboulay procedure.

Umbilical hernia

This is a very common condition with visceral protrusion because of failure of the normal cicatricision process evident in the first few weeks after birth. There is a marked racial variation for reasons that are obscure but affecting with up to 5% of West African children. Other predisposing factors include omphalitis and increased intra-abdominal pressure (e.g. chronic cough), and congenital hypothyroidism.

Clinical features

The umbilical defect is usually circular and the skin protrusion conical (larger examples may resemble an elephant's trunk). The actual fascial defect varies but may be >5 cm. Although not present at birth, they become apparent in the first month of life. Thereafter, >90% reduce gradually over time and close spontaneously, usually by the age of 2 years. Although there is a low risk of complication (e.g. obstruction), this can occur in ~7% of cases.

Surgical closure is indicated to improve cosmesis and for symptoms (Box 5.21).

Box 5.21 Operation – repair of umbilical hernia

- The defect is approached, via a sub-umbilical semi-circular incision. The sac is separated from the skin (can be densely adherent) and the defect defined.
- Horizontal closure using absorbable fascial sutures (e.g. Vicryl®2/0). The often redundant skin should usually be tacked back to fascia but left to shrink with time and growth.
- Umbilicoplasty may be performed for gross examples of redundancy.

Complications

- Seroma (5%), recurrence (2%)

Femoral hernia

The femoral canal is a physiological triangular space medial to the femoral vein allowing for normal changes in venous distension. It transmits lymphatic channels and contains a lymph node (of Cloquet).

Anatomically, its base is the ileo-pectineal fascia overlying bone, medially the sharp lacunar ligament (of Astley–Cooper) which continues anteriorly as the inguinal ligament. Typically there is a narrow incompressible neck, with a more rounded fundus.

Epidemiology

Less than 1% of all groin hernias in children.

Clinical features

There is usually an intermittent groin swelling and, typically in children, the recent wound of a negative inguinal exploration. Careful physical examination is required to distinguish from an inguinal hernia. The palpable key is the pubic tubercle – femoral hernias are below and lateral; inguinal hernias are above and medial.

Management

Although most surgeons' experience in children is small, surgery is usually entirely successful (Box 5.22). Laparoscopic repair has also been reported.

> ### Box 5.22 Operation – repair of femoral hernia (Lockwood 'low' approach)
>
> Skin crease femoral incision. A palpable hernia typically has multiple fascial layers with only a relatively small sac. Dissect to the neck, transfix and reduce above canal. The canal can be closed by approximating inguinal ligament to the base with non-absorbable sutures, being careful to avoid narrowing the femoral vein.
>
> A retroperitoneal approach (McEvedy), has also been described for the acutely obstructed femoral hernia consisting of a dissection in the transversalis fascia behind the rectus muscle, approaching the neck from above, with the option of opening the peritoneum and visualizing the trapped bowel.

Further reading

Inguinal hernia

Ein SH, Njere I, Ein A. Six thousand three hundred sixty-one pediatric inguinal hernias: a 35-year review. *J Pediatr Surg* 2006;**41**:980–6.

Ron O, Eaton S, Pierro A. Systematic review of the risk of developing a metachronous contralateral inguinal hernia in children. *Br J Surg* 2007;**94**:804–11.

Hydrocele

Davenport M. ABC of general paediatric surgery: inguinal hernia, hydrocele and the undescended testis. *BMJ* 1996;**312**:564–7.

Lee SL, Dubois JJ. Laparoscopic diagnosis and repair of pediatric femoral hernia: Initial experience of four cases. *Surg Endosc* 2000;**14**:1110–113.

Umbilical hernia

Brown RA, Numanoglu A, Rode H. Complicated umbilical hernia in childhood. *S Afr J Surg* 2006;**44**:136–7.

Cilley RE. Disorders of the umbilicus. In: Grosfeld JL, O'Neill JA, Fonkalsrud EW, Coran AG (eds). *Pediatric Surgery*. Philadelphia, PA: Mosby, 2006, pp1143–56.

Femoral hernia

De Caluwé D, Chertin B, Puri P. Childhood femoral hernia: a commonly misdiagnosed condition. *Pediatr Surg Int* 2003;**19**:608–609.

Lau ST, Lee Y, Caty MG. Current management of hernias and hydroceles. *Semin Pediatr Surg* 2007;**16**:50–7.

Radcliffe G, Stringer MD. Reappraisal of femoral hernia in children. *Br J Surg* 1997;**84**:58–60.

Oncology

General principles

Though rare (~1500 new cases per annum in the UK and Ireland), in developed countries cancer kills more children than any other single cause. The commonest malignancies are leukaemia and tumours of the central nervous system. The other common childhood tumours are described in chapters in this section.

Differences from adult cancers

- Mostly embryonal tumours and sarcomas, carcinoma is rare
- Aetiology is genetic, environmental causes are rare
- Most are highly chemosensitive
- More children are cured

Overall long term survival rates now exceed 70%, ranging from >90% for Hodgkin's lymphoma, retinoblastoma, Wilms' tumour, stage 1 and 2 neuroblastoma, and gonadal germ cell tumours to <30% for stage 4 neuroblastoma.

Genetics

Certain syndromes predispose to cancer but these are rare, e.g. Costello syndrome for rhabdomyosarcoma, Denys–Drash syndrome and sporadic aniridia for Wilms' tumour. A genetic cause is only demonstrable in 2% in Wilms' tumours with loss of heterozygocity on chromosome 11p13 (*WT1* gene). This genetic abnormality is, however, associated with 20% of relapsed Wilms' tumours.

The *Myc-N* oncogene in neuroblastoma is associated with a worse prognosis when amplified and is now a component of risk stratification and a determinant of treatment.

Cytogenetics for diagnosis, e.g. t11:22 for PNET and DSRCT and t12:13 for alveolar rhabdomyosarcoma.

Organizations

Because children's cancers are rare, clinical trials and their statistical analysis must be multicentre and international. The national organization for the UK is the Children's Cancer and Leukaemia Group (CCLG). Collaborative trials exist with the main European group - International Society of Paediatric Oncology (SIOP) and the North American, Children's Oncology Group (COG).

Children's Cancer and Leukaemia Group

- 22 regional centres with a lead paediatric surgeon in each centre
- Supra-regional centres for certain tumours (e.g. bone, eye, liver)
- Multidisciplinary teamwork is highly evolved in the regional centres. Surgeons must develop close working relationships with their colleagues in oncology, radiology, and pathology

Treatment paradigm

- i.e. set of practices that define a scientific discipline

Most solid tumours are treated in the following sequence:

Biopsy → chemotherapy → surgical resection of primary tumour → complete chemotherapy (± radiotherapy for certain tumours, e.g. alveolar rhabdomyosarcoma or if incomplete resection).

Exceptions

- Surgery alone, e.g. neonatal tumours and teratomas
- Primary surgery without biopsy, e.g. (para)testicular tumours (rhabdomyosarcoma and teratoma)
- Diagnosis without biopsy, e.g. germ cell tumours with raised serum α-fetoprotein
- Complete response to chemotherapy obviating the need for surgical resection, e.g. lymphoma, some rhabdomyosarcomas

Role of the surgeon

Diagnosis

Initial consultation, clinical examination, and assessment of imaging with paediatric oncologist.

Biopsy

- Must be prompt and adequate for diagnosis. An inadequate or non-diagnostic biopsy is a serious adverse event
- Usually open incisional; multiple core needle samples suffice in certain cases. Plan incision so that it may be excised at the time of resection
- Laparoscopic or thoracoscopic techniques may be used
- Tissue must be received immediately and unfixed by the paediatric pathologist
- Fine needle aspiration cytology is not adequate, except possibly for parotid and thyroid tumours
- Cytology of ascites or pleural effusions may be diagnostic in the ill child with non-Hodgkin's lymphoma

Central venous access

Often performed at same time as biopsy if clinical diagnosis and need for chemotherapy is reasonably certain

Resection of primary tumour

- Most protocols specify precise timing. The surgeon should plan ahead at the time of diagnosis.
- Ensure fitness for operation. ?Need for GCSF. Platelet count should be >80 × 10^9/L.
- Post chemotherapy, pre-operative cross-sectional imaging should be studied in detail with the radiologist and be available in the operating theatre.
- Except for stage III and IV neuroblastoma, extracapsular section with a 1–2 cm margin of normal tissue is required.
- The specimen should be carefully orientated for and received fresh by the pathologist.
- Consider primary re-excision before starting chemotherapy in patients who have had inadequate or non-diagnostic initial surgical procedures (usually in a district general hospital), e.g. in rhabdomyosarcomas of the paratestis or limb and trunk.

Adjunctive surgery

- Transposition of ovaries or testes out of radiotherapy field
- Displacement of small bowel from pelvic radiotherapy field by absorbable mesh or tissue expander
- Insertion of brachytherapy ports
- Prophylaxis, e.g. thyroidectomy in MEN 2B

Metastasectomy

Occasionally indicated but only when primary tumour controlled. Commonest indication is pulmonary metastases from osteosarcoma, usually by wedge resection using linear stapler. *Thoracoscopy is contra-indicated* as manuality is essential to detect those metastases not demonstrated on CT scan.

Further reading

CCLG website: http://www.ukccsg.org/ (accessed 15 July 2008).

COG website: http://www.childrensoncologygroup.org/ (accessed 15 July 2008).

SIOP website: http://www.siop.nl/index.html (accessed 15 July 2008).

UK oncology survival statistics

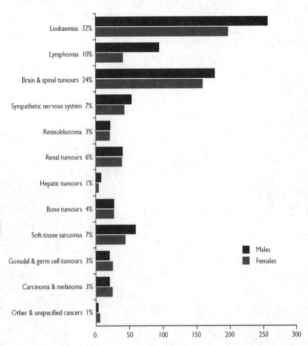

Fig. 6.1 Annual average number of cases by diagnostic group and sex, ages 0–14 years. Great Britain 1989–98. Reproduced with permission from Toms JR (ed). *CancerStats Monograph 2004*. London: Cancer Research UK, 2004.

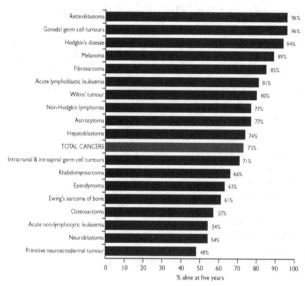

Fig. 6.2 Percentage of patients still alive five years after diagnosis, Great Britain, 1992–6. Reproduced with permission from Toms JR (ed). *CancerStats Monograph 2004*. London: Cancer Research UK, 2004.

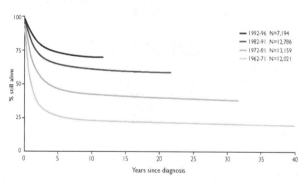

Fig. 6.3 Survival of childhood cancer patients diagnosed in successive periods, Great Britain 1962–96. Reproduced with permission from Toms JR (ed). *CancerStats Monograph 2004*. London: Cancer Research UK, 2004.

Glossary of oncology and genetics

Chromosome nomenclature

Forty-four autosomes (ranging from largest Ch1 to smallest Ch21) + 2 sex chromosomes. Each subdivided according to position of centromere into short (p = petit) and long (q) arm. Visible (by staining, typically Giemsa (G)) regions numbered from the centromere to the end. Further precision is given by various bands and sub-bands. (e.g. *TSC1* gene for tuberose sclerosis – 9q34, i.e band 4, region 3 of long arm of Ch9).

Centromere

Chromosome point of movement during mitosis, attached to cell microtubules. Metacentric (in middle), submetacentric (favouring one side) or acrocentric (at one end) used to discriminate chromosomes.

Telomere

The end of each chromosome, composed of highly repetitive DNA. Each division results in some loss of telomeric length and is associated with cell ageing.

Human genome
- Estimated 3 billion base pairs and 20–25,000 genes

Base pairs
- **A**denine binds **T**hymine (uracil in RNA) and **G**uanine binds with **C**ytosine

5′ and 3′ ends (of DNA, RNA)
- Pronounced 5 and 3 'prime'
- Nucleotides have a ribose backbone which varies at each end depending on a free OH^- or phosphate group (at 3 or 5 position). Conventionally sequence is read from 5′ to 3′.

Codons
- Combination of three base pairs coding for specific amino acids
- Start and stop codons begin and terminate sequence

m-RNA (messenger)

Sequenced from unwound DNA (transcription) and encodes for amino acid sequence (hence protein) at ribosomes.

Single nucleotide polymorphism (SNP – 'snip')
- A DNA sequence variation consisting of a single nucleotide base pair
- Should occur in at least 1% of population to be considered an SNP
- May be entirely silent, if in the non-coding part of the genome

Sense and antisense
- The portion of single-strand DNA which is read by mRNA, while the opposite strand sequence (antisense) is not taken further, but may have a regulatory role
- Novel antisense drugs (e.g. fomivirsen for CMV retinitis) may have a role in future

Homeobox (e.g. **Hox gene**)

- DNA gene sequence within gene and involved in regulation of embryonic development. Four clusters in humans (*HOXA*, *HOXB*, *HOXC*, and *HOXD*).

Ploidy

Aneuploidy is addition or subtraction of entire chromosomes.

Loss of heterozygosity (in cell)

- Lack of function of one set of parent chromosomes
- Leaves remaining tumour suppressor gene exposed to mutation and loss of function
- Classic example is retinoblastoma, LOH leads to flawed expression of RB1

MYC

- Proto-oncogene first discovered in Birkitt's lymphoma, where translocations involving chromosome 8 are frequent
- Normally involved in cell growth and proliferation
- Over-expression or mutation leads to oncogenesis
- Binds with enhancer box sequences
- *Myc-N* = neuroblastoma (avian)-derived

P53 (aka protein 53)

- A transcription factor (MW 53 KDa) which regulates the cell cycle, and functions as a tumour suppressor (the 'guardian of the genome')
- May activate apoptosis and initiate DNA repair
- Encoded by gene *TP53* (on Ch 17)
- Inherited defects in *TP53* found in Li-Fraumeni syndrome

Southern blot

- Named after Edwin Southern, when professor of biochemistry at Edinburgh
- Technique used to determine DNA length variations after restriction enzyme digestion

Northern blot (who says biochemists lack humour!)

- Electrophoretic gel technique used to determine RNA length variations after endonuclease digestion and hybridization probing

Western blot

- Electrophoretic gel technique used to separate native or denatured proteins

FISH (fluorescent in-situ hybridization)

- Technique used to identify gene deletions using probe attached to fluorescent molecule

PCR (polymerase chain reaction)

- Technique developed by Nobel prize winner Kary Mullis in 1983 and used to amplify (replicate) lengths of DNA, either for identification or quantification

RT-PCR
- Reverse transcription PCR is used to amplify a piece of RNA (via its cDNA)

Gel electrophoresis
Proteins, RNA and DNA can be separated on the basis of their mass (usually) and/or electric charge by running a current through an agarose gel. Various 'lanes' are set containing molecules of known mass or charge to compare. Molecules need to be visualized in a separate process (by UV fluorescence, autoradiography etc).

DNA microarray ('Gene Chip®')
- Arrangement of thousands (typically) of DNA oligonucleotide sequences unique for known genes on a matrix, to study levels of gene expression

Surgical complications of oncological treatment

Chemotherapy (CT) and radiotherapy (RT) cause severe tissue damage, either directly or by marrow toxicity. They may also be synergistic as in the liver damage seen with the combination of RT and actinomycin D.

Chemotherapy

Infection

Neutropenic patients (<1000/mm^3) pose special problems:

- abscesses – pus does not form so traditional incision and drainage is not appropriate. Needle aspiration for microbiology, broad-spectrum antibiotics and administration of granulocyte colony-stimulating factor (GCSF) are indicated
- necrotizing fasciitis – rapidly spreading infection typically of synergistic organisms (e.g. aerobic organisms such as Gp A *streptococcal* spp., *staphylococcal* spp., *Klebsiella*, together with anaerobic species such as *bacteroides* spp. and *clostridial* spp.) Clinically there is gas formation (crepitation), and rapidly progressive gangrene of the overlying skin. Requires early diagnosis, broad-spectrum antibiotics and typically aggressive debridement
- ecthyma grangrenosum – this starts as painless, red macules which turn pustular and develop a gangrenous eschar. It occurs particularly on the perineum, and is associated with pseudomonas sepsis. It requires aggressive antibiotic therapy
- compartment syndrome – usually lower limb, characterized by severe pain and limitation of movement. Also associated with pseudomonas. Requires appropriate antibiotic therapy and fasciotomy.

Opportunistic infections

Surgical involvement is most commonly required for fungal lung lesions (usually *aspergillus* spp.) either for diagnosis (bronchoscopy or biopsy), or occasionally for treatment (lung resection).

Ileus and constipation

These are specifically caused by vincristine. Standard treatments suffice.

Pancreatitis

A number of drugs may predispose but the commonest are corticosteroids and L-asparaginase. Treatment is medical, though occasionally surgery may be needed for pseudocyst or abscess.

Haemorrhagic cystitis

Associated with the alkylating agents, cyclophosphamide, or ifosfamide. Cystoscopy may be needed to confirm diagnosis. Prevention is by hydration and Mesna®. Severe cases may require bladder irrigation, cystoscopy and diathermy, instillation of intravesical 1% alum, 1% formalin or prostaglandin F$_2$, cystotomy or rarely cystectomy.

Neutropenic enterocolitis

May be extensive or patchy, most commonly involves the caecum (typhlitis). Initially mucosal, but may progress to be transmural and cause perforation or stricture requiring surgery. Presents with abdominal pain and distension, vomiting, and diarrhoea with bleeding. Ultrasound is helpful in confirming the diagnosis and management is conservative with broad-spectrum antibiotics including anti-pseudomonal agents and metronidazole. The condition usually resolves once the neutrophil count recovers, spontaneously or with the aid of GCSF.

Tumour lysis syndrome

This is seen particularly in association with non-Hodgkin's lymphoma particularly but also in chemosensitive hepatoblastoma and stage IV neuroblastoma. It occurs in rapidly growing tumours responding to induction therapy and may be precipitated by surgical procedures. It is caused by rapid release of purines, potassium, and phosphorus causing hyperuricaemia, hyperkalaemia, hyperphosphataemia, and secondary hypocalcaemia. Acute renal failure may occur but can be prevented by pre-hydration and allopurinol (or one of its newer analogues e.g. Rasburicase – recombinant uric oxidase). However, once established, haemofiltration may be needed.

Gastrointestinal bleeding

May be due to peptic ulcer (e.g. steroids) or gastritis. Endoscopy is diagnostic and potentially therapeutic.

Hepatic veno-occlusive disease, is associated with actinomycin D ± radiotherapy, thioguanine, and has a high incidence following stem cell tranplant. In its acute form it may present with tender hepatomegaly and ascites but chronically it can lead to lead to portal hypertension and variceal bleeding.

Radiotherapy

Causes acute inflammation followed by a chronic fibrosing process. If surgical procedures are needed after radiotherapy they should be timed to be after the former has settled but before the latter has developed, usually about 8 weeks after completion of radiotherapy.

Prevention and treatment of complications of abdominal RT

- Temporary displacement of organs from the radiotherapy field; testes, ovaries (laparoscopy is ideal), or small bowel which may be displaced from the pelvis by absorbable mesh or a tissue expander
- Diversion – sigmoid colostomy may be needed for radiation proctitis
- Treatment of radiation enteritis should be conservative as far as possible, as surgery carries a high complication rate, but may be unavoidable for obstruction or fistula

Bone marrow transplant (BMT)

All CT complications may occur in BMT patients, but some have an increased incidence, e.g. pancreatitis and opportunistic infection.

Graft versus host disease (GVHD)

Can affect any organ but commonly skin, and a biopsy may be needed. The GI tract is also commonly affected and the surgeon may be involved in the differential diagnosis of GVHD from opportunistic infections such as cytomegalovirus and Herpes simplex virus. Depending on clinical localization, biopsies may be oral or by upper or lower GI endoscopy. Intestinal GVHD is managed medically with corticosteroids. Perforation and late stricture formation are indications for surgery.

Surgery

Marrow suppression may compromise surgery. Platelet count should be 50 $\times 10^9$/L (depending on procedure). GCSF may be needed peri-operatively.

Miscellaneous

Intussusception

Ileo-ileal intussusceptions may occur in the early postoperative period after retroperitoneal tumour resections (e.g. Wilms' tumour and neuroblastoma). If suspected, laparotomy is indicated.

Adhesive obstruction

This may occur in any child who has had an intra-abdominal tumour resection, indeed in good-prognosis tumours such as Wilms' tumour, delayed diagnosis and treatment of adhesions is now the commonest cause of surgical mortality. Give written information regarding the serious significance of bile vomiting to all patients before they are discharged from surgical follow-up.

Further reading

Arul GS, Spicer RD. Surgical complications of childhood tumours. In: Carachi R, Azmi A, Grosfeld JL (eds). *The Surgery of Childhood Tumours*. London: Arnold, 2008, pp497–519.

Wilms' tumour

Wilms' tumour (WT) (synonym nephroblastoma) is named after the German surgeon Max Wilms (1867–1918), who first described the characteristic histological features in 1897. The management is one of the success stories of paediatric oncology as cure rates have risen to >90%. Current research is now focused on dose reduction to reduce long term treatment-related morbidity.

Incidence
- 6% of all paediatric malignancies
- 1 in 10,000 children
- Commonest childhood renal tumour

Epidemiology
The peak incidence is between 1–3 years. About 5% have associated syndromes.

Aetiology
WT arises from failure of the metanephric blastema to develop normally, and in some cases it may progress via a premalignant stage of nephrogenic rests. These are found adjacent to 30% of tumours and in the syndromic diseases. The term nephroblatomatosis refers to the presence of multiple nephrogenic rests. WT has offered researchers an insight into the molecular genetics of tumourogenesis and has largely supported the 'two-hit' theory. Research with WT families have allowed identification of some of the genes responsible. Common associations are listed in Table 6.1. The importance of WT in these syndromes relates to the higher incidence of bilateral disease (4–15%) and the earlier age of onset. At-risk individuals should therefore be screened. Other, less well-defined abnormalities include the loss of p53 tumour suppressor gene in most cases and an association with changes in chromosome 1p and 16q and a poor prognosis. Despite this, the genetic basis of sporadic WT remains elusive.

Clinical features
Sporadic WT typically presents as an asymptomatic abdominal mass. Symptomatic cases are characterized by intermittent pain (33%), haematuria (25%), hypertension (10%) and systemic symptoms of malaise, lethargy, fever, and anaemia (20%). The mass, if palpable, arises from the loin, is usually non-tender and may be ballotable.

Investigation
US is the first-line investigation and may be diagnostic, and is the best modality to evaluate intra-caval extension. CT scanning is used to define anatomy, and exclude contralateral disease and lung metastases. The role of MRI is not clear but it may replace CT in some centres.

Although WT can be diagnosed by a combination of history and imaging, with an accuracy approaching 95%, neuroblastoma may mimic the radiology. Hence urinary catecholamines and neuron-specific enolase are still important excluders. Other primary renal tumours (e.g. mesoblastic nephroma in infants; renal cell carcinoma, and sarcomas in older children) may have to be considered. Finally, xanthogranulomatous pyelonephritis can mimic WT but urine cultures, infection markers, and imaging should differentiate.

Table 6.1 Genetic associations and syndromes

Name	Gene defect	Features
WAGR	Ch 11p13 (*WT1*), gene deletion (*WT1* – Wilms', *PAX6* – aniridia)	• **W**ilms' tumour
		• **A**niridia
		• **G**enitourinary malformation
		• Mental **R**etardation
Denys–Drash	Ch 11p13 (*WT1*)	• Genitourinary abnormalities
		• Glomerulopathy (renal failure <10 years)
		• Wilms' tumour
Beckwith–Weidemann	Ch 11p15 (*WT2*)	• Macroglossia
		• Hemihypertrophy
		• Exomphalos
		• Ear abnormalities
		• Wilms' tumour
Familial Wilms'	Ch11, (*FWT1* q17) (*FWT2* q19)	

Staging

The UK staging conforms with current SIOP protocols with the addition of a biopsy. The details are listed in Table 6.2. Classical WT histology is 'triphasic' consisting of blastema, stromal, and tubular elements. The proportion of each component, together with the degree of anaplasia allows tumours to be categorized into low, intermediate, or high risk. Note that, unlike in North America, SIOP histology includes the tumour response to chemotherapy.

Management

There are major differences in treatment philosophy between North America, Europe, and the UK. In the former, primary nephrectomy is the mainstay of treatment, followed by therapy guided by the pathological staging. SIOP supports adjuvant chemotherapy based on imaging, then additional treatment based on the pathology. In the UK the majority of patients with suggestive imaging will undergo percutaneous biopsy followed by two courses of chemotherapy and re-imaging. They will then undergo surgical resection and pathological staging, which will take into account the tumour response to chemotherapy. Dependent on the stage and histology, further treatment might include: no treatment, further chemotherapy; escalation of the chemotherapy and or radiotherapy. Despite such major differences, no one strategy has actually been shown to have a survival advantage over another.

Table 6.2 SIOP Staging of WT – pathological staging following neo-adjuvant chemotherapy

Stage	Features	Comments
I	Tumour limited to the kidney, completely excised	Kidney confined or within fibrous capsule, no tumour rupture, no residual tumour apparent beyond margins of resection. No sinus vessel involvement (intrarenal possible). No pelvic/ureteric wall involvement
II	Tumour extends beyond kidney, completely excised	Regional extension of tumour; vessel infiltration; local spill of tumour confined to flank. No residual tumour apparent at or beyond margins of excision
III	Residual non-haemtogenous tumour confined to the abdomen	Lymph node involvement of hilus, periaortic nodes, or beyond, diffuse tumour still, residual disease remaining due to infiltration of vital structures
IV	Tumour deposits beyond stage III	i.e. lung, liver, bone, brain
V	Bilateral disease at diagnosis	

Controversies

Primary nephrectomy versus adjuvant chemotherapy

The former allows accurate staging at the time of diagnosis with immediate confirmation of histology, while the latter downstages the tumour with resultant under-treatment, reduced surgical morbidity, and tumour spill. The UK group continues to use precutanous biopsy, which allows tissue diagnosis prior to treatment but not without risk (bleeding, tumour seeding/spill, and need for emergency nephrectomy).

Surgery

- Surgery for unilateral uncomplicated disease is radical nephrectomy with lymph node sampling.
- Oncological principles apply with a transperitoneal approach and meticulous vessel and tissue control.
- In children with predisposition syndromes or where there is bilateral disease, careful assessment for the possibility of nephron-sparing surgery is required in the hope of delaying renal replacement.

Specific complication

- Tumour spill

Outcomes

Overall survival approaches 90% and treatment reduction has been the focus of recent trials in order to minimize morbidity for the majority of patients. Further improvements in survival will require identification of high-risk tumours and the optimization of treatment escalation for this group; this will be the challenge for oncologists over the next few years.

Further reading

Arya M, Shergill IS, Gommersall L *et al*. Current trends in the management of Wilms' tumour. *BJU Int* 2006;**97**:899–900.

Brown KW, Malik KT. The molecular biology of Wilms' tumour. *Exp Rev Mol Med* 2001;**3**:1–16.

Scott RH, Stiller CA, Walker L, Rahman N. Syndromes and constitutional chromosomal abnormalities associated with Wilms' tumour. *J Med Genet* 2006;**43**:705–15.

Liver tumours

Incidence

- ~2% of all childhood cancers
- 1–1.5 per million children per year

Typically liver tumours are malignant but benign lesions may account for one-third of tumours (e.g. haemangioendothelioma, mesenchymal hamartomas, adenoma, and focal nodular hyperplasia, and various types of cysts).

There are two key types:

- hepatoblastoma (HPB) – 80%, younger
- hepatocellular carcinoma (HCC) – 20%, older.

(Embryonal sarcoma and rhabdomyosarcoma occur but are rare.)

Epidemiology

The ratio of HPB to HCC varies around the world from 6:1 in the USA to 1.6:1 in developing countries. Embryonal sarcoma is seen in older children. Rhabdomyosarcoma is predominantly a lesion of the extrahepatic bile ducts.

Aetiology

About 50% of HPB have an associated genetic influence (e.g. Beckwith–Wiedeman, hemihypertrophy, and familial polyposis coli syndromes) and an association with low birth weight. This may be due to inactivation of the APC tumour suppressor gene (found in about 80% of cases). HCC is associated with environmental factors and co-existing liver disease (e.g. tenfold increase in risk in HBV carriers in endemic areas). There is also an increased risk in HCV and HIV infection and in certain metabolic liver disease (e.g. tyrosinaemia, progressive familial cholestasis). Nevertheless, only about one-third have cirrhosis of the liver as opposed to adults where up to 90% have cirrhosis.

Clinical features

These usually present as an abdominal mass or, less commonly, with evidence of malignant malaise and metastases. Jaundice is a feature of rhabdomyosarcoma only, unless the tumour involves both right and left hepatic ducts.

Liver biochemistry is usually normal in HPB, although anaemia and thrombocytosis are common. Most HPB and >65% of HCC have raised alpha-feto protein levels.

Management

For HPB, this is well developed, predominantly through international studies (e.g. SIOP) with a well-defined disease-assessment system of pre-treatment extent (PRETEXT) of disease staging into four categories depending on the number of liver sectors involved (Fig. 6.4). Radiological imaging in the form of ultrasound scanning, CT, and MRI define the extent of disease. Chest x-ray is done to exclude pulmonary metastases.

In principle, all patients have pre-operative chemotherapy (typically adriamycin and cisplatin) with excision of the tumour about two-thirds of the way through the programme.

For HCC, the response to chemotherapy is often poor and primary resection is the treatment of choice.

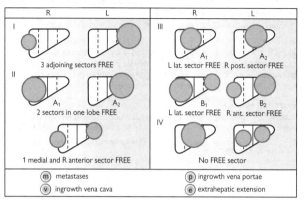

R	L	R	L
I	3 adjoining sectors FREE	III	A_1 L lat. sector FREE A_2 R post. sector FREE
II	A_1 A_2 2 sectors in one lobe FREE		B_1 L lat. sector FREE B_2 R ant. sector FREE
1 medial and R anterior sector FREE	IV	No FREE sector

(m) metastases   (v) ingrowth vena cava   (p) ingrowth vena portae   (e) extrahepatic extension

Fig. 6.4 PRETEXT classification of hepatoblastoma (I to IV). Stage I (three sectors free of tumour); stage II, (two adjacent sectors free); stage III (one sector or two non-adjoining sectors), and stage IV (no free sectors).

Surgery

- The aim is complete surgical removal of the tumour.
- If this cannot be achieved through surgical resection due to all sectors being involved by the primary tumour, multifocality or involvement of portal veins, then total hepatectomy with transplantation may be indicated, provided there is no residual tumour evident outside the liver after chemotherapy.

The outcome of transplantation as primary treatment is currently considerably better than as rescue treatment for local recurrence after resection. Thus, criteria for transplant would be: unresectable tumour, complete removal obtained only by total hepatectomy, i.e. no extra-hepatic disease, chemotherapy-sensitive tumour, and clearance of extrahepatic metastases.

Radiotherapy may be required in rhabdomyosarcoma for any residual tumour.

Outcome

- More than 80% of HPB tumours become resectable after chemotherapy.
- Overall survival for HPB is >75%.
- Survival with HCC is poor ~30% at 5 years.

In HPB, the histological fetal subtype has a better prognosis with mixed, macrotrabecular, and anaplastic the worst. Five-year survival after transplantation is >60%. Sarcomas have a generally worse prognosis than HPB, but results have improved with better chemotherapy.

Further reading

Austin MT, Leys CM, Feurer ID et al. Liver transplantation for childhood hepatic malignancy: a review of the United Network for Organ Sharing (UNOS) database. *J Pediatr Surg* 2006;**41**:182–6.

Stringer MD. The role of liver transplantation in the management of paediatric liver tumours. *Ann R Coll Surg Engl* 2007;**89**:12–21.

Intestinal tumours

Tumours of the gastrointestinal tract are rare in childhood, with a spectrum from benign to malignant pathology. Predisposing factors include the hereditary syndromes and those lesions arising from metaplastic changes secondary to chronic exposure to irritants (e.g. chronic gastroesophageal reflux, Barrett's oesophagitis, or after caustic injury).

Clinical features

Dyspepsia, vomiting, weight loss, intestinal obstruction, or upper/lower GI bleeding. Anaemia can be a presenting feature in children with foregut pathology (e.g. GIST). Investigations should include contrast studies, ultrasound, gastrointestinal endoscopy, and biopsy with CT imaging of the primary site and metastastes.

Hereditary syndromes

Peutz–Jeghers syndrome

- Autsomal dominant (1 in 80,000 live births), mutation of *STK11/LKB1* on Ch19.
- Multiple hamartomatous polyps found throughout GI tract. Nonetheless, they have increased risk of intestinal (oesophageal, stomach etc) cancer. About half of patients will have died from malignancy by 57 years of age.
- Pigmented muco-cutaneous macules are characteristic (lower lip, gingival).
- Enterosocopy (surveillance/therapeutic polypectomy) can be utilized to limit intestinal resection and risk of short gut syndrome.
- Associated with extra-intestinal malignancies – thyroid, uterine, breast, testicular, and ovarian tumours.

Familial adenomatous polyposis (FAP)

- Autosomal dominant (1 in 5–17,000 live-births), mutation of *APC* gene located on Ch 5q21; 80% have family history.
- Multiple adenomatous polyps within colon. Lesions develop in the first decade of life with 100% malignant transformation by the 30s and 40s.
- Also at greater risk for foregut malignancy (gastric/duodenal/ periampullary cancer) as adults and have other associated tumours, e.g. desmoid, papillary thyroid, and liver tumours.
- Prophylactic proctocolectomy is recommended during adolescence.

Gardner's syndrome (1951)

- FAP and jaw osteomas, odontomas, desmoids, and lipomas

Turcot's syndrome (1959)

- FAP & medulloblastoma/glioma

Gastrointestinal stromal tumours (GIST)

These are rare mesenchymal tumours originating from the interstitial cells of Cajal (i.e. c-kit (CD117) +ve) and tend to have a female predilection. Mostly found in stomach (50–70%) – where they typically have a 'volcano' appearance endoscopically – small bowel (20%), and colon (10%).

Carney's triad (1977)

- GIST, ganglioneuroma, pulmonary chrondroma

Surgical resection is curative. Imatinib mesylate (Gleevec®) – a c-kit inhibitor – is used to treat recurrent or metastatic disease.

Carcinoid tumours

These are rare neuroendocrine tumours arising in various sites and are classified according to origin as foregut, mid-gut or hindgut. These have distinct histochemical and secretory features. Thus, foregut tumours are argentaffin –ve and secrete 5-hydroxytryptophan, mid-gut tumours are argentaffin +ve and secrete serotonin 5-hydroxytryptamine Rarely they may arise outside (e.g. lungs).

- Associated with MEN type 1 syndrome (see page 214)

Carcinoid syndrome

- Occurs with liver metastates and systemic release of various metabolites, causing flushing, watery diarrhoea, bronchospasm but is very rare in children (Box 6.1)

Box 6.1 Common scenario – incidental finding at appendicectomy

Accounts for < 0.2% of appendix specimens. Most are found at the tip and if recognized at surgery, then palpate and sample regional nodes. If negative/unremarkable then simple appendicectomy is curative. If nodes are palpably abnormal, tumour >2 cm, or at base, then consider right hemicolectomy and node dissection.

Urinary metabolites (e.g. 5-HIAA) and specific imaging studies (e.g. OctreoScan®) guide surveillance and follow-up.

Oesophageal neoplasms

- Rare occurrence in childhood; however, corrosive injury, Barrett's oesophagus and history of oesophageal atresia are predisposing factors to adenocarcinoma in adulthood.
- Lifelong surveillance endoscopy ± biopsy is recommended. The role of anti-reflux surgery for prevention is controversial.
- Smooth muscle tumours (leiomyomas, leiomyosarcomas) occur rarely, and tend to be multiple or diffuse at presentation.
- Female predilection.

Lymphomas

- Commonest small bowel malignancy (see page 312)

Solitary rectal polyp/juvenile polyps

These are benign hamartomas, typically found in 4–5-year-old age group. May present with rectal bleeding or a prolapsing 'cherry red' lesion seen on straining/stooling. Autoamputation can occur. The treatment is proctoscopy and polypectomy.

Colorectal cancer

This is sporadic and rare in childhood. Most have advanced disease with aggressive tumour biology at presentation. Some are associated with polyposis syndromes and inflammatory bowel disease. Management includes resection, staging, and multimodal therapies as for its adult counterpart.

Other rare tumours

- Zollinger–Ellison syndrome – caused by gastrinomas in the stomach or pancreas which induce hyperacidity in the normal stomach. Associated with MEN type 1 (see page 214)
- Plexiform neurofibromata/sarcomas can develop throughout the GI tract, e.g. Von Recklinghausen's disease
- Vascular malformations may cause focal or diffuse haemorrhagic lesions; GI bleeding can be massive and life threatening, e.g.:
  - proteus syndrome (1979) – colonic haemangiomata, and multiple GI polyps
  - blue rubber bleb nevus syndrome (1958), consists of both cutaneous and visceral discrete venous malformations
- Desmoplastic 'small round cell' tumours arising in peritoneal cavity and stomach. Tend to be aggressive lesions with a poor prognosis
- Rhabdomyosarcomas – rare and aggressive
- Leiomyomas – mostly benign lesions typically in the stomach, but also found elsewhere. Excision is curative
- Teratomas – see page 184
- Gastric adenocarcinoma is very rare with poor prognosis

Further reading

Adzick NS, Fisher JH, Winter HS, Sandler RH, Hendren WH. Esophageal adenocarcinoma 20 years after esophageal atresia repair. *J Pediatr Surg* 1989;**24**:741–4.

Keshtgar AS, Losty PD, Lloyd DA, Morris AI, Pierro A. Recent developments in the management of Peutz–Jeghers syndrome in childhood. *Eur J Pediatr Surg* 1997;**7**:367–8.

La Quaglia MP, Heller G, Filippa DA et al. Prognostic factors and outcome in patients 21 years and under with colorectal carcinoma. *J Pediatr Surg* 1992;**27**:1085–90.

Losty P, Hu C, Quinn F, Fitzgerald RJ. Gastrointestinal manifestations of neurofibromatosis in childhood. *Eur J Pediatr Surg* 1993;**3**:57–8.

Miettinen M, Lasota J, Sobin LH. Gastrointestinal stromal tumors of the stomach in children and young adults: a clinicopathologic, immunohistochemical and molecular genetic study of 44 cases with long term follow up and review of the literature. *Am J Surg Pathol* 2005;**29**:1373–81.

Prommegger R, Obrist P, Ensinger C et al. Retrospective evaluation of carcinoid tumors of the appendix in children. *World J Surg* 2002;**26**:1489–92.

Neuroblastoma

This is malignant neoplasm of neuroblasts – cells originating from the embryonic neural crest – normally only present in the fetus. Neuroblastoma may arise in the adrenal medulla or anywhere along the sympathetic nervous system ganglion chain from the neck to the pelvis.

It is responsible for 10% of all childhood tumours and for 15% of all childhood cancer deaths.

Epidemiology

- ~1 in 9000 children
- M:F 1.2:1
- 40% are diagnosed by 1 year
- 75% by 7 years
- 98% by 10 years

Associations

- Other neural crest disorders (e.g. neurofibromatosis, Hirschsprung's disease)
- Beckwith–Wiedemann syndrome and mutations on chromosome 16p12–13

Site

- Adrenal 50%, paraspinal 24%, mediastinal 20%, neck 3%, pelvis 3%

Clinical features

- >50% present with an abdominal mass.

Neck tumours involving the stellate ganglion may produce a Horner's syndrome; mediastinal tumours may cause respiratory symptoms or dysphagia; paraspinal tumours at any level may invade the intervertebral foramina causing cord compression.

Spread may be by direct invasion, regional or distant lymphatic infiltration, or haematogenous metastases most commonly to the liver or bone.

General symptoms of malignany include malaise, weight loss, fever, and anaemia. Hypertension may occur secondary to ectopic catecholamine production. Bilateral periorbital ecchymosis or 'panda eyes' results from metastases to the skull. Multiple skin nodules and hepatomegaly occur in infants with the stage 4S disease.

Plain radiographs may demonstrate paraspinal widening, a mass effect, tumour calcification, or bony metastases.

CT with contrast and MRI are useful to delineate the tumour as well as its relationship to the viscera and vascular structures and to assess intra-spinal extension. Radioisotope scintigraphy with radiolabelled MIBG (meta-iodobenzylguanidine) and technetium can demonstrate the primary tumour and bony metastases.

Urinary levels of catecholamines and their by-products are usually elevated. Tissue diagnosis by needle or surgical biopsy with bone marrow aspirate is essential. This allows the evaluation of tumour biology.

Staging

• International Neuroblastoma Staging System (INSS): see Table 6.3

Table 6.3 International Neuroblastoma Staging System

Stage	Description
1	Localized tumour, completely excised, with or without microscopic residual disease, lymph nodes removed en-bloc may be positive but other nodes negative
2a	Unilateral tumour with incomplete macroscopic excision, ipsilateral and contralateral lymph nodes negative
2b	Unilateral tumour with complete or incomplete macroscopic excision, positive ipsilateral nodes, negative contralateral nodes
3	Tumour infiltrating across midline, or unilateral tumour with contralateral lymph node involvement, or midline tumour with bilateral lymph node involvement or bilateral infiltration (unresectable)
4	Distant metastases
4S	Stage 1 or stage 2 localized primary tumour with metastases to liver, skin, or bone marrow, in infants less than 1 year of age

Pathology

The International Neuroblastoma Pathology Classification (INPC) system categorizes tumours as having either favourable or unfavourable histology on the basis of various criteria including:

• stroma-rich or stroma-poor appearance of tumour
• degree of differentiation
• mitotic karyorrhexis index
• age of patient.

Biology

Several genetic alterations have been found associated with neuroblastoma. Amplification of the oncogene *N-myc* and diploid tumours are associated with a worse outcome, independent of tumour stage.

Management

• Individualized based on INSS stage, age, *N-myc* status, INPC (histology), and DNA ploidy to categorize each patient as low, intermediate or high risk:
  • low risk – complete surgical excision
  • intermediate risk – surgery and standard chemotherapy
  • high risk – intensive combination chemotherapy followed by surgical excision, +/– radiation therapy

Surgery for neuroblastoma

Excision is intended to remove all macroscopic disease (e.g. retroperitoneal clearance for abdominal tumours), although the advantage of tumour debulking has not been proven.

Prognosis

Risk-based management aims to provide the highest chance of cure with the lowest chance of complications.

- Survival:
  - >90% for low risk
  - 70% for intermediate risk
  - 30% for high risk

Screening for neuroblastoma

Testing urinary vanillylmandelic acid and homovanillic levels in children <18 months of age resulted in a large increase in the incidence of neuroblastoma detected in infants, without any decrease in the incidence or mortality of neuroblastoma in children >1 year. It is therefore likely that most cases detected by screening undergo spontaneous regression.

Further reading

Brodeur GM, Pritchard J, Berthold et al. Revision of the international criteria for neuroblastoma diagnosis, staging and response to treatment. *J Clin Oncol* 1993;**11**:1466–77.

Kiely EM, Barker G. Neuroblastoma. In: Ashcraft KW, Murphy JP, Sharp RJ, Sigalet DL, Snyder CL (eds). *Pediatric Surgery*. Philadelphia, Pennsylvania: WB Saunders Company, 2000, pp875–90.

Testicular tumours

- 1–2% of all paediatric solid tumours
- Two peaks – ~2 years and puberty
Divided into (Table 6.4):
- Non-germ cell tumours (Leydig, Sertoli, gonadoblastoma)
- Germ cell tumours (teratoma, yolk-sac (YSK))

Risk factors

Caucasian, intersex, cryptorchidism

Clinical features

Most present with a painless testicular mass. The differential might include epididymitis, hydrocele, hernia, and testicular torsion.

Investigation

- US, CT/MRI retroperitoneum; chest radiograph/CT)
- tumours markers – α-fetoprotein and β-HCG. (AFP is raised if there are yolk-sac elements, a raised β-HCG is rarely found in prepubertal tumours and is more used in adult seminomas.)

Non-germ cell tumours

Gonadal stromal tumours most common in this group. Usually benign and originate from mesenchymal stem cell differentiating into Leydig, Sertoli, or granulosa cells.

Leydig cell tumour

- Peak at 4–5 years. They are encapsulated, yellow-brown and microscopically show eosinophilic cells with granular cytoplasm; ~40% have Reinke's crystals.
- Abnormal production of testosterone causes precocious puberty (irreversible skeletal, muscular, and penile growth). Corticosteroids, progesterone and oestrogens are also produced.

Surgery

Inguinal approach – orchidectomy. Enucleation possible with few recurrences.

Sertoli cell tumour

These are white or yellow with lobulations. Microscopically, they consist of polygonal cells with eosinophilic cytoplasm. Occasionally, they may be associated with Peutz–Jeghers syndrome and Carney complex. Gynaecomastia is possible.

Surgery

In infants, observation only is possible. If treatment is necessary, inguinal orchidectomy with retroperitoneal exploration is carried out.

Gonadoblastomas

These are commonly associated with intersex conditions and can be bilateral in up to one-third of cases. Histologically, they are characterized as large germ cells, sex-cord derivatives, with stromal elements.

Management

- Female-raised gonadal dysgenesis: gonads removed
- Male-raised: undescended testes should be removed; scrotal testes can be observed

Germ cell tumours

Teratoma

Most common in children. Prepubertal mature teratomas are benign. Immature teratomas are less common and can have malignant foci (YSK cells). Histologically consist of endoderm, ectoderm, and mesoderm and tend to be well-encapsulated with cysts. Cartilage, bone, mucous glands, or muscle may be seen.

- Ultrasound features – complex hypoechoic area with surrounding echogenic signals

Management

Radical orchidectomy. Enucleation is possible with no recurrence. Recurrent immature teratomas can be salvaged with platinum-based chemotherapy.

Yolk sac tumours

Typically arise in children under 2 years. Macroscopically are firm and yellow-white. Histologically, they consist of a mixture of epithelial and mesenchymal cells.

- ~90% are confined to the testis
- ~5% metastasize to retroperitoneal lymph nodes
- ~90% AFP elevated

Management

Radical inguinal orchidectomy in all with full clinicopathological staging (tumour markers and imaging).

Table 6.4 Testicular tumours

Tumour classification	Tumour
Non-germ-cell tumour (gonadal stromal)	Leydig cell
	Sertoli cell
	Granulosa cell
	Mixed
Non-germ-cell tumour	Gonadoblastoma
Germ cell tumours	Yolk sac
	Teratoma
	Mixed germ cell
	Seminoma
Supporting tissue tumours	Fibroma
	Leiomyoma
	Haemangioma
Reticulo-endothelial	Lymphomas
	Leukaemias

Further reading

Agarwal PK, Palmer JS. Testicular and paratesticular neoplasms in prepubertal males. *J Urol* 2006;**176**:875–81.

Lymphomas

> Thomas Hodgkin (1798–1866), English physician working at Guy's Hospital, London described his disease in *On Some Morbid Appearances of the Absorbent Glands and Spleen* in 1832.

Incidence
- 3rd most common paediatric malignancy (after leukaemia and brain tumours)
- Divided into two main types:
  - Hodgkin's lymphoma (HL) – 40%
  - non-Hodgkin's lymphoma (NHL) – 60%

All HL are of B-cell origin, and the diagnostic cells are large binucleate cells (Reed–Sternberg cells).

Subtypes of Hodgkin's lymphoma
- Nodular sclerosing >65%
- Mixed cellularity 22%
- Lymphocyte predominance 9%
- Lymphocyte depletion uncommon

Subtypes of non-Hodgkin's lymphoma
- B-cell (CD20 +ve)
- T-cell

Burkitt's lymphoma is the commonest NHL subtype (42%), causing jaw and orbital tumours in its endemic form in Africa. Marked association with Epstein–Barr and HIV infection.

Clinical features
Hodgkin's lymphoma
- Incidence increases with age
- Twice as common in teenagers compared to those <10 years
- Usually (80%) presents with persistent painless cervical adenopathy

About one-third of patients present with 'B symptoms', e.g. unexplained fever >38°C (aka Pel–Ebstein fever), unexplained weight loss ≥10% in previous 6 months, or drenching night sweats. These are regarded as negative prognostic features.

Non-Hodgkin's lymphoma
- Incidence hardly changes between the age of 3 years and 14 years
- All are diffuse and fast growing
- Abdominal lymphomas are usually B-cell NHL

Abdominal lymphoma may present as a mass, bowel obstruction, intussusception, ascites, or hepatosplenomegaly.

Most primary mediastinal lymphomas are of T-cell origin (thymus) and may cause respiratory symptoms and/or superior vena caval syndrome.

Differential diagnosis

- Acute lymphoblastic leukaemia
- Infectious mononucleosis
- Atypical/typical mycobacterial infection
- Cat scratch disease (caused by intracellular bacteria *Bartonella* spp.)
- Lymphadenitis
- Toxoplasmosis (protozoal infection again from cats – *Toxoplasma gondi*)
- HIV/AIDS

Investigations

- Bloods – FBC (and differential), biochemistry (including Ca^{2+}, Mg^{2+}, PO_4^{2-}), liver function tests
- CXR pa/lat, lateral nasopharyngeal XR
- Abdominal US
- Abdominal MRI/CT – disease sites measured in three dimensions for later comparison (Fig 6.5)
- PET scan – may help determine need for radiotherapy in HL
- Lumbar puncture and bone marrow/trephine
- Lymph node/mass biopsy
- Dependent on scenario (bone scan, testicular US, Head/spine MRI/CT, cardiac echo, and creatinine clearance)

Staging

- Modified Ann Arbor (Cotswold modification for HL, St Jude modification for NHL)

Surgical guidelines at diagnosis

Hodgkin's lymphoma

Remove entire node and send fresh to assess histopathological node architecture, immunohistochemistry, and molecular analysis. If the disease is localized to single node mass in an otherwise well patient, then resection should be attempted, providing this does not involve extensive surgery (and may allow treatment in lower-risk group).

Staging laparotomy is no longer required.

Non-Hodgkin's lymphoma

Use least-invasive procedure that provides a precise diagnosis. Primary resection in abdominal disease is only indicated for localized disease. Intussusceptions should be resected and mesenteric nodes sampled.

Secondary surgery

A residual mass may need to be resected or biopsied for diagnosis, not treatment.

Mediastinal lymphoma

These tumours can cause grave problems with airway management and need a planned approach. After hydration and allopurinol therapy, assess if pleural effusion or ascites are present which could be tapped and used to confirm diagnosis. If a GA is not thought safe and biopsy is not practical under LA, then pretreatment with steroids ± vincristine to allow shrinkage is preferable.

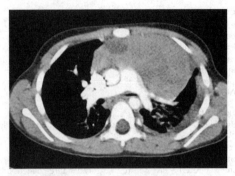

Fig. 6.5 CT showing airway compression by mediastinal mass.

Management
- Essentially multi-agent chemotherapy ± radiotherapy

Examples
- HL – OEPA ± RT ± COPP or COPDAC
- NHL (heterogeneous group)
  - B-cell – COP then COPADM + CYM (5–7 cycles)
  - T-cell – extended leukaemia-type protocol
  - Anaplastic large cell lymphoma – methotrexate-based chemotherapy

Complications of treatment
- Tumour lysis syndrome (NHL)
- Second malignancy(HL)
- Cardiomyopathy
- Infertility

Prognosis
- Hodgkin's lymphoma with risk-adapted therapy has 5-year survival of >90%.
- NHL is a more heterogeneous group but survival ranges from >90% (good risk Burkitt's lymphoma) to 64 % (3-year survival) in poor-risk anaplastic large-cell lymphoma.

Further reading

Paxton V, Dickson MD, Andrew M. Malignant neoplasms of the head and neck. *Semin Pediatr Surg* 2006;**15**:92–5.

Pizzo PA, Poplack DG. *Principles and Practice of Pediatric Oncology* (5th edn). Lippincott, Philadelphia 2005.

Rhabdomyosarcoma

Rhabdomyosarcoma (RMS) is a malignant tumour arising from primitive mesenchymal cells with the potential for differentiation into skeletal muscle. The benign equivalent (rhabdomyoma) occur typically within the tongue or cardiac muscle.

Incidence
- ~5% of all childhood malignancy
- 55 new cases per year in the UK

Clincal features
Age at presentation is 3–5 years with various anatomical sites:
- head and neck (35%), e.g. orbital, parameningeal and non-parameningeal (i.e. ENT, sinuses etc)
- genitourinary tract (25%), e.g. bladder, prostate, paratesticular, vagina, uterus
- extremities (20%)
- other sites (20%), e.g. heart, lung, gastrointestinal and biliary tracts.

The clinical picture depends on the site. Thus, orbital tumours may present with proptosis, chemosis, conjunctival or an eyelid mass. GU tumours present with urinary obstruction, a pelvic, or scrotal mass. Tumours of the extremities present as mass lesions. The initial presentation may be a distant metastasis.

Some RMS have a relationship with various genetic syndromes (e.g. Li Fraumeni, Costello, Beckwith, neurofibromatosis).

Pathology
Rhabdomyoblasts (retaining cross-striations and positive expression for vimentin, desmin, actin, myogenin, etc), divide into embryonal (55%, tend to be younger) or alveolar (20%), depending on degree of differentiation. Two distinct subtypes of embryonal RMS are recognized:
- botryoid (Greek – bunch of grapes) variant is a descriptive term for an RMS arising in association with a mucosal surface (e.g. vaginal and biliary)
- spindle-cell variant arises typically in the paratestis.

Pleomorphic RMS tends to occur only in adults.

Histological types are closely linked to prognosis:
- favourable (embryonal) – orbital, all head and neck (exceptions), all gu (exceptions), biliary
- unfavourable (alveolar) – extremity, trunk, parameningeal, bladder, and prostate.

Prognosis
Prognostic risk groups (low, standard, high, very high) are based on histology, site, patient age, initial size of tumour (<5 cm versus >5 cm) and lymph node disease.

Management

Multi-modality involving surgery, chemotherapy, and radiotherapy targeted to the needs of the individual patient. The treatment plan is guided by the prognostic risk group.

Surgery

The role of surgery must be decided by the multidisciplinary team.

Biopsy

Adequate tissue must be obtained to allow pathological characterization. Specimens must be transported fresh and rapidly to the pathologist. The minimum requirement is multiple needle core biopsies. Fine needle aspiration is inappropriate

Surgical resection

There is no place for mutilating surgery in an attempt to remove large lesions. There is no role for 'debulking'. As this is a chemosensitive tumour, surgery should be reserved for small tumours <5 cm, and for tumours that have achieved maximum response to either chemotherapy, radiation therapy, or both. In such cases the aim should be to achieve complete microscopic excision through an appropriate approach

Primary re-excision

Indicated when there are histologically positive resection margins that are amenable to resection and when achieving complete microscopic resection would avoid the need for intensification of adjuvant treatment.

Chemotherapy

Based on risk group:
- **low risk** – vincristine, actinomycin D
- **standard risk** – ifosfamide, vincristine, actinomycin D (IVA)
- **high risk** – IVA ± doxorubicin (IVADo)
- **very high risk** – IVADo + maintenance therapy

Radiation therapy

This is restricted to patients in standard risk groups with residual disease after excision and all those in high- or very-high-risk groups.

Outcome

Predicted 3-year survival:
- 30–40% for localized very-high-risk tumours
- ~ 90% for low-risk tumours

Further reading

Newton WA Jr, Gehan EA, Webber BL *et al.* Classification of rhabdomyosarcomas and related sarcomas. Pathologic aspects and proposal for a new classification – an Intergroup Rhabdomyosarcoma study. *Cancer* 1995;**76**:1073–85.

Soft tissue tumours

These constitute a diverse group defined according to the tissue of origin (ectoderm or mesoderm). Common pathology encountered in paediatric surgical practice is highlighted.

Congenital epulis/'fibrous tumour'/Neumann's tumour

Granular cell tumour arising from the anterior maxilla in newborn girls (8:1). Resection is curative.

Adipose tissue tumours

Common lesions include lobulated lipomas (~94%), lipoblastomas (~5%), and the rare liposarcomas. Many of these lesions are slow growing and excision is curative. Liposarcoma require chemotherapy where excision may be incomplete.

Desmoid tumours

These are locally invasive tumours arising from musculo-aponeurotic elements. The typical sites are the abdominal wall, retroperitoneum, and skull. They can be associated with Gardner's syndrome. Abdominal lesions may prove challenging to resect due to risk of damage to vital structures. Management may incude radiotherapy and chemotherapy (vinblastine, methotrexate), α-interferon, and imatinib mesylate (Gleevec®) have been deployed to control disease/achieve remission.

Infantile myofibromatosis (multiple synonyms)

Benign fibrous tumour (single or multiple) usually presenting in children <2 years. Typical sites include the head, neck, and torso, but may affect retroperitoneum and extremities. Spontaneous involution may occur (?following massive apoptosis). Although excision is 'curative', postoperative surveillance is recommended as there is a risk of local recurrence (~5%).

Generalized myofibromatosis variants and a rare association with visceral involvement may indicate a poor prognosis with ~70% mortality (cardiovascular/GI complications).

Aggressive ' destructive'/non-resectable lesions – role for chemotherapy (vincristine, actinomycin D, cyclophosphamide), steroid injections, interferon or radiotherapy.

Neurofibromas

These are benign tumours secondary to abnormal proliferation of Schwann cells and accompanying perineural fibroblasts (distinct from Schwannomas). They can be solitary (well-delineated, shiny, and white), or less commonly plexiform (myxoid, 'bag of worms').

Associations

- Von Recklinghausen's disease (NF1, 1 in 3000, autosomal dominant) – café-au-lait spots, acoustic neuromas, gliomas, Lisch iris nodules
- MEN syndromes (type 2B – mucosal neurofibromas, phaeochromocytoma, and medullary thyroid carcinoma)

Occasionally sarcomatous transformation (4% risk in NF1) may occur, indicated by rapid change in tumour size etc.

Management is directed by genetic counselling/screening (patients and family), imaging studies (CT, MR, US), and resection/debulking procedures. There may be a limited role for chemotherapy, immune-targeted treatment and radiotherapy.

Primitive neuroectodermal tumours (PNET)

These can be found in the CNS (e.g. medulloblastoma) but are of more relevance to paediatric surgeons as peripheral tumour and are highly aggressive 'small round blue cell' tumours. These share a common genetic heritage with Ewing's sarcoma of bone.

Genetics
- >90% have characteristic chromosomal translocation (t(11;22)(q24q12)), and stain for MIC2 protein (CD99).

Sites
- Chest wall (sometimes known as Askin's tumour)
- Paraspinal regions
- Extremities (especially upper thigh and buttock)
- Kidney, pancreas, adrenal etc

Management
Chest wall lesions require image-guided biopsy, chemotherapy, and delayed resection. Definitive surgery involves wide resection (rib excised with primary tumour together with rib above and below the lesion to ensure 'field clearance'). Reconstruction techniques (e.g. latissimus dorsi flap/prothetic mesh) are used to restore the body wall defect. Radiotherapy is utilized post-operatively for 'positive margins'.
- Event-free survival ~50% at 5 years

Further reading

Gopal M, Chahal G, Al-Rifai Z *et al.* Infantile myofibromatosis. *Pediatr Surg Int* 2008;**24**:287–91.

Shamberger RC, La Quaglia MP, Gebhardt MC *et al.* Ewing sarcoma / primitive neuroectodermal tumor of the chest wall: impact of initial versus delayed resection on tumour margins, survival and use of radiation therapy. *Ann Surg* 2003;**238**:563–7.

Wiswell TE, Davis J, Cunnigham BE *et al.* Infantile myofibromatosis. The most common fibrous tumor of infancy. *J Pediatr Surg* 1988;**23**:315–18.

Endocrine tumours

Endocrine tumours represent only 3–5% of all tumours in this age group. Presentation may be a mass effect, incidental or related to hormone production. Features and associations are shown in Table 6.5.

Adrenal

Adenomas

These benign tumours are uncommon and usually functional, usually presenting with excess steroid production (Cushing's syndrome – virilization, precocious puberty). Treatment is excision once the diagnosis is confirmed.

Adrenocortical carcinoma

Are extremely rare (~0.2% of all tumours) with metastases being common at presentation. Survival is consequently poor with early presentation, and complete resection offers the only prospect of cure.

Phaeochomocytoma (derived from the adrenal medulla)

These tumours are rare and usually recognized for their excess catecholamine production (hypertension, tachycardia, sweats, headache, and nervousness). CT and MRI are useful and ^{131}I-labelled meta-iodobenzylguanidine (MIBG) can identify active tissue. Pre-operative stabilization with α-blockade over a period should allow correction of fluid and electrolytes with the addition of β-blockade if required. Complete resection should be curative, with chemotherapy and radiotherapy reserved for metastatic or non-resectable disese.

Thyroid

Thyroid carcinoma (follicular and papillary)

A disease of the second decade, this has a strong association with radiation exposure. There has been a reduction in incidence correlating with reduction in therapeutic irradiation, while clusters of tumours are associated with radiation accidents (e.g. Chernobyl disaster). Presentation is commonly a neck mass with cervical lymph node involvement already present in ~75%. Imaging with US can identify nodes and CXR is useful as the lung is a site of early metastasis (~6%). Treatment is surgical (with attention to the recurrent laryngeal nerve and the preservation of parathyroid tissue) followed by radioiodine treatment. Disease-free survival is associated with age (>12 years) and histology (follicular > papillary) and ranges from 83% to 97%. Late recurrence (20 years) is recognized in up to one-third, and long-term follow up is mandatory.

Medullary carcinoma of the thyroid

These represent only 5% of thyroid tumours. The importance of the condition lies with its familial associations, aggressive nature, and early presentation. Survival requires early surgery prior to metastasis. In families with MEN 2A or familial medullary thyroid carcinoma (FMTC), where the *RET* mutations can be demonstrated, a prophylactic thyroidectomy is advocated before the age of 5 years. In families with MEN 2B, the tumour is even more virulent and surgery before 1 year is the current advice.

Parathyroid (see page 213)

Tumours of the parathyroid are rare, presenting with abnormalities of calcium metabolism. Solitary adenomas are most common; however, diffuse hyperplasia of the four glands is a feature of MEN 1 and found in around 30% of MEN 2A patients. Surgical exploration and removal of the affected gland is commonly curative for adenomas, but total resection and limited heterotopic autotransplant may be required in hyperplasia.

Table 6.5 Features and associations of endocrine tumours

	Genes	Syndromes
Thyroid		
Papillary	*RET*	
Follicular	TSH receptor	
Medullary	*RET*	MEN 2A, MEN 2B, FMTC
Adrenal		
Adenoma		
Adrenocortical carcinoma	p53, *CHEK2*	Li-Fraumeni
	p57	Beckwith-Weidemann
Phaeochromocytoma	*VHL*	Von Hippel-Lindau, neurofibromatosis, tuberosclerosis, Sturge–Weber, MEN2A, MEN 2B
Parathyroid		
Adenoma		
Hyperplasia		MEN 1, MEN 2A

Common operations

Circumcision

History
Considered to be the most widely performed operation in the world. Its origins lie are in prehistoric era. Two of the three Abrahamic world religions require circumcision as part of the faith. Circumcision on the eighth day of life is a tenet of the Jewish faith (*Bris Milah*) and is performed by a *mohel*, often a vocation that is passed from father to son. In order to emulate the prophet Mohammed, Muslims also perform circumcision, and, though the timing is less strict, it is usually done well before puberty.

Contraindications
Hypospadias, buried penis, megameatus intact prepuce (MIP) syndrome

Surgical procedure
There are a number of alternative methods, including some non-surgical techniques (e.g. Plastibell® Hollister, Gomko clamp®, Allied Health products).

Freehand method
Retract foreskin completely, stretching phimosis if necessary. Separate all adhesions and clear away all smegma. Reduce the foreskin and press down on the suprapubic fat pad to identify the full length of the penis and the level of the planned skin incision at the level of the coronal groove. Mark this circumferentially and symmetrically. Hold the foreskin with artery forceps (ventral and dorsal in midline) and excise outer skin either by cutting along a cross-clamp (traditionally 'bone-cutters') distal to the glans (and therefore protecting it), or by sharp dissection beginning with a dorsal slit with scissors or scalpel (Fig. 7.1). Trim 'mucosal' layer of skin leaving a narrow (3–4mm) cuff around the base of the glans and angled up towards the frenulum.

Retract the penile skin fully, identify all bleeding vessels and achieve haemostasis – using bipolar (only) diathermy. Suture skin to 'mucosa' around the corona, using absorbable (e.g. 5/0 or 6/0 Vicryl®) interrupted sutures. Place figure-of-eight suture at frenulum to achieve satisfactory cosmesis and secure frenular artery. A circumferential subcuticular suture is also possible (ensure it is not too tight!).

Postoperative management
Always controversial, Most leave the child without any form of dressing to avoid the trauma of its removal. Covering suture line with Vaseline® or chloramphenicol ointment may reduce scabbing and aid healing. Regular baths after 48 h may aid healing and help with uncomfortable voiding.

Complications (more common in community circumcision)
- Bleeding – may requiring re-exploration and haemostasis (if persistent think of possibility of coagulopathy or platelet diathesis)
- Infection – treat with oral antibiotics (IV if cellulitis), newly exposed glans prone to secondary *Staphylococcus* infection
- Meatal stenosis – particularly a risk of BXO is present (~5%). Treat initially with topical betamethasone (0.1%) cream. Meatal dilatation may be required
- Not enough (may require revision) or too much (painful erections)
- Altered sensitivity of glans (controversial)

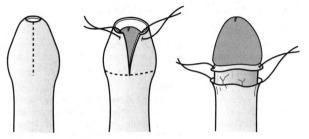

Fig. 7.1 Circumcision. The first stage is a slit at the back of the foreskin.

Skin and soft tissue abscess

Indications and timing

Pus formation comes at the end of an inflammatory process – drainage shouldn't be attempted too early. The hallmark sign is fluctuance.

Causative organisms

Principally *Staphyloccoccal* spp. (MRSA included), occasionally *Steptococcal* spp. but also consider *Coliform* spp. *Klebsiella* etc, in perianal abscesses for instance. Chronicity and atypical behavior in a neck abscess may suggest atypical mycobacteria (e.g. *Mycobacterium avium intracellulare*). Unusual sites may suggest unusual organisms (e.g. scalp abscess, aka kerion, caused by fungal infection). Multiple or recurrent abscesses may suggest underlying host-defence predisposition (e.g. Job syndrome, aka hyperimmunglobulinaemia E; chronic granulomatous disease where host neutrophils lack the capacity to complete phagocytosis), or regional problem (e.g. hidradenitis suppurativa, pilonidal abscess).

Contraindications

High risk of damage to surrounding or deep structures – e.g. large blood vessels. Needle aspiration and antibiotics may be safer in some circumstances.

Anaesthetic

Usually general anaesthesia is needed in the child, but older children may tolerate this procedure with adequate local anaesthesia.

Surgery

Use either a single straight incision parallel with the skin fold (Langer's) lines or a cruciate incision in a large abscess. It is important to gain good separation of the skin edges to prevent primary healing and recurrence.

Procedure

Incise the skin overlying the abscess. Once the cavity is entered, take a swab and ideally collect some pus in a syringe to send for microscopy, Gram staining, and culture. Open the cavity widely, ensuring the skin edges are well separated. Drain all the pus and break down any loculations with gentle curettage. Debride the edges of the cavity with a curette. Wash out the cavity with normal saline and achieve haemostasis with bipolar diathermy as necessary. Consider the need for a 'wick' within the cavity to keep the skin edges apart. While useful, these are often painful to remove. You can use ribbon gauze or paraffin gauze for a wick and remove it after 24 h.

Postoperative antibiotics are not usually required, unless there is evidence of cellulitits, systemic illness, or host immunodeficiency.

Complications

- Nerve damage to adjacent/deep structures
- Haemorrhage – erosion of adjacent vessel
- Recurrence of abscess – especially if edges heal prematurely or if there is an underlying commonication (e.g. fistula-in-ano, branchial or pyriform sinus fistula).

Common nerves at risk

Head and neck (Fig 7.2)

Parotid

Facial nerve (cranial nerve VII) – motor nerve to muscles of facial expression. Exits skull via the stylomastoid foramen, small branch to digastric, occipitalis and stylohyoid, and then becomes enveloped by superficial and deep parts of the parotid gland, where it divides into five branches (temporal, zygomatic, buccal, mandibular, cervical).

- Nerve injury – asymmetry of face, failure to close eyelids, failure to keep food in mouth while chewing

Submandibular triangle (posterior and anterior digastric via hyoid bone, body of mandible)

Submandibular branch of Vth nerve – motor nerve to lower part of orbicularis oris. From parotid, passes inferiorly to just behind angle of jaw. Swings forward to pass superficial (~1 cm in front of angle) to the body and reach the lower lip.

- Nerve injury – drooping of lower lip

Posterior triangle (sternomastoid, trapezius and middle third of clavicle)

Accessory nerve (cranial nerve XI) – motor nerve to sternomastoid and trapezius. Exits skull at jugular foramen, to pass deep to upper third of sternomastoid, and reach the posterior triangle. It is very exposed and passes down across the triangle to reach the deep aspect of the trapezius.

- Nerve injury – limitation of shoulder movement and shrugging deficit. 'brushing hair test'

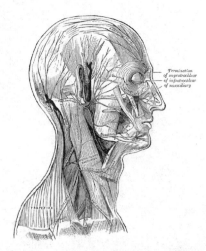

Fig. 7.2 Anatomy of head and neck. Image first published in Gray's Anatomy: Descriptive and Surgical 1858. Reproduced with permission of Elsevier.

Upper limb

- **Median nerve** – motor nerve, supplying flexors of wrist, small muscles of hand. Descends with brachial vessels on medial side of arm to enter antecubital fossa. Leaves between two heads of pronator teres and descends forearm between wrist and digital flexor tendons to pass through carpal tunnel, beneath flexor retinaculum. Gives off important ('million dollar nerve'), but superficial, recurrent branch to thenar eminence as it reaches the palm
- **Ulnar nerve** – sensory and motor nerve, to pre-axial aspect of limb. Descends on medial aspect of triceps, and passes posterior to medial epicondyl of humerus. Enters flexi carpi ulnaris and descends through anterior compartment to join ulnar artery. Passes within Guyon's canal to reach palm
- **Radial nerve** – sensory and motor nerve, to posterior aspect of limb (triceps and extensors). Leaves brachial plexus with profunda brachial artery to gain posterior compartment via triangular space. Winds round back of humerus and passes anterior to lateral epicondyle. Leaves deep to brachioradialis. Supplies extensors and passes posterior to wrist only as sensory nerve

Lower limb

- **Common peroneal nerve** – motor to dorsiflexors of foot, sensory to anterolateral aspect of leg and foot. Leaves popliteal fossa between biceps and gastrocnemius and winds round the neck of fibula to lie on peroneus longus. Divides into deep peroneal nerve (supplies tibialis muscle, extensors) before passing in front of ankle as cutaneous nerve to 1st web) and superficial peroneal, which is mainly sensory but also supplies peroneal compartment
- Nerve injury – foot drop, high-stepping gait. Sensory deficit varies with level, from small patch over distal hallux (deep peroneal), to more extensive strip overlying anterior ankle and up to level of knee (superficial peroneal)

Inguinal hernia

Anatomy

Canal is bounded inferiorly by inguinal ligament ('rolled' lower edge of external oblique, superiorly by overarching conjoint tendon (from internal oblique/transversalis), anteriorly by external oblique aponeurosis, and posteriorly by transversalis fascia. It runs between deep inguinal ring to superficial inguinal ring (triangular deficit with base on pubis, and pubic tubercle lateral.

Inguinal hernias in children are almost invariably indirect (i.e. through both rings), but direct hernias can be seen typically in preterm infants with a grossly stretched deep ring. This usually requires some kind of posterior wall repair (e.g. Bassini, McVay) in addition to the herniotomy.

Open inguinal herniotomy

Indications

Timing is important – the risk of incarceration is highest at <6 months of age, and should prompt early repair. Older children can wait for elective repair as long as the parents are warned to present urgently if there are signs of incarceration. In girls, if ovarian prolapse into a hernia is suspected, repair should be performed as soon as possible due to the risk of ovarian ischaemia. Following reduction of an 'irreducible' hernia, surrounding tissues are usually bruised and oedematous, and the prudent will defer repair for at least 48 h.

Incision

- Skin crease, roughly centred over the deep inguinal ring

Procedure

- Divide subcutaneous tissues and Scarpa's fascia, exposing the external oblique aponeurosis and inguinal ligament.
- Most surgeons split the fibres of the external oblique and enter the canal, which removes one layer of spermatic fascia to dissect through, and avoids the ilioinguinal nerve.
- Next identify the hernial sac by splitting the cremasteric fibres, and pick up the anterior-lying sac with non-toothed tissue forceps. Gently separate the fascia and posteriorly placed vas (medial) and vessels (lateral) and adjacent fascia from the sac, until it is possible to go all the way round. Care and patience are required to do this successfully without damaging structures and while keeping the sac intact.
- Define whether the fundus of the sac is visible or whether it carries on into the scrotum. Divide at the level of dissection between clips. Now, clear adhesions off the sac back to visualize the deep inguinal ring (epigastric vessels medial border). Transfix the sac with 3/0 or 4/0 suture and remove the remainder of the sac.
- Ensure the testis sits in the bottom of the scrotum (consider orchidopexy).

If the sac is inadvertently opened all is not lost! Care and precision are required to successfully complete repair. Either isolate the sac more proximally or place small artery forceps on all free edges of the sac and perform a purse-string-type repair at the deep ring.

Can't find the vas deferens? Look harder, but consider unrecognized cystic fibrosis, or renal agenesis on that side.

In girls, open the sac and inspect contents ensuring the ovary (if visible) is normal. Reduce the contents, transfix, and divide the sac. If the ovary appears abnormal, consider biopsy and rare androgen insensitivity syndrome (aka testicular feminization). Sliding hernias are only a real problem in female hernias – where the medial wall is contiguous with meso-ovary and Fallopian tube. This requires careful dissection to free the whole structure, allowing return and probably closure under direct vision.

Complications

- Synchronous recurrence – risk ~2%. Related to acute repairs, prematurity, underlying abdominal factors (e.g. ascites, VP shunt)
- Metachronous recurrence – risk ~7%; boys = girls, left > right
- Testicular atrophy (1%) – higher risk if previously incarcerated. Presents >6 months
- Damage to vas deferens (incidence not known)
- Chronic pain – perhaps related to ilioinguinal nerve damage

---

Names to impress

- **Littre's (1658–1726) hernia** – sac contains Meckel's diverticulum
- **Amyand's (1680–1740) hernia** – sac contains appendix (first case also allowed the world's first deliberate appendicectomy!)
- **Richter's (1742–1812) hernia** – sac contains less than the whole circumference of the bowel

Laparotomy (aka coeliotomy)

Skin incision (Box 7.2)

Abdominal access requires appropriate exposure. In comparison to adult practice, where midline and paramedian approaches used, most access in infants and children is via a muscle-cutting transverse incision – either above or below the level of the umbilicus.

Specific operations may use a specific approach (e.g. Lanz muscle splitting for appendicectomy; Pfannenstiel* rectus splitting for bladder surgery etc); however, it may be difficult to do much else beyond the wound confines.

> **Box 7.2 Karl Langer (Austrian anatomist 1819–1887)**
>
> Developed concept of cleavage lines, based on experiments involving stabbing corpses with circular implements and finding that the resultant wounds were actually elliptical. They correspond to collagen fibre alignment in the dermis.

Anatomy (Fig 7.3)

Superficial fascia of the abdominal wall is in two layers (Camper's and Scarpa's) – there is no deep fascia as such. The wall is trilaminar with opposed muscle direction. External oblique muscle becomes aponeurotic anteriorly with junction along a line from the tip of 9th rib to the anterior superior iliac spine. Internal oblique and transversus are muscular throughout to the paramedian position of the rectus sheath. This encases two recti, running from the xiphoid to the pubis. The nerve supply runs between IO and transverses. The inferior epigastric runs from medial to the deep inguinal ring to gain access to the posterior rectus sheath, joining with the internal mammary artery from above. Dermatome – umbilicus = T10.

Abdominal wall opening

Muscle-cutting transverse laparotomy

- Incise skin, divide subcutaneous fat and Scarpa's fascia
- Divide anterior rectus sheath – pass tissue forceps under muscle fibres of rectus allowing you to lift these fibres upwards off underlying sheath. Divide with diathermy providing haemostasis
- Enter peritoneum under direct vision between clips avoiding damage to abdominal contents
- Complete division of lateral muscles with diathermy under direct vision. If crossing midline, ligate ligamentum teres (4/0, 3/0 Vicryl®) and divide

Abdominal wall closure

- Technique – mass versus layer:
  - choice often arbitrary – mass or 'all layers' closure typically uses interrupted absorbable (e.g. 3/0 or 4/0 Vicryl in neonates; 2/0 or even 0 Vicryl in older children), suture as 'figure of eight' or 'far and near'
  - layered closure is probably quicker, the suggested guideline for suture: wound length is 4:1

---

* Hermann Johannes Pfannenstiel (1862–1909) – German gynaecologist

- Technique – absorbable versus non-absorbable:
  - latter rarely needed in paediatric practice (possible exception – liver transplantation)
  - choice for former usually between Vicryl® (polyglactin) and PDS® (polydiaxanone); 'wound support' is ~30 and 60 days respectively. Intra-abominal infection probably warrants latter material
- Skin closure – suture versus glue:
  - typical closure would use subcuticular absorbable material (e.g. Vicryl® ~30 days; Vicryl rapide® ~10 days; Monocryl® 20 days), but full- thickness interrupted skin closure may be required in some circumstances (e.g. preterm infants with bowel necrosis and peritoneal soiling due to NEC)
  - advent of topical adhesives (e.g. Dermabond® octocyanoacrylate), has allowed faster skin closure and maybe a lower incidence of wound infection

Complications
- Wound failure
- Wound infection

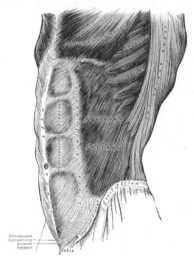

Fig. 7.3 Image first published in *Gray's Anatomy: Descriptive and surgical* 1858. Reproduced with kind permission of Elsevier.

Intestinal anastomosis

Indications
Restoration of intestinal continuity as an elective (e.g. during stoma closure) or emergency (e.g. following resection of irreducible intussusception or NEC) procedure.

Relative contraindications
- Intra-abdominal sepsis and/or widespread inflammation (e.g. acute NEC)
- Ischaemic bowel
- Unrelieved distal obstruction

Procedure (Fig 7.4)
- Division of mesentery
- Bowel-end preparation – ensure no ischaemia, divide with diathermy.
- Full-thickness stay sutures – although 180° is often quoted, if a lesser angle is used this allows the posterior wall to fall away (cf 'triangulation' in vascular anastomoses)
- Anterior wall – commonest method is single-layer seromuscular (Fig. 7.4) using absorbable suture (e.g. 5/0, 6/0 PDS® for neonates, 4/0, 5/0 Vicryl® for infants etc). Knots on outside. Take care at corners – commonest leak points
- Posterior wall – reverse stay sutures to bring to front and complete anastomosis. Knots on outside
- Mesenteric closure

A stapled anastomosis is acceptable in older children and adolescents, and may be considered for some esoteric procedures in older infants (e.g. STEP procedure for bowel lengthening). The pelvis is a difficult area to hand suture in – stapled side–side anastomosis is typically done as part of Duhamel pull-though (GIA-II or ENDO GIA®, Autosuture), or end-to-end anastomosis using a circular stapler (e.g. EEA®, Autosuture) in low anterior resections in adolescents.

Complications
- Early leakage (<2 days) is a technical fault, and if recognized should prompt urgent re-exploration.
- Late leakage – this may be recognized by symptoms of impaired resolution of ileus, increased abdominal pain, and unstable/swinging pyrexia, and if untreated leads to local (sometimes generalized) peritonitis and intra-abdominal abscess formation. X-rays may show a soft-tissue mass and/or pneumoperitoneum, Some can be treated conservatively, particularly if drainage of intestinal content is achieved (perhaps spontaneously through the wound or via an intra-abdominal drain).
- Anastomotic stricture – late complication, often at the site of previous leakage. Presents as bowel obstruction and may need surgical revision.

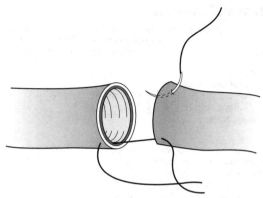

Fig. 7.4 Small bowel anastomosis. Seromuscular sutures pick up two of three layers, and tend to lead to an everted appearance. Use opposite stay sutures to approximate wall.

Further reading

Thornton FJ, Barbul A. Healing in the gastrointestinal tract. *Surg Clin North Am* 1997;**77**:549–73.

Intestinal stomas

Stomas may be formed in the ileum (ileostomy) or colon (colostomy) and occasionally in the jejunum (jejunostomy). In children they are usually temporary, but permanent stomas are required for some conditions.

Indications

Diversion of faecal stream:
- distal obstruction (e.g. Hirschsprung's disease, anorectal malformations)
- distal inflammation (e.g. NEC, colitis)
- distal anastomosis

Incision

Stoma position is important – consider both anatomy and function. Someone (invariably not you) will have to place a stoma bag every day – avoid bony points and skin creases. 'Top of hill, not bottom of valley'.

If stoma is formed as part of a full laparotomy – ?separate stoma or as part of surgical wound (typically these would be temporary).

Procedure

Arguments about the merits of end-stoma over loop are largely spurious if based upon 'overspill' of contents into distal end.
- End stoma (mucous fistula or leave stapled/oversewn distal end within abdominal cavity):
  - excise disc of skin, consider same for muscle
  - mesenteric window – preserving vessels. Divide bowel either with point diathermy or GIA stapler. Control contents with non-crushing clamps if former. Ensure enough bowel can be brought through wall without tension
  - fix to abdominal wall in layers (peritoneum and muscle), then to the skin. Evert mucocutaneous junction by including 'bite' of serosa as well as full-thickness mucosa. Colostomies can be left flush with the skin but aim to form 'spout' in ileostomy (so-called Brooke ileostomy). This protects skin and allows close-fitting appliance
- Loop stoma:
  - classically requires skin bridge. Use 'V' or inverted 'W' skin incision to achieve this
  - mesenteric window, avoid marginal artery (of Drummond) in transverse colon
  - fix both limbs to anterior abdominal wall in layers. Pass the 'V'-shaped bridge through the mesenteric window
  - incise antimesenteric border of the colon, evert edges of stoma, and suture these to the skin incision.

If a stoma is formed using abdominal incision, ensure *secure* interrupted suture closure of muscle layer – wound failure with a stoma leaking intestinal contents is a disaster.

Complications (20–30%)

- Necrosis – look at stoma closely in early postoperative period – most have some degree of oedema and venous engorgement. Overt necrosis suggests devascularization, too much tension, or not enough abdominal wall defect
- Stomal prolapse – typically transverse colostomy – if recurrent consider revision and suture of entry limb to underside of abdominal wall.
- Stricture – associated with ischaemia
- Retraction – associated with ischaemia and tension
- Skin excoriation – jejunostomy > ileostomy > colostomy. Consider use of skin protection e.g. Cavilon® spray
- Parastomal hernia – failure of muscle layer, needs revision
- Fluid loss and electrolyte imbalance – especially in small infants with an ileostomy. Oral NaCl supplements and regular monitoring of urine Na$^+$ levels (aim for >20 mmol/L)

Appliances

- One-piece versus two-piece, e.g. Stomahesive wafer and flange/ Natura® closed bag (ConvaTec)
- Closed versus drainable bags

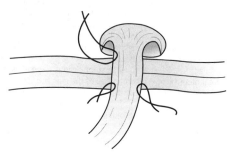

Fig. 7.5 Eversion ileostomy. Suture the internal serosa to the peritoneum and muscular layer to fix the stoma. Evert edge by taking three 'bites' with mucocutaneous suture.

Further reading

ConvTek UK http://www.convatec.co.uk/UK/ (accessed 16 July 2008).

Millar AJ, Lakhoo K, Rode H et al. Bowel stomas in infants and children. A 5-year audit of 203 patients. S Afr J Surg 1993;**31**:110–113.

Nour S, Beck J, Stringer MD. Colostomy complications in infants and children. Ann R Coll Surg Engl 1996;**78**:526–30.

Posterolateral thoracotomy

This is the typical approach for most lung and oesophageal procedures. In the older child, selective bronchial intubation may be desirable for unilateral procedures.

Positioning

Full lateral with legs flexed; arm on operative side lies forward and upwards and may require support. A small bolster placed under the chest may open the opposite rib space and improve exposure. Supports and adhesive strapping are required to prevent rolling.

Incision (Fig 7.6)

- Skin marking of ribs or tip of scapula may help orientation. Gentle upward curve from anterior axillary line, 1 cm below tip of scapula, to border of erector spinae muscles.
- Conventional – muscle cutting (latissimus dorsi and serratus anterior) in line of skin incision to reach subscapular plane. Protect long thoracic nerve (C5, 6, 7) running on anterior border of serratus anterior.
- (Alternative but preferred by senior author – muscle splitting. Develop superior and inferior skin flaps. Identify anterior border of latissimus dorsi and separate adjacent and underlying serratus along intermuscular plane. Stretch both muscles to reach subscapular plane.)
- Elevate scapula, count down from uppermost rib (should be 2nd) to identify desired rib space (typically 3rd/4th for OA and TOF; 4th/5th for upper lobectomy, 5th/6th for lower lobectomy or diaphragm.
- Divide intercostal muscles (keeping to upper border of rib avoiding damage to neurovascular bundle.
- Extrapleural approach – use moist swab or peanut to gently sweep away parietal pleura from the underside of the ribs and intercostal muscles posteriorly. Continue until azygous vein and apex of lung are exposed.
- Transpleural approach – open avoiding underlying lung.

Use suitable rib retractor (e.g. Finochietto) to maintain exposure. Two are required for the muscle-splitting approach.

Closure

Consider need for local anaesthesia into intercostal muscles and chest drain. Place absorbable (e.g. 3/0 – neonates, 2/0 – older infants and children, Vicryl®) sutures around ribs for approximation (not too tight). Anatomical repair of muscles. Close fascia and skin.

Specific complications

- Damage to nerve supply to serratus anterior (long thoracic nerve) results in winging of scapula.
- Incision over scapula may cause adhesions resulting in restricted movement and unsightly scar.
- Tight closure of ribs (especially in infant) may affect development of chest wall and cause scoliosis in severe cases.

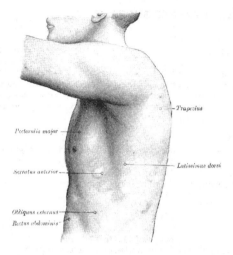

Fig. 7.6 Landmarks of thorax. Image first published in Gray's Anatomy: Descriptive and surgical 1858. Reproduced with kind permission of Elsevier.

Minimal access surgery

General considerations

MAS is a relatively new development in paediatric surgery with the first paediatric laparoscopic appendicectomy reported in 1991 and laparoscopic fundoplication in 1993. Most procedures can be successfully completed using a minimal access approach, but the widely reported applications include: diagnostic laparoscopy, appendicectomy, gastric fundoplication, cholecystectomy, splenectomy, inguinal herniorrhaphy, pyloromyotomy, bowel resection, nephrectomy, and pyeloplasty.

Advantages

- Smaller incisions, reduced wound complications, better cosmesis
- Reduced tissue trauma – decreased inflammatory response
- Magnification of the operative field
- Reduced postoperative pain, shorter hospital stay

Disadvantages

- Carbon dioxide insufflation
- Two-dimensional image and lack of tactile feedback
- Greater expense – initial cost and consumables,
- Technically difficult to perform, longer duration of operations, increased difficulty with haemostasis
- Learning curve

Training

MAS is particularly amenable to simulation training. Simulators range from simple self-constructed boxes to advanced computer programs that deliver realistic tactile feedback for a range of operations.

Pre-operative considerations

Patient selection

Some patients may be unsuitable for MAS because of:

- decreased respiratory function
- anatomical anomalies, e.g. severe kyphoscoliosis
- adhesions from previous surgery
- small size (>2.5 kg for therapeutic laparoscopy).

Consent

In general, the risks and complications are similar to the equivalent open procedures with the addition of:

- conversion to open procedure
- risks of carbon dioxide insufflation, e.g. gas embolus
- damage to internal organs

Bowel preparation

- Give as per any regime used for the equivalent open procedure
- For upper GI surgery, consider giving an enema 2 h pre-operatively, to improve visibility by deflating the transverse colon

Anaesthetic room considerations

- Minimize bag/valve/mask ventilation

- Minimize use of nitric oxide
- Early gastric decompression with a naso- or orogastric tube
- Empty the urinary bladder with a catheter or the Crede manoeuvre

Operative considerations
- Patient positioning – see Fig. 7.7
- The skin is prepped and draped over an area which will permit unhindered conversion to an open procedure if necessary
- Many surgeons prefer insertion of the first port by an 'open' technique over Verres needle insufflation, to minimize the risk of visceral injury(Box 7.2)
- Port positioning – see Fig. 7.8

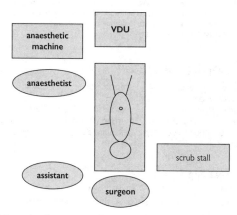

Fig. 7.7 Principles of patient positioning in MAS. The patient and equipment are positioned so that the operating surgeon faces the visual display straight on, while allowing appropriate access for monitoring and intervention by the anaesthetist.

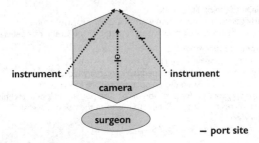

Fig. 7.8 Port positioning in MAS. Working ports are positioned to facilitate ergonomic manipulation of the instruments and triangulate with the centre of the camera view. The camera should face in the same direction as the surgeon to avoid the difficulty of paradoxical movements.

Box 7.2 Open (Hasson) access

- Replaced previously popular Veress needle technique, as it is intrinsically safer
- Subumbilical curved incision – expose linea alba and base of umbilicus. Insert 2/0 Vicryl 'J' suture to lift midline into wound. Incise, longitudinally, through linea. Blunt dissection through parietal peritoneum.

Further reading

Davenport M. Laparoscopic surgery in children. *Ann R Coll Surg Engl* 2003;**85**:324–30.

Zitsman JL. Pediatric minimal access surgery: update 2006. *Pediatrics* 2006;**118**:304–308.

Laparoscopic inguinal hernia repair (infants)

Access

- Open (Hasson) insertion of 3 mm or 5mm umbilical port
- 0° endoscope
- Under direct vision, make a 3 mm stab incision laterally in the flank just above the level of the umbilicus and insert a 3 mm tissue grasping forceps directly through the incision without a port
- Repeat on the contralateral side but insert a 3 mm needle driver loaded with a 4/0 monofilament non-absorbable suture on a 17 mm round-bodied needle cut to a length of 10–12 cm
- The suture should be loaded onto the needle holder by grasping the suture itself 2–3 cm behind the needle and applying not more than two clicks of the needle holder ratchet mechanism

Procedure (Fig 7.9)

- Inspect the genitalia in girls and examine the degree of hernial defect on both sides. Reduce contents if possible.
- Pick up the peritoneum forming the neck of the sac with the forceps and close the defect with one or two sutures. A purse string, Z-stitch or a combination of both may be used.
- Avoid the vas deferens medially and the testicular vessels inferiorly. Both should fall away from the peritoneum as it is picked up.
- Some surgeons incise the peritoneum laterally at the neck of the sac and resuture it to stimulate a more-intense inflammatory response and increase scarring.
- A contralateral PPV (or hernia) may be closed in an identical fashion without changing instruments or position.

Complications

- Synchronous recurrence ~2–8%
- Testicular atrophy ~1%
- Damage to vas deferens (incidence not known)

Laparoscopic fundoplication

Positioning

Patient

- Infants and small children 'frog-legged' at the foot of the operating table
- Older children – legs apart at the end of the table (?abductable leg plates or Lloyd–Davies stirrups). Avoid lithotomy poles
- Post-port insertion – reverse Trendelenberg (head up) position
- Use large orogastric Maloney bougie

Surgeon

- 'French position', i.e. between the patient's legs

Ports

- Sub-umbilical 5mm port (for camera)
- Hypochondial 3 mm or 5 mm working ports (×2) – to provide a 60° angle in relation to the hiatus
- 4th port (below and lateral to the left hypochondrial port) used to retract fundus or a loop of tape around the distal oesophagus
- Also – left lobe of the liver is best retracted using a Nathanson retractor, of appropriate size, placed through a small stab wound just below the xiphisternum

Procedure (Fig 7.9)

- Retract the fundus of the stomach caudally using grasping forceps. Open the lesser omentum using a diathermy hook to the right of the oesophagus. Continue dissection across phreno-oesophageal ligament to the left side of the oesophagus, expose left limb of the crura
- Short gastric vessels may be divided at this stage or left intact according to the surgeon's preference
- Create posterior window behind the oesophagus by blunt dissection to identify posterior vagus. Aim to achieve a good length (2–3 cm in an infant, 3–4 cm in an older child) of intra-abdominal oesophagus
- Approximate two limbs of the crus behind the oesophagus – 2/0 Ethibond suture on a ski needle. Advance the bougie to ensure that the hiatal closure is not too tight
- Pass a grasping forcep through the retro-oesophageal window to pull the fundus through to the right side of the oesophagus – if tight then certainly divide short gastric vessels. The 'shoeshine manoeuvre' is performed by grasping the fundus on either side of the oesophagus, and sliding from side to side ensures that a loose symmetrical wrap will be achieved
- Construction of wrap – initially a single 2/0 Ethibond suture (ski needle) approximates the wrap in front. Further sutures are placed on either side the top incorporating the upper edge of the hiatus and the lower the anterior wall of oesophagus to prevent migration. Use bougie to check for tightness

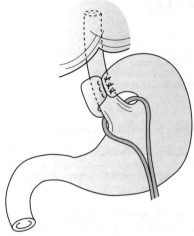

Fig. 7.9 – 360° fundoplication (after Nissen). Sling around GOJ to improve traction and mobilize sufficient distal oesophagus.

Thoracoscopy

Indications

- Oesophageal atresia repair, duplication cyst, Heller's myotomy
- Diaphragmatic hernia repair, plication of diaphragm
- Empyema thoracis, lobectomy, sequestration, lung cysts, lung biopsy
- Aortopexy, PDA ligation, sympathectomy, tumour biopsy, tumour resection, thoracic duct ligation

Positioning

Infant

- Lateral decubitus position – lung biopsies, decortications, lung resections
- Semi-prone position with the affected side slightly elevated – for oesophagus etc
- Supine position with the affected side elevated slightly – for anterior mediastinal structures

Surgeon

- Right or left with the monitor opposite him
- Anterior and the posterior mediastinum – the surgeon stands on the side of approach
- Lobectomy – best place is standing facing the patient
- For some procedures a monitor on either side of the patient is ideal to enable the surgeon to move to the opposite side of the patient if necessary.

Port sites

As the chest wall is rigid and the ribs prevent free mobility of instruments, careful thought as to the position of the ports is required.

For lung biopsies, the camera port may best be placed in the mid-axillary line below the level of the tip of the scapula. Peripheral lesions can often be excised after snaring with an Endoloop®, but if a linear stapler is to be used then care must be taken to place a 12 mm port in the lowest interspace possible and as anterior as possible to prevent undue damage to the ribs and to ensure that there is room to open the device.

Insufflation of CO_2 to a pressure of 6 mmHg is sufficient to deflate the lung. Double-lumen tubes for single lung ventilation are only suitable in older children. A bronchial blocker may be used in younger patients, but positive pressure insufflation of CO_2 is usually satisfactory.

Normal laparoscopic instruments may be used. Lung tissue can be divided and sealed satisfactorily with one of the pulsed bipolar devices such as the PlasmaKinetic® device (Gyrus PLC) or LigaSure® (Valleylab). Intracorporeal suturing in the newborn requires advanced endoscopic skills, as the available space is extremely limited.

Urology

Undescended testes

The most common congenital anomaly in male genitals, with an incidence rate of 2–4% at birth, falling to 1% at 1 year (Fig 8.1).

Classification
- Palpable testis: 80%
  - extracanalicular
  - ectopic
  - intracanalicular
- Non-palpable testis: 20%
  - intra-abdominal
  - absent or atrophic (5%)

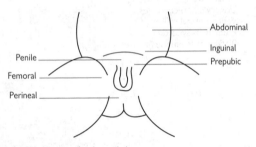

Fig. 8.1 Possible location of undescended testes.

Clinical features

Aim to manipulate the testis into the scrotum if possible. Retractile testes have a normal length of spermatic cord but because of an exaggerated cremasteric reflex have only the briefest stay in the scrotum. These usually have a normally developed hemiscrotum. Those with a short spermatic cord are confirmed as undescended. Ectopic testes have a normal-length spermatic cord but have ended up in an aberrant position.

If nothing can be felt, a groin ultrasound is a reasonable non-invasive investigation and may detect up to 90% of intracanalicular testes, otherwise laparoscopy is indicated in order to distinguish between true absence and an intra-abdominal testis.

> **Warning!**
> Beware the infant with bilateral impalpable testes. This may represent ambiguous genitalia and require early endocrine and genetic evaluation.

Management

Hormonal therapy

Human chorionic gonadotrophin (HCG) or luteinizing hormone-releasing hormone (LHRH) have been used to stimulate testicular descent with a claimed success rate of ~20%.

Surgery

The timing of orchidopexy is controversial but current opinion ranges from 6 to 18 months.

Orchidopexy for palpable testes

The testis is mobilized through an inguinal incision; by division of the distal gubernacular remants, opening the canal, and separating the vas and vessels from the processus, which is ligated at the level of the deep inguinal ring. Further length may be gained by freeing the vessels as they lie in the retroperitoneal space. The now-mobilized testis is placed and fixed in a sub-dartos scrotal pouch.

Intra-abdominal testis

Laparoscopy gives precise visualization of the testis, its size, and quality. If it can be drawn to the contralateral ring it may be suitable for a single-stage orchidopexy – most are not however. Alternatively, a staged Fowler–Stephens procedure may be done, involving a preliminary ligation, clipping, or diathermy to the testicular vessels.

Follow-up

For those boys with retractile testis, an annual follow-up is advised, as at puberty 33% will descend spontaneously, 33% will remind retractile, but 33% will have become truly undesccended and require surgery ('ascending testis syndrome').

Complications and prognoses

Infertility

Alteration in spermatogenesis has been described in boys >6 months. This may affect fertility (sperm count) but not necessarily paternity (possibility of becoming a father).

Cancer

This is a controversial area and the perceived risk has changed over the years from a quoted 40-fold increase in risk to ~6-fold for unilateral UDT and ~10-fold for BUDT, currently. Nonetheless, risk calculation would suggest that of 100 boys treated by a surgeon, one would develop malignancy during their adult years. Parental counselling is advocated.

Further reading

Barthold JS, Gonzalez R. The epidemiology of congenital cryptorchidism. Testicular ascent and orchiopexy. *J Urol* 2003;**170**:2396–401.

Patil KK, Green JS, Duffy PG. Laparoscopy for impalpable testes. *BJU Int* 2005;**95**:704–708.

Acute scrotum

Testicular torsion

Torsion is a surgical emergency with two anatomical types: extravaginal where the twist is outside the tunica and at the level of the spermatic cord and found in neonates, and intravaginal where the twist is within the tunica due to the ('bell-clapper' defect). The peak age of onset in the latter case is during adolescence.

Outside the neonatal period, torsion is an acutely painful event, usually accompanied by vomiting. The scrotum is tender and erythematous, and the testis may have a high, horizontal lie. Doppler ultrasound or radio-nuclide testicular scans have been described but essentially the diagnosis should be established at open operation. The timing of detorsion determines outcome with a >50% testicular loss rate if performed after 6 h, falling to 25% after 12 h. Fixation of the contralateral testis is mandatory.

Torsion of the hydatid of Morgagni

This condition typically occurs just prior to puberty at ~12 years. Clinically the pain and swelling are less severe and the torted remnant may be visible as a 'blue-dot' at the upper pole of the testis. These can be treated conservately if the diagnosis is secure, although surgical operation removes both doubt and the infarcted hydatid.

Epididymo-orchitis

The peak age in childhood is from 3–5 years, with either a viral or an ascending urinary bacterial aetiology. Management is conservative and antibiotics are used in case of bacterial infection; however, if there is *any diagnostic doubt*, surgical exploration should be done. It is important to investigate for underlying congenital urinary anomalies (i.e. ectopic ureter) on confirmation of a bacterial cause.

Testicular trauma

The patient with a history of testicular trauma is presented initially with pain and localized oedema. On physical examination it is important to palpate the testicular consistency, looking for scrotal haematoma and/or testicular damage.

Scrotal ultrasound may give information on the degree of testicular compromise and information about possible testicular rupture. In stable patients with mild trauma (most of the cases) management is conservative (rest, analgesic, scrotal support). Patients with severe trauma should undergo surgical exploration, aiming to repair tissue damage.

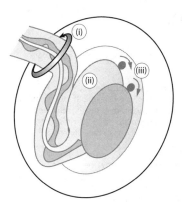

Fig. 8.2 Three common causes of the acute scrotum in children. (i) Intravaginal torsion, (ii) acute epidydmitis, and (iii) torsion of a hydatid of Morgagni (there are two).

Further reading

Davenport M. ABC of general surgery in children. Acute problems of the scrotum. *BMJ* 1996;**312**:1358–9.

Varicocele

Incidence
- 6% of 10 year-year old boys and 15% of adult males

Aetiology
Failure of the venous valve mechanism. About 90% are left-sided and this is suggested to arise from the different mode of entry of the right and left testicular vein into the vena cava or left renal vein. The right junction is acute, whereas the left junction is at 90°. It is rarely associated with a left-sided renal tumour and venous encroachment.

Clinical features
Usually asymptomatic but may be noticed by the patient/parent. Occasionally some complain of a dragging sensation. Boys must be examined in standing position with Valsalva manoeuvre. US (with colour-flow Doppler) should be performed to measure testicular volume and check for renal masses. Varicoceles are graded by severity.

Subclinical varicoceles are impalpable but detected on scanning:
- grade 1 – palpable only on Valsalva
- grade 2 – palpable but not visible at rest
- grade 3 – palpable and visible at rest.

Large varicoceles may cause some discomfort and cosmetic concerns, and hence treatment is indicated, but treatment of asymptomatic varicoceles remains controversial.

> There is an increased incidence of varicocele in infertile men (~30%).

Surgery has been shown to improve sperm counts in some. The testicle on the affected size may be smaller, and surgery in adolescents may result in catch-up growth. Some advocate surgery for all, others reserve intervention for large symptomatic varicoceles and those with poor testicular growth. The risks of conservative treatment must be weighed against the risk of surgery.

Surgery
The principle of surgery is to occlude the venous drainage. This may be achieved by radiographic embolisation or surgical ligation. Ligation may be performed laparoscopically, trans- or retroperitoneal. Open surgical approaches may be high retroperitoneal (Palomo) or within the inguinal canal (Ivanissevich). The testicular vessels are mobilized and the veins ligated (with or without ligation of the testicular artery – in the latter case the blood supply is via vasal vessels).

Ligation of the testicular artery decreases the recurrence rate but is associated with a 5% risk of testicular atrophy and 5% risk of hydrocoele due to ligation of associated lymphatics. Subsequent vasectomy is contra-indicated.

Recurrence
- Varicocele recurrence ~20%

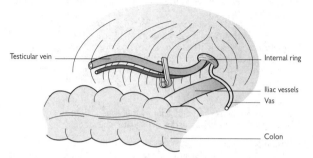

Testicular vein

Internal ring

Iliac vessels

Vas

Colon

Fig. 8.3 Laparoscopic view of the internal ring with tortuous testicular vein. Clip applied to both artery and vein.

Further reading

Diamond DA. Adolescent varicocele: emerging understanding. *BJU Int* 2003;**92**(Suppl 1):48–51.

Madden NP. Testis, hydrocoele and varicocoele. In: Thomas DFM, Rickwood AMKR, Duffy PG (eds). *Essentials of Paediatric Urology*. London: Martin Dunitz, 2002, pp198–201.

Phimosis and paraphimosis

Phimosis may be defined as a condition where the foreskin is unable to be retracted to expose the glans. The word itself is derived from the Greek for 'muzzling' (φιμωσις).

At birth >96% of boys have an adherent, non-retractile foreskin – falling to 50% by 1 year, 10% by 3 years and 1% at 17 years. This can be termed 'physiological' phimosis. This is never obstructive to voiding and rarely requires surgical intervention. Nonetheless, phimosis can be pathological, arising probably as a result of recurrent local infection, inflammation and scarring.

Aetiology

During development, the epithelium of the glans and inner prepuce are fused, natural separation occurring during later childhood.

Clinical features

Voiding difficulty may manifest simply as 'ballooning', but occasionally this can become severe and obstructive with a fine stream. Collections of smegma may predispose to overt bacterial infection. Balanitis implies inflammation of the glans; posthitis, inflammation of the foreskin.

Balanitis xerotica obliterans

This occurs in older boys and adolescents (peak age 11 years) and is much more severe, with dense, whitish tissue affecting not only the foreskin but also the glans and meatus. Aetiology is not really understood but often thought of as a variant of *lichen sclerosis et atrophicus*. It typically requires circumcision, although topical steroids or tacrolimus have also been suggested.

Management

The aim of treatment is to achieve either painless, easy foreskin retraction, or circumcision. There are a variety of non-circumcision options which include topical steroids (e.g. 0.1% betamethasone, applied to the foreskin bd for one month), retraction under anaesthesia, and preputioplasty (Box 8.1).

Box 8.1 Preputioplasty

The foreskin is retracted. There is usually a clear phimotic band which should be divided by multiple small longitudinal incisions which are closed transversely. This increases circumference. Postoperatively, parents are instructed to mobilize the foreskin once the initial oedema has settled. Recurrence is ~20%.

Circumcision is described on page 322.

Paraphimosis

This is a condition where the foreskin is able to be retracted but becomes stuck in that position – invariably resulting in oedema, swelling, ischemia, and pain. (Fig 8.4)

Management

This is a surgical emergency and reduction should be attempted by manual compression of the glans and traction on the prepuce under local, regional, or general anaesthesia (as appropriate). Creation of multiple small holes in the oedematous foreskin with an orange (26g) needle may allow fluid to be squeezed out thereby facilitating reduction (Dundee technique). Occasionally, a dorsal slit to divide the constriction ring and relieve the ischaemia is required. Consideration should be given to later circumcision as cosmesis is usually poor.

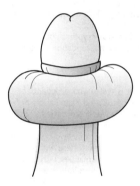

Fig. 8.4 Subcoronal, oedematous preputial band.

Further reading

Davenport M. Problems with the penis and prepuce – ABC of paediatric surgery series. *BMJ* 1996;**312**:299–301.

Elder JS. Circumcision, urethral prolapse, penile torsion, buried penis, webbed penis and mega-lourethra. In: Frank JD, Gearhart JP, Synder HM (eds). *Operative Pediatric Urology* (2nd edn). London: Churchill Livingston, 2002.

Gardiner D. The fate of the foreskin. A study in circumcision. *BMJ* 1949;2(4642):1433–7.

Oster J. The further fate of the foreskin. *Arch Dis Child* 1968;**43**:200–203.

Hypospadias

Hypospadias (*hypo* – under and *spadias* – rent, Greek), the most common congenital abnormality of the penis, has three components:
- ventrally placed urethral meatus
- ventral chordee (downward curvature) of the penis
- ventral deficiency of the prepuce ('hooded' prepuce).

Incidence
- ~1 in 300 males
- Most recent studies suggest an increase in incidence but more data are required to validate these findings

Epidemiology
There are recognized familial risks (up to 20% increased risk with affected father/siblings) and racial differences (white > black, increased incidence in Jewish and Italian families). Unilateral cryptorchidism (~9%) and inguinal herniae (~9%) are not uncommon.

The presence of bilateral cryptorchidism necessitates urgent exclusion of disorders of sexual differentiation (DSD), i.e. karyotype, hormone profile, etc.

Aetiology
Urethral development is testosterone dependent, either by fusion of the genital folds or by apoptosis-led cannulation between 8 and 20 weeks' gestation. The process moves from base to tip, meeting the glandular-ingrowth at the level of the corona (this complex junction may account for the frequency of defects at this level). Some research has postulated that endocrine disrupters may interfere with androgen pathways, but few cases have demonstrable abnormalities in the androgen-signalling systems. Population studies suggest dietary influences (increased incidence in vegetarian mothers) and environmental agents (oestrogens – environmental or phyto-, plasticisers, and pesticides) may play a role.

Clinical features
Hypospadias is commonly diagnosed at birth. Initial evaluation should include a general examination, antenatal history, and specifics of the hypospadias (meatal position, degree of chordee, the appearance of the prepuce and scrotum). Testicular position should also be documented (bilateral cryptorchidism requires emergency endocrine/urology review). The position of the meatus is usually described using the terms in Fig. 8.5. Parents must understand circumcision is contraindicated as the prepuce may be required for corrective surgery.

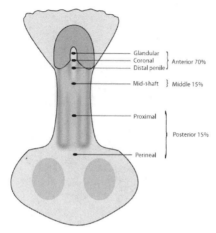

Fig. 8.5 Classification of hypospadias.

Surgery

Contemporary procedures aim to straighten the penis, move the meatus to the tip, and improve the cosmetic appearance. In the UK, surgical repair is generally recommended for all but the most minor defects, but practice does vary worldwide. The operation is often performed in the first year of life; however, more-complex repairs may be delayed until endocrine evaluation and response to testosterone is assessed. The surgical technique is dependent upon patient factors (age, meatal position, chordee, glans size, depth of glanular 'groove', previous surgery etc), and surgeon preference. There is no consensus but surveys suggest the majority of UK and North American surgeons favour the principles of the procedures outlined below.

Tubularized incised (urethral) plate (TIP or Snodgrass)

This technique is commonly used for primary, anterior, or middle repairs, and has gained popularity as it gives good functional and cosmetic results with acceptable complication rates. Having released the skin and demonstrated correction of the chordee, a 'U'-shaped incision around the urethral plate is made and the edges mobilized. A longitudinal midline incision is then made and the edges are tubularized over an appropriate calibre stent (Fig. 8.6). Usually, a further 'waterproofing' layer of tissue is placed over the repair (developed from prepuce or dartos) and the glans is approximated. Depending on the surgeon and parental preference, the foreskin can be reconstructed or excised.

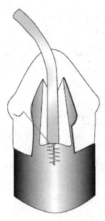

Fig. 8.6 Snodgrass procedure.

Two-stage (Bracka) technique

This is more commonly used in proximal hypospadias with marked chordee and redo procedures. The penis is prepared by excising the abnormal or scarred ventral tissue, correcting the chordee, opening the glans, and preparing the corpora for the graft. A full-thickness graft is harvested (prepuce, buccal mucosa, or post-auricular skin) and sutured onto the prepared ventral surface of the penis. The graft is allowed to mature and after a minimum interval of 6 months, a tubularized urethroplasty is performed.

Postoperative care

Most surgeons use a catheter (urethral or suprapubic) and a pressure dressing to minimize bruising (foam, swab, Tegaderm® etc) for 7–10 days. Oral antibiotics, regular analgesics, and anti-spasmodics are usually given whilst the catheter is *in situ*.

Specific complication

Fistulas (2–15%) require further surgical closure, and stenoses (1–4%) may require dilation or meatotomy. Total disruption of the repair is rare (<1%). Overall, the more severe the lesion the higher the incidence of complication.

Further reading

Baskin LS. Ebbers MB. Hypospadias: anatomy, etiology, and technique. *J Pediatr Surg* 2006;**41**:463–72.

Manzoni G, Bracka A, Palminteri E, Marrocco G. Hypospadias surgery: when, what and by whom? *BJU Int* 2004;**94**:1188–95.

Sharpe RM. The 'oestrogen hypothesis' – where do we stand now? *Int J Androl* 2003;**26**:2–15.

Snodgrass WT. Snodgrass technique for hypospadias repair. *BJU Int* 2005;**95**:683–93.

Disorders of sex development

Definition

Any congenital condition in which development of chromosomal, gonadal, or anatomic sex is atypical.

Clinical features

Presentation might include newborn anatomical gender uncertainty, an apparent sex differing from antenatal karyotype, female virilization, failure of puberty, or primary amenorrhoea.

Enquire about parental consanguinity, family history of early neonatal deaths (adrenal insufficiency), disorders of pubertal development (5α-reductase deficiency), primary infertility, maternal medications in pregnancy (placental transfer of androgens), and evidence of virilization during the pregnancy (androgen-secreting tumour or placental aromatase deficiency).

Look for the presence or absence of gonads, with particular attention to the inguinal orifices. Bilateral undescended testes always require investigation. The degree of virilization can be described in terms of Prader staging, with a measurement of the phallus length, if applicable (Fig. 8.7). The position of urethral and vaginal (if present) openings and the degree of labial–scrotal fusion, rugosity, and pigmentation should also be described. Medical photography is often helpful.

Investigations

- Urgent karyotype
- Baseline and serial electrolytes
- 17-hydroxyprogesterone (OHP) (if congenital adrenal hyperplasia is suspected
- US of the pelvis/urogenital tract (may require expert interpretation)

Further investigation for diagnosis requires specialist multidisciplinary team input including paediatric endocrinologists, urologists, gynaecologists, psychologists, geneticists, and specialist nurses. Where there is doubt, a neonate should not be assigned a sex of rearing, and the registration of the birth of the child should be delayed. Parents need to be supported and reassured that the baby will be given a definite sex assignment.

Further investigations

- FSH, LH, inhibin B, AMH, androstenedione, dehydroepiandrosterone sulphate (DHEAS), testosterone, and dihydrotestosterone
- ACTH, synacthen test with serial cortisol, and 17-OHP measurements, urinary steroid profile
- 3-day and 3-week HCG testing

Management

This is dependent on the diagnosis and the appearance of the external genitalia. Where possible, surgery for cosmetic appearance, rather than function, should be delayed until the affected child can be involved in the decision. Bilateral gonadectomy should be considered for dysgenetic gonads (risk of gonadoblastoma) and testes present in a child with a female sex of rearing (virilization at puberty). The fertility of the child and the need for hormone replacement are also considered. Expert psychological input is required from diagnosis to adulthood.

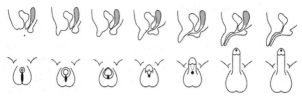

Fig. 8.7 Prader staging system – differential virilization of the external genitalia from normal female (left) to normal male (right). From *Helvetica Paediatrica Acta* 1958; **13**: 5–14.6. With kind permission of Springer Science and Business Media.

Further reading

Lee PA, Houk CP, Ahmed SF, Hughes IA. Consensus statement on management of intersex disorders. International Consensus Conference on Intersex. *Pediatrics* 2006;**118**:e488–e500.

Renal anomalies

Embryology

There are three stages in renal development: (i) pronephros, (ii) mesonephros, and (iii) metanephros. The ureteral bud arises from the caudal end of the mesonephric duct (4th week gestation) and ascends into and is engulfed by the metanephros. There is both true and relative ascent to reach their final position by the 8th week. The arterial supply is serial from adjacent vessels, unlike the descending testis which retains its original supply throughout.

Epidemiology

- ~10% of the general population has some kind of renal anomaly.

Renal agenesis

- 1 in 4000 (bilateral – Potter's syndrome) 1 in 1000 (unilateral), L > R
- Infants with Potter's syndrome, have severe oligohydramnios, may be stillborn (40%), and have a characteristic facies (epicanthic fold extending onto cheek). Those born alive will have fatal respiratory failure

URA is usually associated with absence of ureter and a hemi-trigone on cystoscopy. Genital anomalies (e.g. bicornuate uterus, absence of the vas and seminal vesicle) are also commonly seen; ~30% show extrarenal anomalies (cardiovascular, vertebral etc).

Horseshoe kidney

- 1 in 500, M > F
- Associated with Turner (XO) syndrome, and Trisomy 18 (Edward syndrome)
- Possible predisposition to malignancy (e.g. Wilms')
- Is a variant of renal fusion whereby the lower poles join in the midline (below origin of inferior mesenteric arteryfrom aorta). The renal pelves remain anterior, with the ureter crossing in front of the isthmus

Clinical features

- One-third will be asymptomatic.
- Most problems can be attributed to PUJ obstruction, with consequent urolithiasis.

Management is directed at definition of PUJ obstruction. If surgery is indicated then it is usually advisable to leave the isthmus intact.

Crossed renal ectopia

- 1 in 7000
- A variant of renal fusion whereby the ectopic kidney crosses the midline, leaving its ureter still with a contralateral insertion. Typically, the inferior of the two kidneys is the one that has crossed.

Multicystic dysplastic kidney (MCDK)

- 1 in 4300 live births, M > F, L > R
- There is replacement of normal renal parenchyma by multiple cysts of varying size, and it is possibly due to ureteric obstruction at some point in early fetal life
- ~ 33% of MCDK are palpable
- ~50% have other GU anomalies (e.g. PUJ and reflux). Therefore, it requires further functional studies such as US, MCUG and radio-isotope studies (e.g. MAG3)

Clinical features

- Involution is common and ~20% become non-detectable by 1 year.
- Whether they cause symptoms is actually unclear. Rare possibilities include newborn respiratory distress (if huge), hypertension, and malignant change (handful of cases).

Management is controversial, for the symptomic or palpable, nephrectomy is reasonable but the rest could be left alone.

Cystic kidney disease

This is a complex area with confusing nomenclature:

- **autosomal recessive polycystic kidney disease** occurs in 1 in 6000 live births and is due to a mutation on Ch6p. This causes both renal and hepatic pathology with spongy renomegaly (but rarely gross cystic change), and hepatic fibrosis (which may cause portal hypertension)
  - most affected children will develop end-stage renal failure early in life, if not as newborns
- **autosomal dominant polycystic kidney disease** occurs in 1 in 500 live births, and arises as a result of a mutation(s) of the *PKD1* gene on Ch16 or *PKD2* gene on Ch4. Most children with ADPKD are asymptomatic, but there is a small number who develop life-threatening renal failure. Most, however, go on to adult life. Pathologically there are bilateral macrocysts, and extrarenal involvement can include liver cysts, mitral valve disease, aortic aneurysms, and intracranial aneurysms. More mundane perhaps, but there is also a much higher incidence of inguinal hernias.

Renal cysts

Most are solitary, affect the upper rather than lower pole, and are asymptomatic, requiring little in the way of treatment.

There are a number of rare associations (e.g. tuberous sclerosis, Meckel syndrome, and Von Hippel–Lindau disease), of which cysts in the kidney may be one manifestation.

Urinary tract stones

Only 1–3% of all urinary stones occur during childhood. Importantly though, such stones may indicate the presence of an underlying metabolic disorder or anatomical abnormality, and in some cases may result in significant long-term morbidity (renal failure).

Epidemiology

Highest risk of stone formation is in boys (M:F = 4:1), those with a positive family history of stone disease, associated bladder dysfunction, and children with metabolic abnormalities. Lower urinary tract stones are commoner in developing countries, while industrialized nations have a higher incidence of upper tract stones. The commonest age at presentation is between 5 and 9 years. Metabolic abnormalities predisposing to stone formation include hypercalciuria, hyperoxaluria, hyperuricosuria, and hypocitraturia.

Clinical features

Younger children generally present with a greater stone burden and primarily with renal calculi. Commonest symptoms include urinary tract infection, haematuria, and abdominal pain. In contrast, older children and adolescents present with acute flank pain (renal colic) and babies with non-specific features, such as nausea, 'off colour', weakness, and malaise.

Investigations

- US with a combined IVU/DMSA is the usual pathway of choice in the paediatric age group. Unenhanced spiral CT scan is the current gold standard in diagnosis for adults but has a far more selective role in children
- Serum calcium, phosphate, electrolytes, urea, creatinine and uric acid
- 24-h urine collection – for calcium/creatinine or oxalate/creatinine ratio

Management

Extracorporeal shock wave lithotripsy (ESWL) is the treatment of choice, with excellent stone-clearance rates but does require general anesthesia in infants and young children. For larger stones, percutaneous nephrolithotomy (PCNL) is safe and effective. With the advent of smaller and flexible endoscopes, ureteroscopy allows safe and effective stone clearance of ureteric stones. Open surgery is now reserved for those with anatomical abnormalities, such as PUJ obstruction. Due to the multifactorial causes of stones in children, good long-term outcomes of surgery can only be achieved when combined with the assessment of metabolic abnormalities to prevent recurrence.

Urinary obstruction

Definition

Any restriction of urine flow which, if left untreated, will cause progressive deterioration of renal and/or bladder function. Table 8.1

Lower tract obstruction

This can present with antenatal urinary tract dilatation, voiding, and bladder dysfunction, culminating in urine retention, with occasional haematuria, UTI and even renal failure. In adolescents, there may be symptoms of sexual dysfunction. A bladder may be palpable.

Table 8.1 Urinary obstruction (lower)

Cause	Sex	Associations
Urethral causes		
Meatal stenosis	M	BXO, post-circumcision
Post-hypospadias	M	e.g. Snodgrass repair
Urethral stricture	M	congenital versus acquired (e.g. trauma/catheter)
Urethral polyps	M	
Anterior urethral valves	M	e.g. Valve of Guerin
Syringocele	M	Dilatation of Cowper's duct in anterior urethra
Posterior urethral valves	M, (1 in 5000)	
Pelvic masses or collections		
Hydrometrocolpos	F	i.e. imperforate hymen, vaginal agenesis
Cloaca/urogenital sinus		congenital adrenal hyperplasia
Pelvic tumours	M < F	e.g. sacrococcygeal teratomas, neuroblastoma, rhabdomyosarcoma
Prolapsing ureterocele	M << F	duplex kidney
Bladder or sphincter dysfunction		
Functional bladder outlet obstruction		i.e. detrusor sphincter dyssynergia Down's syndrome
Neuropathic bladder	M > F	e.g. spinal dysraphism, anorectal malformation, and acquired (trauma, ischaemia)
Miscellaneous		
Prune belly syndrome	M	See page 374
Drugs	M	Anticholinergics

Upper tract obstruction

As urinary tract obstruction almost always causes dilatation, it is frequently detected with antenatal US scanning. This now accounts for the majority of cases and the challenge is to identify those cases with true obstruction from the non-obstructed dilated systems. Other symptoms might include UTI, sepsis, abdominal pain, renal colic, abdominal mass, haematuria, and renal failure. Table 8.2

Table 8.2 Urinary obstruction (upper)

Cause	Sex	Associations
Vesico-ureteric junction obstruction (VUJO)	M:F 3:1	Vesico-ureteric reflux
Ureteral stenosis or valves	M > F	Multicystic dysplastic kidney
Pelvi-ureteric junction obstruction (PUJO)	M:F 2:1	Vesico-ureteric reflux, VUJO, multicystic dysplastic kidney
Stones		See p364
Extra-luminal causes		Appendix mass, tumour, e.g. neuroblastoma, rhabdomyosarcoma; retroperitoneal fibrosis, vascular

Clinical features

Acutely there may be signs of pain, sepsis, dehydration, and acidosis. A mass, suprapubic or loin, may be palpable. Look for signs of spinal dysraphism (e.g. meningomyelocele, hairy tuft, skin lesion, buttock wasting, absent anocutaneous reflex, etc).

A standard investigation protocol should include urinalysis, haematology, and biochemistry, with renal imaging such (US and MCUG), spinal imaging (if necessary), together with functional isotope renography. In some cases urodynamics and endoscopy will be needed.

Initial treatment

- Resuscitate and correct electrolyte disturbance and acidosis and treat associated sepsis
- Drainage of infected obstructed system by bladder catheterization (urethral or suprapubic) and ureteric stent or percutaneous nephrostomy insertion for the kidney
- Use subsequent assessment of kidney and bladder function to direct further definitive treatment

Definitive operative approach

See Table 8.3.

Table 8.3

Cause	Treatment
Meatal stenosis, urethral stricture	Dilatation/meatotomy or meatoplasty, optical urethrotomy, urethroplasty
Urethral polyp, anterior urethral valves, syringocele	Endoscopic excision/incision
Posterior urethral valves	Endoscopic incision, vesicostomy, ureterostomy (uncommon)
Hydrometrocolpos	Incise imperforate hymen
Cloaca etc	Surgical reconstruction
Pelvic tumours	Chemotherapy, radiotherapy, surgical excision
Prolapsing ureteroceles	Endoscopic puncture, excision
Functional BOO	Alpha-antagonists (e.g. alfuzosin, tamsulosin)
Neuropathic bladder	Intermittent catheterization, anticholinergics (e.g. oxybutynin, tolterodine), bladder/sphincter reconstruction
VUJO	Stent, ureteric re-implantation
Ureteral stenosis or valves	Excisional ureteroplasty
PUJO	Pyeloplasty (Hynes–Anderson), either open or laparoscopically
Extraluminal causes	Initially endoscopic stenting of ureter/treat mass and ureterolysis

Postoperative assessement

This should consist of both clinical assessment and radiological imaging to ensure there is free drainage of urine. For simple cases such as PUJO, early discharge is possible, but for other causes such as neuropathic bladder and posterior urethral valves, lifelong follow-up is required to monitor renal, bladder, and sexual function.

Complications

Most can be anticipated and described as non-specific (e.g. bleeding, urine infection) or due to recurrence (e.g. strictures). However, some are specific to the condition (e.g. renal failure is seen in ~30% of PUV, bladder obstruction due to formation of flap-valve after endoscopic puncture of a ureterocele).

Further reading

Gearhart JP, Rink RC, Mouriquand PDE (eds). *Pediatric Urology*. (Editors) WB Saunders Company, 2001. Philadelphia

Thomas DFM, Rickwood AMK, Duffy P (eds). *Essentials of Paediatric Urology*. Martin Duntz Ltd, 2002. London

Vesicoureteral reflux

Primary vesicoureteral reflux (VUR) is the most common urological anomaly in children It occurs in 30–50% of children who present with urinary tract infection. It is associated with UTI and renal damage. Parenchymal injury in VUR occurs early (<3 years), and most renal scars are present when reflux is discovered at initial evaluation for UTI.

Epidemiology
• 1–2% of paediatric population
• Higher incidence in siblings (up to 50%) and offspring

Aetiology
The ureterovesical junction (UVJ) acts as a valve and closes during micturition or when the bladder contracts. The main defect in patients with vesico-ureteral reflux (VUR) is believed to involve malformation of the UVJ, in part due to shortening of the submucosal ureteric segment due to congenital lateral ectopia of the ureteric orifice. Since VUR primarily involves abnormalities of the ureter and ureteric orifice, it has been suggested that the timing and positioning of branching of the ureteric bud from the Wolffian duct may be related to VUR. The underlying abnormality could be due to mutations in one or more developmental genes that control these processes.

Management
Controversial. The two main options available for the treatment of VUR are medical or surgical.

Medical
This strategy is based on three important assumptions:
• sterile VUR in most cases is not harmful to the kidneys and has no relevant effect on kidney function
• children can outgrow VUR (at least the lower grades)
• continuous low-dose antibiotic prophylaxis can prevent infection for many years while VUR is still present.

The patient is required to take low-dose daily antibiotics (±bladder training) and anticholinergics together with annual US and MCUG for assessement. However, the International Reflux Study Group has shown that 84% of the children with grade III and IV reflux randomly allocated to medical treatment still have reflux after 5 years. In those with bilateral reflux, 91% had persistence of reflux after 5 years. (Fig 8.8)

Surgery
Anti-reflux procedures
The majority of the open anti-reflux procedures entail opening the bladder and performing a variety of procedures on the ureters such as transvesical reimplantation (Politano–Leadbetter technique) and transtrigonal advancement of the ureters (Cohen technique). These procedures, although effective, involve open surgery and prolonged in-hospital stay and are not free of complications, even in the best hands. Although open surgery achieves a success rate of up to 98% in grade II–IV VUR, the American Urological Association report on VUR reported persistence of VUR in 20% of ureters after re-implantation of ureters for grade V reflux. The rate of obstruction after reimplantation needing re-operation varies from 0.3 to 9.1%.

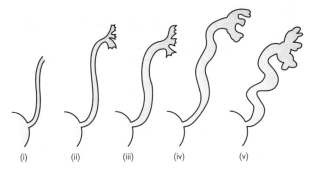

Fig. 8.8 International Reflux Study Group. Grade (i) – non-dilated ureter, not reaching pelvis; (ii) reflux up to pelvis; (iii) dilated ureter with normal pelvicaliceal anatomy; (iv) dilated ureter and abnormal caliceal blunting; (v) gross ureteric tortuosity, and deformation and dilatation of pelvi-caliceal anatomy.

Endoscopic treatment of VUR (Box 8.2)

This has several advantages over other options. In contrast to long-term antibiotic prophylaxis, it offers immediate cure of reflux with a high success rate, its success does not rely on patient or parent compliance, and the procedure is virtually free of adverse side-effects.

Indications
- High-grade primary VUR (grade III–V)
- VUR in duplex renal systems
- VUR secondary to neuropathic bladder and posterior urethral valves
- VUR in failed re-implanted ureters

Box 8.2 Technical notes – endoscopic injection

- Any paediatric cystoscope can be used for this procedure.
- Use either a disposable Puri flexible catheter (STORZ) or a rigid metallic one attached to a 1 mL syringe pre-filled with Deflux®.
- Introduce needle under the bladder mucosa 2–3 mm below the affected ureteral orifice at the 6 o'clock position.
- In children with grade IV and V reflux with wide ureteral orifices, the needle should be inserted not below but directly into the affected ureteral orifice.
- The needle is advanced about 4–5 mm under the mucosa and the injection started slowly. As the Deflux® is injected, a budge appears in the floor of the submucosal ureter. A correctly placed injection creates the appearance of a nipple on the top which is a slit-like or inverted crescent orifice.

Patients are treated as day cases and an MCUG and ultrasound are performed 6–12 weeks after discharge.

Endoscopic subureteral injection of Deflux® is excellent first-line treatment in children, with 87% success in high-grade VUR after one injection.

Further reading

Menezes M. Puri P. The role of endoscopic treatment in the management of Grade 5 primary vesi-coureteral reflux. *Eur Urol* 2007;**52**:1505–10

Puri P, Pirker M, Mohanan M et al. Subureteral dextranomer\hyaluronic acid injection as first line treatment in the management of high grade vesicoureteral reflux. *J Urol* 2006;**176**:1856–60.

Prune belly syndrome

Definition

The typical features include:
- a deficit in abdominal wall musculature
- bilateral cryptorchidism
- dilated urinary tracts.

However, both females and males without all three characteristics also occur. Also known as Eagle Barrett syndrome and the triad syndrome.

Incidence

- ~ 1 in 40,000

Epidemiology

- 97% male with 100% discordance in monozygotic twins

Aetiology

Not known; however, there are a number of hypotheses including transient bladder outflow obstruction, a primary mesodermal defect involving a developmental arrest between the 6th and 10th week of gestation, and an abnormality of yolk sac regression.

Associated anomalies

Include pulmonary hypoplasia, pneumothorax, cardiac defects (tetralogy of Fallot), gastrointestinal anomalies (e.g. malrotation, atresias, anorectal malformation, 'wandering' spleen), and orthopaedic anomalies (e.g. leg deformity secondary to fetal compression, scoliosis).

Clinical features

The antenatal ultrasound may show a dilated urinary tract, but other more common causes exist. The condition should be apparent at birth, with the characteristic floppy wrinkled abdominal appearance and impalpable testes. The abdominal wall allows palpation of the dilated urinary tract but ultrasound confirms the presence of this third feature.

The differential diagnosis might include antenatal causes of urinary tract dilation, including PUVs, severe VUR, and megacystis-microcolon.

The most prognostic feature is the degree of renal dysplasia and associated abnormalities. Some may be stillborn or die soon after birth due to respiratory insufficiency (secondary to oligohydraminos), some may have normal renal function and good urinary tract dynamics and require little intervention. Most, however, are intermediate and require individualized multidisciplinary management.

Management

This includes full assessment for associated abnormalities, CXR, and prophylactic antibiotics. Catheterization or instrumentation should be avoided as there is high risk of urinary tract infection due to stasis of urine. Urological management is rarely urgent, and aims to preserve renal function by preventing infection and, rarely, relieving obstruction. Subsequent close monitoring and management of renal function and infection are required.

Multiple surgical procedures may be required, although routine surgical correction of the dilated urinary tract is controversial. Urinary diversion for recurrent UTIs or deteriorating renal function may be useful. Circumcision may be performed to reduce the incidence of urinary infection. Rare cases with true urethral obstruction will require intervention. Orchidopexy should be performed, although fertility is unlikely. Abdominoplasty may improve cosmesis. One-third will develop end-stage renal failure and require transplantation. Poor bladder emptying may be managed by intermittent catheterization.

Long-term survival depends on the severity of the renal dysplasia, and one-third of infants who survive develop renal failure.

Further reading

Eagle JF, Barrett GS. Congenital deficiency of abdominal musculature with associated genitourinary abnormalities: a syndrome. *Paediatrics* 1950;**6**:721–36.

Skoog SJ. Prune belly syndrome. In: Belman AB, King LR, Kramer SA (eds). *Clinical Pediatric Urology*. London: Martin Dunitz, 2002, pp947–83.

Woodhouse CRJ, Ransley PG, Innes-Williams D Prune belly syndrome – report of 47 cases. *Arch Dis Child* 1982;**57**:856–9.

Bladder exstrophy

Embryology

Bladder exstrophy results following incomplete closure of the inferior, anterior fetal abdominal wall. Within the first 8 weeks of gestation there is failure of migration of mesenchymal cells between the ectoderm of the abdominal and the urogenital and anorectal canals. The aetiology is unknown.

Definition

Classical bladder exstrophy is characterized by a low-lying umbilicus, exposed bladder plate, diastasis of the pubic symphysis, and abnormal genitalia. In males, this constitutes severe penile epispadias and in females anterior vaginal ectopia and bifid clitoris. Anterior anal ectopia occurs in both sexes.

Incidence

- ~ 1 in 40,000 live births
- M:F = 2:1

Associated conditions

Spina bifida and cleft palate, although congenital renal abnormalities are surprisingly uncommon (<2%). Preterm birth and gastrointestinal anomalies may also co-exist.

Clinical features

Antenatal ultrasound may show a permanently empty fetal bladder, normal kidneys, low-lying umbilicus, and in males a short penis with dorsal chordee.

Reconstructive surgery

The aims are to preserve renal function, achieve urinary continence, and create or preserve cosmetically acceptable and functionally normal external genitalia. Controversy, however, exists as to the initial surgical technique.

Staged reconstruction

This includes closure of the bladder plate and posterior urethra soon after birth with delayed epispadias repair (~6–12 months) and bladder-neck reconstruction (modified Young–Dees–Leadbetter procedure) at ~3 years.

Complete primary repair (Schrott and Siegal)

This is a newer technique involving closure of the bladder plate and epispadias repair ±ureteral re-implantation in one stage shortly after birth.

Iliac osteotomy

Controversy also exists as to the use, timing and type of iliac osteotomy. If the diastasis is <4 cm and primary repair is undertaken within 6 days of birth then the pubis can usually be approximated without osteotomy.

Complications

- **Cutaneous fistulae –** (up to 16%), e.g. urethrocutaneous or vesico-cutaneous fistulae, with no real difference if the complete repair is performed.
- **Epididymitis** (up to 30%) – this can be a recurrent problem in older age-groups adults. Occasionally, orchidectomy, vasectomy, or epididymectomy may be required.
- **Bladder stone formation** – stones are common and secondary to chronic infection with urease-producing organisms (e.g. *Proteus* spp.). The incidence is increased post-augmentation (up to 50%). The cause is multifactorial but factors include recurrent infection, stasis, and urinary biochemical abnormalities such as raised oxalate and low citrate.
- **Risk of malignancy** – there is an increased risk of malignancy in both native exstrophy bladders and intestinal augments. Although rarely performed now, the highest risk occurred when urine was diverted into the faecal stream (e.g. ureterosigmoidostomy). Overall risk of neoplasia in adults born with exstrophy has been estimated as ~17% (i.e. 65x that of normal population).

Outcome

- **Renal function** – early series showed poor renal function with 10% of those with ureterosigmoidstomy dying of renal failure. VUR is common (>90%) and probably due to high vesical pressures; detailed evaluation is required to determine whether any deterioration is secondary to lower tract dynamics.
- **Urinary continence** – this is highly variable ranging from 12% to 83%, but mostly achieved with self-catherization (urethral or Mitrofanoff) and bladder augmentation. Care must be taken to avoid high bladder pressures. Important factors quoted for achieving urinary continence include successful initial bladder closure, adequate bladder capacity prior to BNR, female sex, and pelvic osteotomies.
- **Psychosexual development and fertility** – several studies have reported dissatisfaction with genital and body appearance – nonetheless, sexual and genital function is adequate. Males may suffer from ejaculatory problems. Fertility may be variable but assisted reproductive technology offers potential solutions to complex fertility problems.

Further reading

Bladder Exstrophy Family Association. http://www.bladderexstrophy.co.uk/index.html (accessed 16 July 2008).

Gargollo PC. Borer JG. Contemporary outcomes in bladder exstrophy. *Curr Opin Urol* 2007;**17**:272–80.

Smeulders N, Woodhouse CRJ. Neoplasia in adult exstrophy patients. *BJU Int* 2001;**87**:623–8.

Trauma, burns, and blast

General considerations

Epidemiology (UK statistics)

- Accidental injury remains the biggest single cause of death for children (>1 year)
- ~16% of deaths in the 1–4 years age group
- ~40% of deaths in teenagers
- More than 2 million children attend A&E departments each year as a result of injuries
- Boys are more commonly injured than girls

Mechanisms of injury

- Blunt trauma (most common)
- Burns/scalds.
- Penetrating trauma (least common)

A detailed history of the mechanism of injury is essential, including accurate timelines. The possibility of non-accidental injury should always be considered if there is any inconsistency between the history and the nature of the injuries sustained.

Patterns of injury

The anatomy of the child, including the large head and the pliable skeleton means that even relatively minor degrees of force can result in significant internal injury. Solid organs are more vulnerable to the effects of blunt trauma in children than in adults. Head injuries are most common in children <1 year, limb injuries are prevalent in older children. Abdominal injury is rare in infants (if it occurs ?non-accidental injury). Children with thoracic injury will also have significant injuries to other body areas in 85% of cases.

Mortality from injury in UK children remains low, and has been falling for the last 15 years, possibly due to safety features (e.g. car seats, seat belts, and cycle helmets).

- overall mortality ~3.5%
  - head injuries ~7%
  - for multisystem injuries, mortality may reach 50% (especially if the head and thorax are involved)

Organization of trauma care

This should include pre-hospital care, immediate in-hospital response teams, and definitive care strategies including transport systems. In some countries, hospitals are categorized according to their ability to manage trauma patients (level 1–3 trauma centres). The multisystem nature of many injuries means that different teams of specialists may be involved simultaneously; coordination of care and overall responsibility for the patient should be clearly defined. All paediatric trauma victims with a history of a significant trauma should be met and assessed on arrival by a trauma team. A&E departments in non-paediatric general hospitals should have a designated paediatric specialist member in the immediate response trauma team.

Immediate care

Mortality from trauma is significantly reduced if active resuscitation and treatment is commenced within the first hour after injury (Golden Hour®). This is the basis for the principles of treatment employed in the Advanced Trauma Life Support (ATLS) and Advanced Paediatric Life Support (APLS) courses.

Treatment is directed at stabilizing and maintaining the airway, breathing, and circulation (ABC) prior to definitive diagnosis and treatment of other specific injuries.

Initial management

The optimal management of the ABCs in children requires knowledge of normal paediatric anatomy and physiology, which differs from that of the adult. Normal values for paediatric respiratory rate, pulse, and blood pressure vary with age (Table 9.1).

The volume of resuscitation and maintenance fluid required and drug doses are weight dependent.

> Weight (kg) = (age in years x 2) + 8
>
> (alternatively – height/weight nomogram, for example a Broselow tape, can be attached to the side of the trolley)

> Estimated blood volume = 80 mL/kg

If there is any evidence of circulatory compromise, a 20 mL/kg crystalloid fluid bolus should be given. If normal haemodynamic values are not achieved, a second crystalloid bolus is required. Further bolus requirements should be given as whole blood or packed cells to replace blood loss. Maintenance fluids should be given separately and should include 5% dextrose (especially important in infants).

Injury prevention

The majority of childhood injuries are avoidable and could be prevented with appropriate attention to safety measures. Parents should be supported through the treatment of their child without adding further guilt to their experience, but information on appropriate preventative measures should be given prior to discharge. Useful factsheets on the prevention of all types of paediatric injury are available from the Child Accident Prevention Trust in the UK (www.capt.org.uk).

Table 9.1 Normal paediatric physiological values

Age (years)	<1	2–5	6–12	>12
Respiratory rate (breaths/min)	30–40	20–30	15–20	12–16
Heart rate (beats/min	110–160	95–140	80–120	60–100
Systolic blood pressure (mmHg)	70–90	80–100	90–110	100–120

Further reading

Buntain WL (ed). *Management of Pediatric Trauma*. Philadelphia: WB Saunders Company, 1995.

Dykes E. Paediatric trauma. *Br J Anaesthesia* 1999;**83**:130–8.

Eichelberger MR (ed). *Pediatric Trauma: prevention, acute care, rehabilitation*. Chicago: Mosby Year Book, 1993.

Greaves I, Porter K, Ryan J (eds). *Trauma Care Manual*. London: Arnold, 2001.

Thoracic trauma

Incidence

Significant injury to the thorax occurs in 5% of children admitted following trauma. Thoracic injuries are rarely isolated, and most occur in association with injuries to other body systems. The presence of a thoracic injury significantly increases the risk of mortality, particularly in children with an associated head injury (mortality >50%).

Aetiology

Thoracic injuries may be the result of blunt or penetrating trauma. The paediatric chest is particularly vulnerable to blunt trauma due to the incomplete ossification of the rib cage. Severe internal thoracic injury may occur in the absence of rib fractures. In children, the most common cause of thoracic injury is blunt trauma, usually from falls or motor vehicle accidents.

Types of injury

Penetrating trauma

This can result in laceration to any or all thoracic organs, including the pericardium and diaphragm. They may also cross the diaphragm and damage intra-abdominal organs. Look for common injuries such as pneumothorax, haemothorax, or a combination of both. Pericardial or cardiac laceration is rare but may present as cardiac tamponade. Oesophageal or aortic damage may also occur.

Blunt trauma

This can result in compression injury of the lungs and major vessels, even in the absence of rib fractures. Pneumo/haemothorax, pulmonary contusion and aortic rupture should all be considered and excluded in patients with blunt force chest trauma. Diaphragmatic rupture is also possible in severe compression injury.

Clinical features

A low threshold of suspicion for intrathoracic injury should be held if the mechanism of injury indicates the possibility of significant blunt force trauma.

Any abnormality in the airway, breathing, or circulation (ABC) should raise the possibility of intrathoracic injury. Increased rate or work of breathing, tracheal shift, abnormal chest movement, poor air entry, or reduced oxygen saturation are all indicators of significant intrathoracic damage. Hypovolaemia is exacerbated by raised intrathoracic pressure from tension pneumothorax or cardiac tamponade.

Investigations

CXR will demonstrate most pneumo/haemothoraces but signs may be subtle in the supine patient and the films should be examined carefully. Pulmonary contusion may not be evident radiologically in the first few hours after injury. Absence of rib fractures does not exclude the possibility of significant pulmonary contusion. After stabilization, patients with suspected severe thoracic injury may require CT scan ± angiography.

Management

Initial management of all thoracic injuries should follow the ATLS principles of stabilization of the ABCs. Any child with an abnormality in airway, breathing, or circulation should be given 100% oxygen. Suspected or proven pneumo- or haemothorax should be treated by the insertion of an intercostal drain. Acute tension pneumothorax should be initially relieved by the rapid insertion of a thoracostomy cannula in the mid-clavicular line on the affected side, prior to insertion of a chest drain (Box 9.1). Supportive ventilation and adequate chest drainage is the mainstay of management of thoracic injury.

Box 9.1 Insertion of chest thoracostomy tube

- Choose appropriate size for drainage of blood/fluid (e.g. 16–20 Fg, but depends on age/size)
- Mid-axillary line, 5th–6th intercostal space (count down from manubriosternal angle – 2nd rib). Aim to site above 6th rib (avoids neurovascular bundle)
- Local anaesthetic infiltration
- Incision down to intercostal muscles then *blunt* dissection with artery forceps (or finger in adolescent) into pleural cavity
- Insert clamped tube – direct tip to base for fluid and apex for air
- Attach to underwater seal, drain and unclamp. Secure chest tube

Thoracotomy is rarely required following blunt force trauma except for severe persistent bleeding or major vessel injury. Penetrating trauma from gunshot wounds should always be explored and such cases should be referred to a thoracic surgeon without delay.

Further reading

Bliss D, Silen M. Pediatric thoracic trauma. *Crit Care Med* 2002;**30**(11 Suppl):S409–15.

Nakayama DK, Ramenofsky ML, Rowe MI. Chest injuries in childhood. *Ann Surg* 1989;**210**:770–5.

Sartorelli KH, Vane DW. The diagnosis and management of children with blunt injury of the chest. *Semin Pediatr Surg* 2004;**13**:98–105.

Abdominal trauma

Incidence

Significant intra-abdominal injury occurs in approximately 4% of children admitted following trauma. Isolated abdominal injury is common in children (>60% cases) and should have a low mortality, but when combined with head or thoracic injury, the mortality rises steeply.

Aetiology

The majority of abdominal injuries result from blunt force trauma. The intra-abdominal solid organs are particularly vulnerable to blunt trauma in children, due to the relatively poor protection offered by the wide shape and incomplete ossification of the rib cage. The commonest causes of intra-abdominal injury in children are falls and road traffic accidents. Even falls from a low height can cause significant intra-abdominal damage if the child strikes another solid object such as a table during the fall. Penetrating injury is rare in children, but when it occurs there may be damage to many vital structures including the diaphragm. Abdominal injury in children <18 months of age should raise suspicion of non-accidental injury.

Types of injury

Penetrating trauma

Although less common, penetrating injury may occur in children. This includes wounds from a knife, gunshot, fence-posts, etc.

Blunt force trauma

Injuries to the spleen, liver, and kidneys are the usual result of blunt force trauma. The majority are simple contusions, but severe force may cause significant lacerations, fracture, or even avulsion. Compression injuries (e.g. handlebar or seatbelt injuries) can also result in intestinal perforation or pancreatic laceration. Deceleration forces from falls or traffic accidents may cause mesenteric or great vessel tears. Bladder and urethral injuries are rare but may occur with pelvic trauma, even in the absence of obvious fractures.

Clincal features

The history needs to be detailed with respect to mechanism (e.g. seatbelt lap strap may suggest intestinal or pancreatic injury, fall over bicycle handlebar may suggest pancreatic injury) and degree of force sustained.

Careful examination (and re-examination) are vital in assessing the possibility of injury. Tenderness or distension should be considered evidence of injury until proven otherwise. Haematuria (microscopic or macroscopic) should lead to further investigation of the urinary tract.

Investigations

Abdominal US may be useful for the initial assessment of doubtful cases, but CT scan (IV and enteral contrast) remains the standard. Peritoneal lavage is now rarely used in children.

Management

• Initial attention to ABC – as always

Abdominal injuries may result in significant hidden blood loss – any circulatory compromise should raise the possibility of bleeding. Although the majority of solid organ injuries can be treated conservatively, high-dependency or intensive care monitoring is essential in the early stages to ensure there is no further bleeding.

Specific organ injury

Liver trauma

Most injuries are contusions or small subcapsular haemtomas which may be treated conservatively (bed rest ~1 week). Significant lacerations (particularly if they involve the porta hepatis, vena cava, or hepatic vein confluence) may be life-threatening, and management may involve surgery (e.g. partial hepatectomy) or interventional radiology (e.g. embolization) – early consultation with a regional centre is advised. Late complications of conservative management include biliary leakage into the peritoneal cavity and secondary infection of haematomas.

Pancreatic trauma

This typically occurs after innocuous blunt force trauma often in boys, and often involving a bicycle. The neck of pancreas (and its duct) is most at risk as it lies just anterior to the vertebral column and becomes crushed by the application of epigastric blunt force. Hence the child is initially well but later develops abdominal pain and tenderness as traumatic pancreatitis ensues. Serum amylase is invariably raised. Outcome depends usually on whether the duct has been lacerated or not. CT or MR scan will aid diagnosis but ERCP is the only definitive investigation. Management is usually conservative but both endoscopic duct stenting and early open surgery (usually distal pancreatectomy) have been advocated for defined duct trauma.

Splenic trauma

The degree of injury ranges from laceration, to avulsion. Evidence of on-going haemorhage suggests a need for laparotomy – however, in practice, surgical intervention is now uncommonly required. Splenectomy should be avoided wherever possible because of the risks of post-splenectomy sepsis (see page 249)and other techniques of splenic preservation should be considered (e.g. direct suturing, partial splenectomy etc).

Intestinal trauma

May be subdivided into:
• mesenteric injury – haematoma or laceration, followed usually by intestinal ischaemia
• actual traumatic perforation.

Extravisceral air (on x-ray or CT scan) or leakage of oral contrast mandates laparotomy, as delayed diagnosis may result in widespread peritoneal contamination and sepsis. Duodenal rupture may be particularly difficult to diagnose because of its retroperitoneal situation and lack of clear abdominal signs.

Renal trauma

The degree of injury ranges from capsular haematoma to pedicle avulsion and may present as haematuria, or as expanding retroperitoneal haematoma. Renal injury is often seen in multiple injuries.

Pelvic fracture may result in significant intra-abdominal bleeding. Pelvic stabilization and transfusion is the optimal management in this situation. Surgical exploration should be avoided due to the risk of exsanguinating haemorrhage.

Penetrating trauma

In the UK, it is advised that all penetrating abdominal injury should be explored (either open or laparoscopic). Even short implements may penetrate the abdominal wall and cause significant injury to the internal organs if sufficient force is used.

Organ injury scaling

Developed by American Association of the Surgery of Trauma in 1987, as way of grading injury (Table 9.2).

Table 9.2 Organ injury scaling

Organ	OIS grade	Description
Liver	I–VI	From contusion to avulsion
Lung	I–VI	From contusion to avulsion of hilum
Spleen	I–V	From haematoma to splenic devascularization
Kidney	I–V	From contusion to avulsion

Surgery – laparotomy for trauma

There is ongoing debate over what constitutes best practice where there are multiple abdominal injuries. Surgeons have moved from sorting out each and every intra-abdominal injury and courting metabolic acidosis, hypothermia, and coagulopathy etc, to what is now known as 'damage control surgery'. This is much simpler and faster, with the aim of transferring quickly from operating theatre to an ICU where the metabolic defects and haemodynamic problems can be more effectively treated. Its principles are:

- control haemorrhage – identify source, judicious use of packing; leave retroperitoneal and pelvic haematomas alone
- prevent contamination – avoid multiple anastomosis, resect dead bowel, staple off proximal bowel ends
- avoid further injury, e.g. compartment syndrome – consider laparostomy.

Use the second-look laparotomy for reconstruction and intestinal anastomosis after 24–48 h.

Further reading

British Trauma Society. http://www.trauma.org/bts/ (accessed 17 July 2008).

Moore EE, Cogbill TH, Jurkovich MD *et al.* Organ injury scaling: spleen and liver (1994 revision). *J Trauma* 1995;**38**:323.

Trauma.org has a large repository of scenarios, moulage, and information. http://www.trauma.org/ (accessed 17 July 2008).

Burns

Incidence

- ~2% of paediatric injuries in the UK result from burns and scalds.

Types of injury

Scalds result from exposure to hot water or steam and typically affect younger children in the home. Direct heat exposure results from fire, domestic appliances, or electrical current. Non-accidental injury, especially in young children, is a possible cause. Most fatalities result from house fires and are actually caused by smoke inhalation.

Scale of skin injury

This is a product of depth of burn and proportion of body surface area affected.

Depth

- Partial thickness (painful, blistered, typically results from scald)
- Full thickness (may be painless, typically results from electrical and flame burn)

(NB electrical burns may cause necrosis of underlying tissue without extensive skin damage.)

Body surface area (BSA)

The time-honoured 'rule of nines' is a helpful method of estimating surface area in adults and older children (Box 9.2).

> **Box 9.2 Wallace 'rule of nines'**
>
> BSA divided into 11 areas of 9% each:
> - head = 9%
> - arms = 9% + 9%
> - trunk front = 18%, back = 18%
> - legs front = 18%, back = 18%
> - genitalia = 1%

However, body proportions differ considerably in younger children, and specialized charts (e.g. Lund and Browder) are more accurate (Fig. 9.1).

Clinical features

Partial-thickness burns result in painful blistering and erythema, while deeper burning causes white areas of full-thickness necrosis which may be relatively insensitive due to nerve ablation.

Smoke inhalation should be suspected in all cases of flame burns, and its effects tend to progress with time. Look for discolouration of the lips, mouth, or pharynx and evidence of increasing oxygen requirements. In severe cases, airway obstruction may occur early due to laryngeal and tracheal oedema.

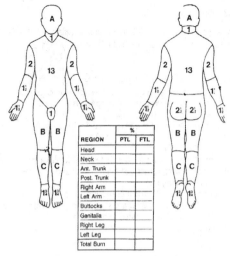

Fig. 9.1 Body surface area calculation (after Lund and Browder).
NB do not count erythema.

REGION	%	
	PTL	FTL
Head		
Neck		
Ant. Trunk		
Post. Trunk		
Right Arm		
Left Arm		
Buttocks		
Genitalia		
Right Leg		
Left Leg		
Total Burn		

Area	Age 0	1 year	10 years	Adult
A = ½ of head	9.5%	8.5%	5.5%	3.5%
B = ½ one thigh	2.75%	3.25%	4.5%	4.75%
C = ½ one lower leg	2.5%	2.5%	3.25%	3.5%

Management

Initial management should follow the ABC principles. The main priorities in initial management are airway protection, fluid replacement, and pain relief. Antibiotics have no place in the initial management of burns.

Intravenous fluid requirements (if >10% BSA in children)

These are directly related to the percentage of body surface area affected by the burn/scald. Intravenous Ringer's/lactate (or Hartmann's) solution should be commenced immediately, taking into account the time that has elapsed since the burn was sustained. In children weighing <30 kg, maintenance intravenous fluids containing glucose should be given in addition to the burn replacement fluid. (Box 9.3)

Sufficient fluid should be given to maintain a urinary output of 1–1.5 mL/kg/h.

Box 9.3 Parkland formula

(4ml crystalloid) × (%BSA burn) × (body weight in kg) = fluid
replacement for first 24 h – half in first 8 h

Criteria for transfer to a burn centre

Optimal management may require transfer to a PICU or burns unit. The
following burns should be referred to a specialist center:
- age < 5 years
- partial thickness (>10% of the total BSA, if <10 years)
- partial thickness (>20% total BSA if >10 years)
- full thickness (>5% BSA)
- involvement of face, eyes, ears, hands, feet, genitalia, or perineum
- circumferential or involvement of major joints and flexures
- additional inhalation injury
- significant chemical or electrical burns, including lightning injury
- children with burn injuries who are seen in hospitals without specialist
  personnel or equipment to manage their care
- non-accidental injury

Further reading

Greaves I, Porter K, Ryan J. *Trauma Care Manual*. London: Arnold, 2001.

Hettiaratchy S, Papini R. Initial management of a major burn I – overview. *BMJ* 2004;**328**:1555–7.

Hettiaratchy S, Papini R. Initial management of a major burn II – assessment and resuscitation.
BMJ 2004;**329**:101–103.

Blast injury

Blast injuries are rare, and occur as a result of accidental or deliberate explosions in confined spaces. Injury to many structures, especially the lungs, may be caused and there are four main types of damage (Table 9.3).

Table 9.3 Blast injury

Type of damage	Common injuries
Primary – direct effects due to pressure changes	Rupture of tympanic membranes
	Pulmonary damage
	Rupture of hollow viscera
Secondary – e.g. effects of fragmentation of explosive device	Penetrating trauma
	Fragmentation injuries
Tertiary – effects of structural collapse and/or body displacement	Crush injuries
	Blunt trauma
	Penetrating injury
	Open or closed head injury
Quaternary – effects of external agents released by explosion	Burns
	Asphyxia
	Effects of toxin inhalation

Explosives can be divided into (i) high order (e.g. TNT, dynamite), characterized by 'detonation', and (ii) low order (e.g. pyrotechnics, black powder), characterized by 'deflagration'. The former has a high-energy high-pressure blast wave capable of causing ear, lung, and intestinal damage, not usually seen in (ii). Proximity to the explosion is important as the pressure diminishes with the cubic root of the distance from its source.

Further reading

Shirley PJ. Critical care delivery: the experience of a civilian terrorist attack. *JR Army Med Corps* 2006;**152**:17–21.

Transplantation

Introduction

Although classical antiquity and the miracle of the early Christian saints records examples of transplantation between individuals, the first solid organ transplant was performed by Joseph Murray (1919–), a surgeon at the Peter Bent Brigham Hospital in Boston, who implanted a kidney between identical twins in 1954. This work was the culmination of the development of safe vascular anastomoses by the French surgeon, Alexis Carrel (1873–1944) and recognition of the immune background to rejection by the British scientist, Sir Peter Medawar (1915–1987). Notably, all three were awarded Nobel prizes.

General principles

- Autograft – movement of tissue within oneself (e.g. skin graft)
- Allograft – transfer of tissue to genetically dissimilar individual
- Xenograft – transfer of tissue between species

Immune response to transplantation

Recognition

Individual genetic identity occurs because of the presence of series of specific antigens on Ch6 termed the human leucocyte antigen (HLA). There are two series, namely class I (i.e. HLA A, B, and C) and class II molecules (e.g. DR, DQ and DP) which are inherited as a co-dominant haplotype. In addition, there are minor histocompatibility antigens (e.g. HY-A1, HA-1) present on other chromosomes, which can cause problems specifically with stem cell transplants.

Response

- Hyperacute (minutes) – caused by blood group mismatch and due to preformed antibodies.
- Acute rejection (3 days onwards), occurs when antigenic material is recognized as 'non-self'. The process involves antigen-presenting cells (typically of donor origin), which interact with naïve CD4+ T-cells within regional lymph nodes. This sets up alloreactive effector (classically) CD8+ T-cells, which migrate and initiate donor organ tissue damage, along with an influx of mononuclear cells, leucocytes etc.
- Chronic rejection (months) is an immune-mediated reaction typically causing a vasculopathy and characterized by fibrosis, deposition of extracellular matrix, and atrophy (vanishing bile duct syndrome – liver; bronchiolitis obliterans – lung). It can be difficult to treat effectively and is a potent cause of long-term organ loss (especially renal and lung).

Cardiac transplantation

Incidence

About 375 (M = F) transplants annually worldwide.

Aetiology

- Congenital heart disease
- Arrhythmia (e.g. sustained supraventricular tachycardia)
- Tumors (e.g. rhabdomyoma)
- Muscle abnormalities (e.g. endocardial fibroelastosis, viral myocarditis, glycogen storage disease)
- Cardiomyopathy (CMP) (e.g. dilated, hypertrophic, restrictive)
- Haematologic (e.g. thalassaemia, hyperviscosity syndrome)
- Metabolic (e.g. carnitine deficiency)
- Cardiotoxic (e.g. doxorubicin, anthracycline)

Indications for transplant

- End-stage cardiomyopathy (45%) and CHD (45%)
- Dilated CMP – most frequent subgroup transplanted (75%)
- Non-operable structural defects, failed palliation e.g. hypoplastic left heart syndrome (HLHS), 'failing' Fontan
- Refractory arrhythmias.
- Retransplantation (e.g. graft vasculopathy, rejection with ongoing graft loss at 2–3%/year)

Pre-operative management

Recipient

- Absolute contraindications (i.e. uncontrolled infection, malignancy, systemic disease limiting life expectancy, major CNS abnormalities)
- Catheterization – transpulmonary gradient (≤15 mmHg), pulmonary vascular resistance (≤6 Wood's units)
- Immunologic – ABO type, panel reactive antibody. (NB ABO mismatch is possible in infants)
- Serology (i.e. CMV, EBV, HIV, hepatitis B and C)

Donor

- Brain death (cerebral blood flow, apnoea test)
- Echocardiogram (EF >40%, no MR, wall motion abnormalities)
- ABO matched or compatible.
- Size (≤3x greater in weight).
- Laboratory: viral serology, bacterial cultures, toxoplasma
- Management: maintain BP (adequate filling, use of vasopressin)

Surgery

Donor

- Median sternotomy and inspect heart
- Heparinize (3 mg/kg), then ligate and divide SVC
- Clamp IVC at diaphragm and cross-clamp ascending aorta and give 4°C cardioplegia solution
- Divide IVC, pulmonary veins, aorta, pulmonary artery, and mediastinal tissue posterior to the atrium

Recipient
- Median sternotomy
- Aortobicaval cannulation/initiate cardiopulmonary bypass at 32°C
- Cross-clamp aorta
- Cardiectomy
- Anastomoses – left atrium, aorta, pulmonary artery, IVC, SVC. Bi-atrial technique (alternative in small infants)

Deep hypothermic circulatory arrest for arch reconstruction (e.g. HLHS)

Postoperative management
- Coagulopathy (prolonged bypass)
- Optimize haemodynamics – inotrope (e.g. adrenaline), chronotrope (e.g. isoprenaline), phosphodiesterase inhibitor (e.g. milrinone), atrioventricular pacing
- Pulmonary hypertension (e.g. nitric oxide)
- Immunosuppresion ('triple therapy' i.e. calcineurin inhibitor (ciclosporin/tacrolimus), antiproliferative agent (mycophenolate mofetil), and corticosteroids (avoid chronic usage if possible)

Specific complications
- Acute rejection – diagnose by endomyocardial biopsy and ECHO with treatment including IV steroids, adjusting immunosuppression and antithymocyte/lymphocyte globulin
- Cardiac allograft vasculopathy – diffuse concentric myointimal proliferation. Treatment – retransplantation. Potent cause of late graft loss (10–20% at 5 years)
- Infection – highest risk in first 6 months. Causative agents – *S. aureus, E. coli, Pseudomonas* spp. Opportunistic – Herpes zoster, *Pneumocystis carini*, aspergillosis, and CMV
- Immunosuppressant-related hypertension, renal dysfunction, hyperlipidaemia, diabetes
- Others – lymphoproliferative disease, tumours

Outcomes
- Overall survival – 50% at 10 years
- 90% having no activity limitation at 5 years

Further reading
Boucek RJ, Boucek MM. Pediatric heart transplantation. *Curr Opin Pediatr* 2002;**14**:611–19.

Canter CE, Shaddy RE, Bernstein D *et al*. Indications for heart transplantation in pediatric disease. *Circulation* 2007;**115**:658–76.

Smith RR, Wray J, Khaghani AM *et al*. Ten year survival after paediatric heart transplantation: a single center experience. *Eur J Cardiothorac Surg* 2005;**27**:790–4.

Liver transplantation

The first ever liver transplant was attempted in March 1963, in Denver, Colorado by Thomas Starzl in a child born with biliary atresia. The child died on-table, of complications related to bleeding.

Indications

Liver disease has generally been underestimated as a cause of death in children. Transplantation should be considered in all cases of acute and chronic disease (~2 /million/year).

The most common indications are:

- biliary atresia (~40 %)
- metabolic diseases (~15%) – such as α_1-antitrypsin deficiency, tyrosinosis, cystic fibrosis, and hyperoxaluria
- acute liver failure (~15%)
- hepatitis (~5%) – both autoimmune and viral causes
- tumour (~2%)
- retransplantation (10–15%).

There are few absolute contraindications, but extra-hepatic malignancy, severe co-morbid systemic disease, fixed pulmonary hypertension, and active AIDS make consideration difficult. Timely referral for assessment is important, as the debilitating effects of liver disease impact negatively on surgical morbidity and mortality.

Pre-operative management

The child and family are fully assessed and counselled. The diagnosis is confirmed and the health status of the patient, the severity of the liver disease, and its vasculature are assessed with laboratory tests of clotting profile, liver biochemistry, and imaging with USS, CT and MRI. Treatment of liver disease and portal hypertension is adjusted as required. Viral screening includes hepatitis A, B, C, EBV, CMV and HIV. Immunization status is updated. Nutritional management is most important.

Living-related donation should also be discussed as an option due to severe donor shortage.

Surgery

Donor operation

Cadaveric donation occurs as part of a multi-organ retrieval procedure. Stable donors aged <45 years are preferred. Donors as young as one month have also been used. Organs are perfused with cold preservation solution (e.g. University of Wisconsin solution) and stored in ice at 4°C. Cold ischaemic times should be kept to <12 h. Size matching is important, and larger donor livers can be reduced in size up to a factor of 20:1 by back-table dissection using the segmental anatomy of the liver so as to preserve vascular and biliary integrity of the graft. Adult livers may be split into two functioning units (Fig 10.1). Living donors are being increasingly used due to the shortage of cadaver donors. The left lobe (segments II/III usually) from a parent are preferred. Living donor morbidity is ~20%, and mortality 0.3% for paediatric recipients.

Recipient operation

This is often a complex operation taking several hours and is approached in three stages – (i) explantation of the native diseased liver, (ii) an anhepatic phase, and (iii) graft reperfusion following completion of hepatic vein, portal vein, and hepatic artery anastomosis. The donor bile duct is drained into a Roux-en-Y loop in most cases.

Postoperative management

Meticulous care is essential, with daily Doppler US for vessel patency, and early diagnosis of both acute rejection and infection using daily FBC, liver biochemistry, and regular liver biopsy. Immunosuppressive agents are routinely administered and include anti-CD25 monoclonal antibodies (daclizumab or basiliximab), a calcineurin2 inhibitor (tacrolimus), and an anti-metabolite (azathioprine or mycophenolate mofetil). Technical complications of vascular thrombosis, venous outflow obstruction, bile leak, or abdominal compartment syndrome tend to occur early and require immediate corrective surgical or radiological intervention.

Outcome

Current 5-year survival is >85%. Long-term complications are those related to toxicity of the immunosuppressive therapy (renal, bone marrow suppression, and steroid side-effects), infective causes (e.g. CMV, EBV, adenovirus), and post-transplant lymphoproliferative disease and lymphoma together with other malignancies as a result of prolonged immunosuppression. Chronic rejection, *de novo* hepatitis, and disease recurrence in patients with autoimmune disease occur and must be excluded if there are any liver biochemistry test abnormalities. However, the overall outlook is excellent with good catch-up growth and an excellent quality of life. Nonetheless re-transplantation may be required in up to 15% of cases.

Further reading

Millar AJ, Gupte GL. Small bowel transplantation in children. *Br J Hosp Med* 2007;**68**:19–23.

Millar AJ, Spearman W, McCulloch M et al. Liver transplantation for children—the Red Cross Children's Hospital experience. *Pediatr Transplant* 2004;**8**:136–44.

Tiao G, Ryckman FC. Pediatric liver transplantation. *Clin Liver Dis* 2006;**10**:169–97.

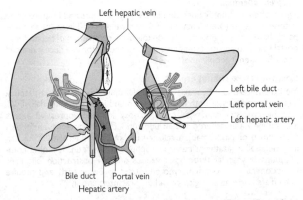

Fig. 10.1 An adult liver graft divided into two functioning units. The smaller graft (segments II/III) for an infant or child and the larger right lobe (segments IV–VIII) for an adult. The division of the graft and allocation of the vessels depends on the recipient size and local anatomy. In a living donor for a child, the graft procured would be a left lateral segment (II/III) as depicted. From *A Companion to Specialist Surgical Practice. Transplantation Surgery: Current Dilemmas*, 2nd edn 2001 W. B. Saunders Harcourt Publishers Ltd 2001 Ed. John LR Forsythe, with permission.

Intestinal transplantation

Introduction

Parenteral nutrition (PN) remains the current standard of care for infants and children with intestinal failure, with a >90% 1-year and 75% 5-year survival. However, outcomes of transplantation of the intestine alone or liver and intestine in patients with intestinal failure-associated liver-disease (IFALD) have recently improved with a near-comparable survival and quality of life.

Indications

Causes of intestinal failure in the paediatric age group are:
- short bowel syndrome, e.g. gastroschisis, NEC, intestinal atresia, mid-gut volvulus
- dysmotility, e.g. intestinal aganglionosis, pseudo-obstruction, degenerative intestinal leiomyopathy, megacystis-microcolon-hypoperistalsis syndrome
- congenital diarrhoeal disease, e.g. microvillous inclusion disease, and tufting enteropathy

Management

Transplantation is only indicated in patients with irreversible intestinal failure (IF) and potentially lethal complications of PN; namely loss of central venous access due to thrombosis of central veins, PN-induced cholestasis and liver failure, and life threatening episodes of central line-related sepsis. Patients with short bowel syndrome but with an expectation of good intestinal adaptation and eventual enteral tolerance but with early-onset severe IFALD may undergo liver transplantation only.

Contraindications

Complete loss of central venous access, immune deficiency syndromes, and severe systemic co-morbidities.

Pre-operative management

Pre-transplant assessment is the same as for other organ transplants, with a focus on preservation of central venous patency, ensuring adequacy of foregut motility, and identification of urinary tract anomalies.

Surgery

The donors should be size- and blood group-matched. There is immunologic advantage of tissue-type matching, but circumstances rarely permit this due to the shortage of donors.
- Isolated intestine – liver function in the recipient is preserved and no portal hypertension
- Liver and intestine – these may be 'en bloc' as a composite graft of liver and hepatoduodenal complex with small bowel, but might include the colon or even the stomach

These latter composite grafts may be reduced in size (liver and intestine partial excision) for them to be accommodated within the often-compromised abdominal domain of the recipient. The proximal gut is sutured in continuity, the foregut portal venous system decompressed by portacaval shunt, and the distal end brought out as a stoma for postoperative effluent volume monitoring and as access for biopsy rejection surveillance.

Postoperative management

Intense immune suppression is required to prevent rejection and maintain the health of the graft (e.g. steroids, tacrolimus, anti-thymocyte, or anti-CD25 globulins). During this time the patient is at risk for infection. All possible prophylactic measures are taken using antibiotics, antiviral and antifungal agents. Enteral feeding is commenced within the first week, and most are on full enteral feeds by 3 weeks. Viral infections, particularly EBV and CMV, are closely monitored. PTLPD occurs in up to 15% of cases. Graft-versus-host disease (GVHD) is uncommon, despite the high lymphocyte load of the graft. Surgical complications include graft ischaemia, abdominal compartment syndrome (staged closure of the abdomen may be required), intestinal perforation, adhesive obstruction, pancreatitis, bile sludge, wound and stoma problems. Post-transplant in-hospital care is usually around 6 weeks.

Outcome and quality of life

Current long-term survival is >50% at 5 years. Chronic rejection does occur and is mostly avoided by close adherence with medication. Quality of life for the survivors is excellent, with most on full enteral feeding and normal activities. Those patients who have not eaten prior to transplant need intense psychological training and speech therapy to help with restoration of normal oral feeding.

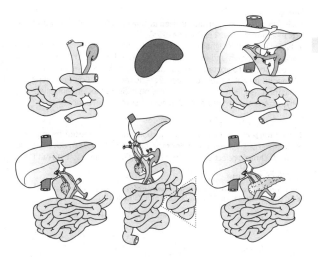

Fig. 10.2 Various types of intestinal transplants + isolated liver transplant. Based on drawings by Jean de ville de Goyet.

Renal transplantation

Renal replacement is needed in children with end-stage renal disease and renal failure (typically with GFR <15 mL/min/(1.73 m^2)). There are clear problems in the very small, and many centres have a minimum weight (>10 kg) and age requirement (>21 months).

Indications

- Glomerulonephritis (30%)
- Cystic/hereditary/congenital (25%)
- Interstitial nephritis (9%
- (NB commonest indication in adults is diabetes, ~40%.)

There are many differences compared to adults; children with ESRF are more likely to be on peritoneal dialysis, and more likely to undergo transplantation. Living-donor transplantation is also more common in children. Unlike in adults, there are relatively few contraindications, but these might include recent malignancy and HIV infection.

- ~ 22% of transplants in UK will be pre-emptive (i.e. the patient will not have been on dialysis). This may allow better growth, and may have a positive effect on graft survival.
- ~16% of transplants in UK will be from living donors (usually parents).
- NB the rate is Scandanavia is up to 80%!

Donor organs are age-restricted from 5–50 years. The median waiting time from listing in the UK, according to most recent statistics (2004), was 214 days.

Recipient operation

- Usually a midline approach is used in small children, with an extraperitoneal one in older children (>20 kg).
- Typically a donor right kidney is placed in left iliac fossa (and vice versa), leaving the pelvis and ureter anteriorly placed. The arterial anastomosis is performed to aorta or iliac, as appropriate. An extravesical, submucosal tunnel is used for most ureteric reconstruction (±stenting).
- Bilateral recipient nephrectomy may be indicated for uncontrolled hypertension, persisting renal infection, severe proteinuria. etc.

Specific complications

The commonest complication is rejection, which is reduced by improved HLA matching. Acute rejection may be treated by high-dose steroids although chronic rejection is more problematic and can result in graft loss.

Further reading

Rees L, Shroffa R, Hutchinson et al. Long-term outcome of paediatric renal transplantation: follow-up of 300 children from 1973 to 2000. *Nephron Clin Pract* 2007;**105**:c68–c76.

Associated specialties

Gynaecology

Although serious gynaecological pathology in children is rare, gynaeco-logical symptoms are relatively common and the following conditions may present to paediatric surgeons.

Pre-puberty

Labial fusion

This affects 1–2% of girls and is probably due to mild vulvitis associated with a lack of oestrogen stimulation.

Clinical features

This is usually evident from the age of one year. The appearance is typical, with fusion of the labial skin extending from the posterior vaginal introitus towards the urethra. A clearly visible thin membranous line in the midline is present, and in severe fusion the urethral opening is visible as a pinhole opening. Although most are asymptomatic, occasionally there may be urine pooling behind the adhesions leading to post-micturition dribbling.

Spontaneous resolution is common and treatment is unnecessary if asymptomatic. If symptomatic, treatment is with oestrogen cream (e.g. Ovestin® (estriol 0.1%)) applied to the labia in the midline daily for a period not longer than six weeks. Surgical separation is rarely needed unless urinary symptoms are severe and persistent. Recurrence is common after treatment.

Vulvovaginitis

This affects up to 5% of prepubertal girls and may be due to poor perineal hygiene combined with a lack of oestrogen stimulation together with the anatomical features of the pre-pubertal vulva. Symptoms are exacerbated by chemicals present in soaps such as bubble bath.

Clinical features

There may be a persistent offensive vaginal discharge and/or vulval irrita-tion. The appearance is typical with a reddened 'flush' around the vulva and anus. The skin may be excoriated, and discharge may collect at the posterior fourchette. Vaginal bleeding is not a sign of simple vulvovaginitis.

Vaginal swabs may be normal, but if positive the commonest organisms are group A beta-haemolytic *Streptococci* and *Haemophilus influenzae*. Treatment is conservative with an emphasis on vulval hygiene. Broad-spectrum antibiotics can be helpful but recurrence is common.

Post-puberty

Ovarian cysts

These are common and can occur at any age, with the most frequent being functional cysts which are usually follicular in nature. Benign ovarian teratomas also occur, which are usually small and can be bilateral (up to 15%). Serous and mucinous cystadenomas are uncommon in children but can occur in older adolescents. Malignant ovarian tumours are rare and are usually of germ cell origin in this age group.

Clinical features

Follicular cysts can present acutely with pain due to haemorrhage and pre-dispose to ovarian torsion. Benign and malignant ovarian tumours tend to have a less-acute presentation with abdominal discomfort, distension and pressure symptoms.

Many follicular cysts resolve spontaneously and are managed conservatively with ultrasound follow-up. Surgical intervention is needed if the patient is acutely unwell or in severe pain. Ovarian cystectomy can be done laparoscopically. Ovarian tissue should be conserved if possible unless torsion has already occurred. Complex ovarian cysts require careful evaluation and imaging with referral on to the appropriate specialist team to achieve a cure and maintain fertility.

Menstrual obstruction

This is rarely seen but may be caused by an imperforate hymen or, less commonly, a transverse vaginal septa.

Clinical features

There is abdominal and pelvic pain becoming more severe in the absence of the onset of menstruation. The pain is initially cyclical but eventually becomes continuous. A pelvic mass is often palpable. If the hymen is imperforate it can be seen as a blue bulge at the vaginal introitus.

A pelvic ultrasound will confirm the presence of a haematocolpos.

Imperforate hymen is easily treated by incision and drainage, but more-complex septae require specialized imaging and surgery within a specialist unit.

Sexually transmitted infections and pregnancy

At least one in four girls in the UK is sexually active before the age of 16 years, and conditions such as ectopic pregnancy and pelvic inflammatory disease must not be forgotten. A sensitive history as to sexual activity should be sought in all girls after puberty. Urinary pregnancy tests are accurate and quick and should be performed if pregnancy is a possibility. Chlamydia in particular may present with pyrexia, generalized abdominal pain, and tenderness over the liver due to perihepatic inflammation (Fitz-Hugh–Curtis syndrome).

Further reading

Hayes L, Creighton SM. Prepubertal vaginal discharge. *The Obstetrician and Gynaecologist* 2007;**9**:159–63.

Wellings K, Nanchahal K, McDowell W *et al.* Sexual behaviour in Britain: early heterosexual experience. *Lancet* 2001;**358**:1843–50.

Cleft lip and palate

Embryology of facial development
- Critical period – 4th–8th gestational week
- Fusion of five facial prominences:
  - paired mandibular processes (from 1st branchial arch)
  - paired maxillary processes (from 1st branchial arch)
  - frontonasal process (medial and lateral nasal processes)
- Failure of fusion results in orofacial clefts

Clefts of lip and palate
- Most common facial anomaly (~1 in 700 in UK)
- **Cleft lip** – failure/disruption of fusion of the medial nasal and maxillary processes
- **Cleft palate** –failure of elevation and fusion of palatal shelves (medial outgrowths of the maxillary processes)

NB cleft lip with or without cleft palate and isolated cleft palate are two distinct conditions.

Cleft lip (± cleft palate) – 60% of referrals

Incidence
- Overall ~1 in 1000 live births
- Racial variation – ~1 in 750 in the Caucasian population, higher in Chinese (~1 in 500) and lower in African-Caribbean (~1 in 2000)

Epidemiology
- Male predominance (2:1)
- Isolated cleft lip – 25%
- Unilateral cleft lip and palate – 25%
- Bilateral cleft lip and palate – 10%

Aetiology
- Multifactorial – genetic and environmental
- Familial association – 30% concordance in monozygotic twins
- Genetics – the risk of clefting rises to 3–4% if one child or parent has a cleft

Syndromic (5–15%)
- Van der Woude
- Chromosomal, e.g. trisomy 13
- CHARGE syndrome
- Ectrodactyl, ectodermal dysplasia, clefting syndrome (EEC)

Environmental
- Maternal diabetes
- Alcohol
- Medications – phenytoin, steroids, diazepam
- Folic acid deficiency
- Parental age (possible effect of increasing parental age for cleft lip ±cleft palate)

Isolated cleft palate – 40% of referrals

Incidence
- Overall ~1 in 2000 live births
- No racial variation

Epidemiology
- Female predominance (2:1)

Aetiology
Environmental
- Alcohol
- Medications

Possible paternal age effect

Genetics

Before considering recurrence risks a possible underlying syndrome must be excluded.

Syndromic (up to 60%)
- Van der Woude syndrome
- Stickler's syndrome
- Velocardiofacial syndrome (22q11 microdeletion)

Other forms

Microform clefts of the lip (forme fruste) or palate (submucous cleft palate) are easily missed. Features of the latter are bifid uvula, central lucency in the soft palate, and bony defect/notch in the hard palate. They may present with nasal regurgitation or hypernasal speech.

Problems associated with CLP/CP

Lip
- Cosmetic – lip and nose
- Feeding – usually normal
- Speech – impairment of production of bilabial sounds (pa, pi), if unrepaired

Soft palate
- Feeding – oronasal communication means the baby is unable to suck adequately. Use of a soft plastic bottle squeezed with constant pressure to squirt milk into mouth and oropharynx overcomes this.
- Speech – abnormal insertion of muscles on the side of the cleft results in soft palate malfunction and velopharyngeal incompetence (VPI). This may result in hypernasality, nasal emission and backing/glotttal/pharyngeal speech (secondary, compensatory phenomenon).
- Middle ear effusion – soft palate muscle malposition results in eustachian tube dysfunction and may cause glue ear and conductive hearing loss from otitis media.

Hard palate
- Dental irregularities (if there is alveolar involvement)
- Teeth – missing/supernumery/abnormal shape
- Maxillary growth
- Compromised, especially if the cleft involves the palate. Scarring from surgery is a major cause, another is an intrinsic problem in the maxilla

Management

Within a multidisciplinary team – specialist nurse, surgeons (plastic, ENT, maxillofacial) paediatrician, speech therapist, audiologist, dentist, orthodontist, clinical psychologist, and clinical geneticist.

Diagnosis (Fig 11.1)

Antenatal
- Cleft lip (>60% of cases)
- Cleft palate alone would not usually be detected
- Parent(s) seen by surgical team in antenatal period

Postnatal
- Parent(s) and neonate seen within 24–48 h

Goals
- Normal speech
- Minimal facial disfigurement
- Normal hearing
- Normal dentition
- A happy, well-integrated child
- A well-balanced, socially adept adult

Timing of surgery/assessment

See Table 11.1.

Table 11.1 Timing of surgery/assessment for cleft lip and palate

Age	Procedure/intervention
3 months	Repair lip, nose, and anterior palate
6 months	Repair soft palate (± grommets if required)
18 months and 3 years	Speech assessment
3+ years	Secondary speech surgery (if required – 5–30%)
8–9 years	If alveolar cleft – pre-operative orthodontics, alveolar bone graft
10+ years	Definitive orthodontics
17–18 years	Rhinoplasty (if required)
17–20 years	Maxillary osteotomy (if required)

Surgical techniques

Lip, nose and anterior palate (3 months)

- **Lip** – radical subperiosteal mobilization of tissues on the cleft side with repair of the orbicularis oris muscle and tension-free skin closure
- **Nose** – separation of congenital adhesions between the alar cartilage on the cleft side and the overlying skin and underlying mucosa (McComb and Andel). Repositioned structures maintained by various methods of fixation
- **Anterior (hard) palate** – unlined turnover flap from the nasal septum (vomerine flap)

Repair palate (Sommerlad) (6 months)
- Radical mobilization of mucoperiosteal flaps of the hard palate
- Repositioning of soft palate muscles (using operating microscope)
- Closure of oral and nasal mucosa

Alveolar bone graft (Boyne and Sands) (8–9 years)
- When canine root two-thirds formed (mixed dentition)
- Local flaps to ensure a mucosal seal
- Bony defect filled with cancellous bone (iliac crest)

Follow-up
- Care should continue to adulthood
- Outcome audited at 5, 10, 15, and 20 years

Cleft Standards Advisory Group report (CSAG)
(1998 recommendations on provision of cleft services)
- Centralization of care to 8–15 units in the UK, treating at least 80–100 new babies per year with each surgeon operating on at least 40 babies per year
- Definitive training for interested trainees in high-volume, high-quality units
- All patient information to be made available for audit and research
- Common database for all patients
- Improved collection of cleft birth recording

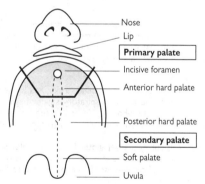

Fig. 11.1 Palatal anatomy.

Otorhinolaryngology

Choanal atresia

This may be a cause of respiratory emergency as neonates are preferential nasal breathers. Suspect bilateral atresia if there is acute respiratory distress after birth that resolves with crying (mouth open) or if there is difficulty passing a nasal catheter. Unilateral atresia may be asymptomatic or present with unilateral nasal obstruction/discharge. (NB 50% have other congenital abnormalities.)

Management

- Urgent taped-in oropharyngeal airway, establish orogastric tube feeding
- Assess posterior choanae with CT scan (atresia may be bony, membranous, or mixed)
- Cardiac echo, hearing test and renal ultrasound to exclude CHARGE association
- Aim for definitive repair as soon as possible if bilateral (unilateral repair delayed until later childhood) – usually endoscopic transnasal approach. Nasal stenting and revision surgery is often required

Obstructive sleep apnoea

Defined as episodes of upper airway obstruction during sleep, associated with hypoxia. Has a multifactorial aetiology including soft tissue lesions (adenotonsillar hypertrophy, macroglossia), craniofacial abnormalities, neuromuscular, and metabolic disorders.

Management

Polysomnography (combination of EEG, oculogram, muscle sensors, and pulse oximetry) to assess severity. The treatment options include adeno-tonsillectomy, nasopharyngeal airway, continuous positive airway pressure (CPAP), craniofacial surgery, and even tracheostomy if severe.

Laryngomalacia

This is the commonest cause of congenital stridor, and is due to soft and immature cartilages of the larynx. Inspiratory stridor begins in the first weeks of life, and is worse when supine or agitated but resolves spontaneously by 2 years. The cry is usually normal (suspect other pathology if not).

Endoscopy reveals tall, tight aryepiglottic folds and an elongated omega-shaped epiglottis, which prolapses into the larynx with inspiration. There is increased incidence of gastro-oesophageal reflux due to high negative intrathoracic pressures.

Management

Intervention only if severe and associated with failure to thrive or respiratory distress (<5% cases). Confirm diagnosis with awake flexible fibre-optic laryngoscopy if possible, or laryngobronchoscopy under GA. Treat hypoxaemia with supplemental oxygen, manage gastro-oesophageal reflux, provide nutritional support, and consider CPAP. Surgical options include aryepiglottoplasty, epiglottoplasty, and, rarely, tracheostomy.

Vocal cord palsy

This has many possible causes including CNS and cardiovascular pathology, trauma, inflammation, and metabolic disorders. Some are idiopathic (~40%). Consider left vocal cord palsy if child is hoarse after thoracic surgery (particularly PDA ligation). Bilateral palsy (~50% cases) may present with respiratory distress, stridor, aspiration, and a weak cry.

Management

A unilateral palsy does not usually require intervention as the contralateral vocal cord compensates, but speech and language therapy input is beneficial.

Bilateral palsy requires tracheostomy for airway protection in more than half of cases, but a minimum of 12 months' observation is recommended before further surgical intervention because of the possibility of spontaneous recovery (>50%). Definitive laryngeal surgery to allow decannulation needs to balance airway improvement against the risks of aspiration and impaired voice. Procedures include laser cordotomy/partial arytenoidectomy, cordopexy, and arytenoidopexy.

Subglottic stenosis

This is defined as a cricoid diameter of <3.5 mm in a newborn.

Congenital stenosis (less common) is often due to cricoid malformation or trapped 1st tracheal ring.

Acquired stenosis is usually seen following endotracheal intubation for management of prematurity. The child may present with failed extubation, stridor, prolonged, or recurrent croup. Laryngoscopy and bronchoscopy allows assessment and grading of severity.

Management

- Watchful waiting for mild stenosis (symptoms may resolve as cricoid cartilage and subglottic lumen enlarge with growth)
- Soft stenosis may respond to balloon dilatation or anterior cricoid split
- Tracheostomy may be required to provide an airway while waiting for the child to grow
- Definitive surgery may be endoscopic or open. Laryngotracheal reconstruction using costal cartilage as anterior ± posterior graft for established stenosis (Fig. 11.2), with partial cricotracheal resection an option for the most severe cases.

Paediatric tracheostomy

Procedure should be performed electively using conventional midline dissection technique. The percutaneous approach is not suitable for children because the airway is small, the trachea is soft, flexible, and very mobile, landmarks are difficult to palpate, and a displaced tube may not be easy to replace quickly. It is prudent to use non-absorbable stay sutures on either side of the vertical tracheotomy opening (Fig. 11.3) to assist with insertion of the tube. These sutures should be labelled and left until the first tube change at one week to assist in replacement of a dislodged tube before a stable fistula tract becomes established. Training of carers is crucial to avoid morbidity and mortality (~0.5%) from a displaced or obstructed tube.

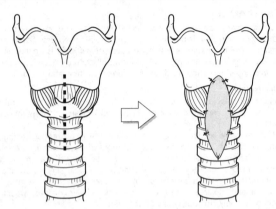

Fig. 11.2 Laryngotracheal reconstruction.

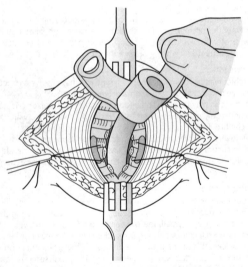

Fig. 11.3 Paediatric tracheostomy. From Spitz L, Coran AG (eds). *Operative Paediatric Surgery* (6th edn). © 2006 Edward Arnold (Publishers) Ltd. Reproduced by kind permission of Edward Arnold (Publishers Ltd).

Further reading

Bailey CM. Paediatric tracheostomy. In: Spitz L, Coran AG (eds). *Operative Paediatric Surgery* (6th edn). London: Hodder Arnold, 2006.

Graham JM, Scadding GK, Bull PD (eds). *Paediatric ENT*. Berlin: Springer-Verlag, 2007.

Orthopaedics

The limping child

Pain involving the lower limbs is one of the most common reasons for children presenting to the doctor. Pain often is associated with a limping gait. Common causes are shown in Table 11.2.

Table 11.2 Common causes for limping gait in children

(Age years)	Common causes
1–5	Dislocated hip (M:F = 1:4)
	Toddler's fracture of the tibia or other trauma (bones, soft tissues)
	Transient synovitis of the hip
	Bone and joint infection
	Juvenile idiopathic arthritis (F>M)
5–10	Trauma
	Transient synovitis
	Bone and joint infection
	Legg–Calve–Perthes disease (M:F = 5:1)
10–15	Slipped capital femoral epiphysis (M:F = 1.5:1)
	Trauma
	Bone and joint infection
	Neoplasm

Clinical evaluation of the limping child
- Asymmetry (atrophy, leg length)
- Presence of deformity
- Erythema, swelling, effusion
- Limited range of joint motion (internal rotation of the hip is a sensitive test for hip pathology such as synovitis)
- Scoliosis, midline dimples, and hairy patches (spinal pathology)
- Neurological assessment of lower limbs is essential

Diagnostic tests
- Plain radiographs (consider pelvis AP if presenting symptom is knee pain)
- Ultrasound of joints and soft tissues (for septic arthritis, subperiosteal abscess in bone infection, myositits)
- Full blood count, CRP, ESR
- MRI (if diagnostic findings remain unclear, this has high diagnostic yield for spinal pathology)
- Bone scan (sensitive but not specific, therefore useful if results of other tests remain unclear)
- Aspiration if joint effusion or subperiosteal abscess are present on ultrasound (investigate aspirate for cell count, gram stain, culture)

Transient synovitis

This is often associated with a recent history of URTI and is most commonly seen in the hip. Usually the radiograph is normal except for indirect signs demonstrating joint effusion. Ultrasound confirms the presence of joint effusion.

Treatment includes bed rest and NSAID, with gradual improvement of symptoms noted and complete resolution within a few days. The differential diagnosis includes septic arthritis of the hip or Legg–Calve–Perthes disease (look for subchondral fracture line of proximal femoral epiphysis of the hip on axial radiograph).

Septic arthritis and osteomyelitis

This is difficult to diagnose in its early stages, with typical features including pain, fever, and a limping gait with restricted movement of the affected extremity (the hip is typically held in external rotation and abduction). Radiographs can be normal in the early stage and bony changes not evident for 14–21 days. Ultrasound is useful to rule out subperiosteal abscess (which requires drainage). MRI can require sedation but is a sensitive test for bone and joint infection.

Joint aspiration is the definite diagnostic procedure and if considered, should not be delayed (most common pathogen in the child is *Staphylococcus aureus*). Treatment includes systemic antibiotic treatment with possible drainage and debridement.

Developmental dysplasia of the hip (DDH)

There are several affected age groups which must be distinguished with regard to diagnosis and treatment. The most-severe form is congenital dislocation of the hip with an incidence of 1–1.5 per 1000 live births.

Risk factors

Girls born in the breech position are most at risk (incidence 70–120/1000). These should all have ultrasound screening. Others include a positive family history of DDH and foot deformities such as congential clubfoot.

Clinical features

In the neonate, a Barlow +ve hip (i.e. hip is located but can be dislocated on clinical examination) is considered a finding that does not warrant treatment for the first two weeks, but treatment should be considered if the hip does not improve. However, a hip that is Ortolani +ve (i.e. hip is dislocated and can be reduced on clinical examination) requires immediate confirmation by means of ultrasound and treatment.

A Graf alpha angle of ≥50° as determined by ultrasound is normal in the neonate, but follow-up at 6 weeks is warranted to ensure improvement of the hip sonographically (normal alpha angle >60°).

Clinical signs beyond the neonatal period include limited hip abduction (compare both hips – is there symmetry?); leg length inequality (flex hips to 90° and compare the levels of both knees); hip instability; and in walking children a limp.

The treatment of DDH is complex and depends on many factors including age, severity of DDH, and compliance of parents. In general, treatment of hip dysplasia and treatment of hip dislocation must be distinguished. Neonates tend to be treated conservatively with a harness while the older the child at diagnosis, the higher the likelihood for surgical procedures (e.g. closed or open reduction).

Marino Ortolani (1904–1983) an Italian paediatrician, first described the test for CDH in 1936. Barlow modified it in 1962.

Legg–Calve–Perthes disease (LCPD)

Definition
- Idiopathic, self-limiting avascular necrosis of the proximal femoral epiphysis, with four radiographic stages (condensation, fragmentation, reossification, healing)

Clinical features
The age at onset can range between 2 and 12 years (early onset – better prognosis) with male predominance (5:1). Presents with unilateral knee pain and/or hip pain in association with limping gait. The hip range of motion (specifically internal rotation) is restricted when compared to the unaffected side (due to synovitis). In the very early stages, pelvis AP and frog-leg lateral radiographs show widening of the joint space and possibly a subchondral fracture line in an axial view. In later stages, fragmentation of the proximal femoral epiphysis is evident.

There is no causal treatment. Treatment is largely symptomatic (e.g. rest and NSAID if acute pain is present). Maintaining a good range of motion of the affected hip is the key principle of the management of LCPD. Surgical interventions include osteotomies around the hip to restore containment of the femoral head within the acetabulum, or soft tissue surgery in case of severe joint contractures. There is limited evidence that surgical treatment improves long-term outcomes.

- Arthur Thornton Legg (1874–1939) American surgeon
- Jacques Calvé (1875–1954) French surgeon
- Georg Clemens Perthes (1869–1927) German surgeon and pioneer in x-rays, both diagnostic and therapeutic

Slipped capital femoral epiphysis (SCFE)

Definition
- Slippage (usually posterior and inferior) of the proximal femoral epiphysis on the metaphysis (femoral neck) occurring through the epiphyseal plate

Clinical features
Has a typical onset in early adolescent growth spurt (most common hip disorder in adolescents), being more common in black or Polynesian children and slightly more common in boys (60%) than in girls; 25% are bilateral.

It often presents with knee, thigh, or groin pain rather than hip pain! Typically the hip is externally rotated in flexion at presentation. However, this is not always present in the early stages and therefore radiographs are mandatory.

Pelvis AP and frog lateral radiographs of both hips should be performed (look for asymmetry of growth plates, location of epiphysis, and their contact to metaphysis; Klein's line, the line along the superior aspect of the femoral neck, on AP view).

Stable slips must be distinguished from unstable slips.

If the child is able to weight-bear (stable SCFE) then they need to be placed on crutches or in a wheelchair (does not constitute treatment, since the epiphysis invariably continues to slip!). If unable to weight-bear, (unstable SCFE), immediate surgical treatment is required. Definitive treatment ideally should be performed within a few days, and the goals of treatment are to prevent further slippage and to achieve closure of the physeal plate by surgical means.

Further reading

Roposch A, Wright JG. Increased diagnostic information and understanding disease: uncertainty in the diagnosis of developmental hip dysplasia. *Radiology* 2007;**242**:355–9.

Cardiology

Patients with structural congenital heart disease (CHD) will frequently undergo non-cardiovascular surgery because of the strong association between CHD and other anomalies. The increasing trend towards early surgical repair of structural CHD with normalization of the patient's haemodynamic status has reduced the number of children undergoing other forms of surgery with unrepaired or palliated CHD. Despite this, co-existing CHD continues to be a major cause of morbidity and mortality in patients undergoing non-cardiovascular surgery. Reduction of this risk requires both the identification of children at greatest risk and implementation of strategies directed towards minimizing the risks.

Incidence
- 5/1000 live births (term) (i.e. 1 in 175 births)
- 12/1000 (preterm)

Table 11.3

VSD	31%	ASD	11%	AVSD	4%
Aortic stenosis	8%	Coarctation of aorta	6%	PDA	5%
Pulmonary stenosis	7%	Pulmonary atresia	3%	Transposition of great arteries	5%
Tetralogy of Fallot	5%	Hypoplastic left heart	4%		

Identification of high-risk patients
- Neonatal surgical emergencies frequently associated with CHD:
  - imperforate anus
  - tracheo-oesophageal fistula
  - diaphragmatic hernia
- Neonate requiring urgent non-cardiovascular surgery with duct dependent systemic or pulmonary blood flow:
  - systemic, e.g. hypoplastic left heart, interrupted aortic arch, coarctation, transposition of great arteries (TGA)
  - pulmonary e.g. pulmonary atresia ±VSD, critical pulmonary stenosis
- Neonate after recent cardiac surgery: either palliative (e.g. systemic to pulmonary shunt procedure) or after repair (e.g. arterial switch operation for TGA) requiring non-cardiovascular surgery
- Premature infant with haemodynamically significant patent ductus arteriosus duct (PDA) requiring non-cardiovascular surgery (e.g. for NEC)

Investigations
- Establish/confirm diagnosis of CHD
- Evaluate significance of underlying CHD (e.g. PDA size in NEC)
- Assessment of myocardial function
- Check side of aortic arch in tracheo-oesophageal fistula

Management

- Prioritize surgical intervention (cardiovascular versus non-cardiovascular)
- Stabilize underlying CHD (prostaglandin infusion, balloon atrial septostomy)
- Non-cardiovascular surgery in tertiary centre with cardiac anaesthetist
- Endocarditis prophylaxis

Congestive cardiac failure (beyond the neonatal period)

Clinical features might include shortness of breath, poor feeding and poor weight gain, recurrent chest infections, sweating, and abdominal pain with findings of cyanosis, cardiomegaly, tachycardia, tachypnoea, weak pulses, and cool peripheries, gallop rhythm, and hepatomegaly.

Causes

In infancy this is usually due to increased pulmonary blood flow (e.g. VSD, PDA, AVSD) and in childhood is more commonly due to reduced myocardial contractility (e.g. cardiomyopathy, post-cardiac repair with reduced function).

Investigations

- Define underlying structural CHD if present
- Assessment of myocardial contractility

Management

In principle, treat the underlying cause before non-cardiovascular surgery, if possible (e.g. VSD repair etc). In an emergency, consider optimization of medical management (e.g. diuretics, vasodilators, inotropes). It is important to ensure that intensive care support is available and ensure endocarditis prophylaxis.

Central cyanosis (Box 11.1)

This is defined as the presence of at least 5 g/dL of reduced haemoglobin within the circulation.

Causes

Include non-cardiac causes (e.g. diaphragmatic hernia), unrepaired/palliated CHD (including Eisenmenger syndrome), undiagnosed CHD, and acyanotic CHD in severe CCF.

Box 11.1 Specific risks associated with a cyanosed child

- Paradoxical embolus in unrepaired/palliated CHD (including cerebral abscess)
- Polycythaemia (increased risk of thrombosis)
- Bleeding (increased tissue vascularity and thrombocytopenia)
- Haemoptysis (in patients with established pulmonary vascular disease)

Investigations

The pre-operative assessment must include haematocrit and renal function, together with full cardiac assessment to establish a diagnosis (if not known), fitness for surgery, and potential risks of non-cardiovascular surgery.

Management

Should include adequate hydration pre-operatively, with consideration of pre-operative haemodilution and meticulous care to avoid entrainment of air in IV tubing as well as endocarditis prophylaxis.

Arrhythmias

These may occur in the absence of CHD, but structural CHD is commonly associated with arrhythmias. Frequently, these can be anticipated with knowledge of the underlying cardiac abnormality. Occasionally, they may be the presenting feature of structural CHD and may be precipitated by anaesthesia. Commonly encountered rhythm abnormalities include:

- supraventricular tachyarrhythmias (atrial enlargement, e.g. Ebstein's anomaly, previous atrial surgery, e.g. AVSD repair, Senning operation)
- ventricular tachycardia (previous cardiac surgery including ventriculotomy for tetralogy of Fallot, presenting feature of long QT syndrome)
- complete heart block (1st- and 2nd-degree heart block rarely compromise haemodynamic status). Can be caused by complex forms of structural CHD (e.g. congenitally corrected TGA, left isomerism sequence) or be maternal antibody mediated in newborns (Anti Ro, Anti La antibodies) where there is a normal cardiac structure, but maybe associated functional myocardial impairment.

Investigations

- Establish nature of arrhythmia (12-lead ECG, ±adenosine)
- exclude underlying CHD if undiagnosed

Management

Tachyarrhythmia
- Undiagnosed – chemical or electrical cardioversion
- Previously diagnosed – continue maintenance therapy pre-operatively and restart early postoperatively

Bradyarrhythmia
- Use of chronotropic agents (e.g. atropine, isoprenaline)
- Temporary transvenous pacing in compromised patients

> Patients who are pacemaker dependent with indwelling permanent pacing systems will require pacing box reprogramming before elective surgery.

Endocarditis

Infective endocarditis (IE) is associated with significant mortality and morbidity and remains one of the most feared complications of structural CHD. The newly revised American Heart Association (AHA) guidelines are based on the premise that bacteraemia from daily activities is more likely to cause IE than bacteraemia from invasive dental procedures. Current patient groups for whom IE prophylaxis is indicated include:

- prosthetic cardiac valve(s),
- previous IE,
- unrepaired cyanotic CHD (including shunts and conduits)
- completely repaired CHD using prosthetic material/device for 6 months post surgery/catheter

- repaired CHD with residual lesion close to a prosthetic patch or device that might impair endothelialization
- cardiac transplant recipients who develop valvulopathy.

Antibiotic prophylaxis for IE is recommended for the above groups of patients undergoing procedures on the respiratory tract, or when procedures are undertaken through infected skin or tissues. It is no longer recommended for genitourinary or gastrointestinal procedures.

- Standard prophylaxis 30–60 min before procedure: amoxicillin/ampicillin 50 mg/kg po or IV (max 2 g)
- Penicillin allergic: clindamycin 20 mg/kg po or IV (max 600 mg)

Conclusions

Non-cardiovascular surgery in patients with structural CHD continues to be associated with increased morbidity and mortality. Knowledge of patient groups at high risk, and identification of clinical presentations that adversely affect outcome will reduce unexpected problems and improve results. The cumulative impact of problems involving multiple organ systems cannot be overstated and needs to be considered when counselling parents about surgical results.

Elective non-cardiovascular surgery needs planning with adequate provision for pre-operative investigations and close liaison between surgeon, cardiologist, and anaesthetist. Ideally, all surgery in this group of complex patients is best undertaken in tertiary centres.

In one European study, the 4-year survival rate was 72% for a live-born child with CHD.

Further reading

Tanner K, Sabrine N, Wren C. Cardiovascular malformations among preterm infants. *Paediatrics* 2005;**116**:e833–8.

Wilson W, Taubert KA, Gewitz M et al. Prevention of infective endocarditis. Guidelines from the American Heart Association. *Circulation* 2007;**116**:1736–54.

Congenital vascular abnormalities

Most are benign vascular lesions of childhood and are usually managed within a multidisciplinary team. Vascular malformations may be classified according to histopathological and clinical features into two principal groups, namely vascular tumours (haemangiomas and others) and vascular malformations (functionally divided into low versus high flow). Most lesions are isolated developmental abnormalities; however some may have a genetic basis and may be part of a genetic syndrome (Table 11.4).

Table 11.4 Associated syndromes

Syndrome	Associated anomaly	*MIM number
Sturge–Weber	CM	185300
Klippel–Trenaunay	CM, VM, LM	%149000
Parkes–Weber	CM, VM, LM	#608355
Blue rubber bleb naevus	VM	%112200
Maffucci (familial)	VM, LVM	#166000
Turner's	VM, LM	%313000
Trisomy 13, 18, and 21	LM	
Roberts and Noonan	LM	#163950
Osler–Rendu–Weber	AVM	%601101
Glomovenous malformations	VM	#138000

Key

CM – capillary malformation; VM – venous malformation; LM – lymphatic malformation;
LVM – lymphovenous malformation; AVM – arteriovenous malformation.

*MIM number – Mendelian Inheritance in Man

http://www.ncbi.nlm.nih.gov/sites/entrez (gateway to online M/M)

Vascular tumours

Infantile haemangiomas (common)

Incidence
- ~10 % full-term Caucasian babies at 1 year of age with increase seen in prematurity (≤ 30%), less common in infants with pigmented skin (1%)
- About 20% are multiple

Epidemiology
- Female predominance (3:1)

Pathogenesis
- True neoplasms that grow by endothelial proliferation

Clinical features
- Not always present at birth but there may be a flat red area or pale patch in ~40%
- Most (~80%) are noticed within the first 3 weeks of life, with ~60% in the head and neck region
- Superficial haemangiomas are strawberry red while deeper lesions are purple or blue. They may be localized or diffuse
- Have a 3-stage cycle with characteristic histological features:
  - rapid proliferating phase – 5–8 months
  - Prolonged involuting phase – 9 months to 7 years
  - Involuted phase – 5–9 years (90% regressed by 9 years)

Complications
- Large size (in proliferating phase) – distorting vital structures, especially on the face
- Multiple/large visceral lesions causing high-output cardiac failure
- Obstruction of vital structures (airway, orbit, external auditory canal)
- Persistent ulceration/bleeding

Investigations
- Soft-tissue US and Doppler flow studies
- Abdominal ultrasound (if >5 exclude visceral, in particular hepatic, lesions)
- Echocardiogram (for large haemangiomas or if there is liver involvement)
- MRI (if the haemangioma is at a site that could interfere with vital structures, e.g. airway, or if there are any neurological complications)
- Histology – GLUT-1 positive, irrespective of phase (glucose transporter protein is a specific tissue marker)

Management
- Expectant – requires parental support, serial photographs, skin care, and wound care (if ulcerated)
- Active intervention – typically indicated in complicated lesions, often in combination

Patching
- Uninvolved eye when periocular haemangioma is threatening amblyopia

Steroids (first-line therapy)
- Intralesional (for localized, cutaneous lesions), e.g. triamcinolone 2 mg/kg, every 4–6 weeks
- Systemic, e.g. prednisolone 2–3 mg/kg/day up to 5 to 6 months of age to cover the active growth period with later reducing dose, but beware of rebound growth

Vincristine (second-line therapy)
- 1 mg/m²/day increasing to 2–3 mg/m²/day according to response – given initially weekly via a central line, length of treatment 5–10 weeks, but can be extended under careful supervision).

Embolization
- For bleeding, high-output cardiac failure etc

Surgery
Indications
- **Emergency/urgent** – tracheostomy (airway obstruction), excision of intra-orbital lesions (vision threatened)
- **Intermediate** – minimize deformity from attenuation of vital structures (eyelids, nasal margin, lips)
- **Late** – excision fibrofatty residue/reconstruction

Other vascular tumours (rare)
- Rapidly involuting congenital haemangioma (RICH)
- Non-involuting congenital haemangioma (NICH)
- Kaposiform haemangioendothelioma (KHE) or related tufted angioma – (associated with Kasabach–Merrit phenomenon)
- Infantile myofibroma

Vascular malformations

Classified according to flow characteristics and vessel type into capillary, venous, lymphatic, arterial, or mixed.

Epidemiology
- M = F

Pathogenesis

Structural anomalies resulting from an error in vascular morphogenesis between 4 and 10 weeks of gestation.

Clinical features

Present at birth, do not involute. Growth stimulated by haemodynamic or hormonal changes.

Investigation
- Radiology (typically US with Doppler flow studies, MRI (including MRA and MRV)

Low-flow lesions

Capillary malformations (aka port wine stains)
Incidence
- Most common vascular malformation (~0.5% of newborns)

Clinical features

Pink, macular patch which becomes purple with age. They can occur anywhere on the body, but most commonly on the face (where they may correspond to the dermatomes of the trigeminal nerve). Secondary soft tissue and bony hypertrophy, skin nodules, and an increased incidence of pyogenic granulomas are also seen.

Management
- Pulsed-dye laser
- Surgery – excision nodules/correction deformity from secondary soft tissue/skeletal hypertrophy

Associations
- Sturge–Weber syndrome (may be associated with neurological problems)
- Cutis marmorata telangiectatica congenita

Venous malformations
Clinical features

Blue, compressible soft tissue masses which fill when dependent and empty on elevation. They may occur anywhere and are usually asymptomatic but may cause disfigurement, or aching, or be complicated by bleeding. Larger/extensive lesions may result in localized/disseminated intravascular coagulopathy (raised D-dimers/low serum fibrinogen).

Management
- Compression garments/NSAIDS
- Anticoagulation (to interrupt clotting cascade)
- Sclerotherapy (e.g. ethanol, Ethibloc®, sodium tetradecyl sulphate)
- Surgery (for small, localized lesions/debulking post sclerotherapy

Associations
- Familial venous malformations (*TIE2* deficiency)
- Glomovenous malformation (glomulin gene)

Lymphatic malformations
Clinical features
- Microcystic – small, raised cutaneous vesicles, full of lymphatic fluid
- Macrocystic – aka cystic hygroma
  - larger, soft subcutaneous swellings which typically transilluminate
  - they may be combined and are most commonly seen on the neck, axilla, and chest
  - skeletal distortion/soft tissue hypertrophy is common and may be complicated by infection or intralesional haemorrhage

Management
- Complicated lesions – analgesia, rest, compression, antibiotics
- Macrocystic:
  - sclerotherapy (STD, OK-432, doxycycline)
  - surgery (debulking/staged excision)
- Microcystic:
  - sclerotherapy (not as effective as for microcystic)
  - surgery (excisional)

High-flow lesions

Arteriovenous malformations
Clinical features

Aggressive, progressive deformity with potential for systemic complication. There is a characteristic nidus with arterial feeders, arteriovenous y fistulae and enlarged veins. They are often quiescent at birth but stimulated by hormonal changes/trauma. Present with throbbing pain, ulceration with bleeding, and cardiac failure. Occasionally a pulsatile mass with a bruit is found.

Schobinger classification

Four progressive stages have been described:
- I = quiescent, stable
- II = expansion, enlargement and tortuous veins
- III = destruction with pain, bleeding, and ulceration
- IV = decompensation with cardiac failure.

Management

According to stage (III–IV) – aggressive treatment:
- **combined embolization** (ethanol, cyanoacrylate, coils and polyvinyl particles), 24–48 h prior to excisional surgery ± reconstruction. Typically difficult/recurrent
- **periodic embolization –** when lesion is in sensitive sites (intracranial/intraorbital)

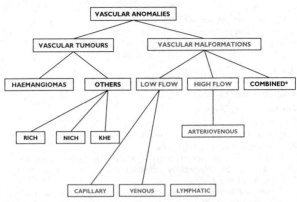

Fig. 11.4 Classification of vascular anomalies – based on International Society for Study of Vascular Anomalies (ISSVA 1996).

Key

RICH – rapidly involuting congenital haemangioma; NICH – non-involuting congenital haemangioma; KHE – kaposiform haemangioendothelioma.

*Combined/syndromic. CLVM – capillary, lymphatic, venous malformation (Klippel–Trenaunay syndrome); CAVM – capillary, arteriovenous malformation (Parkes–Weber syndrome), SWS – Sturge–Weber syndrome.

Further reading

Elluru RG. Azizkhan RG. Cervicofacial vascular anomalies. II. Vascular malformations. *Semin Pediatr Surg* 2006;**15**:133–9.

Harper JI, Oranje A, Prose N. *Textbook of Pediatric Dermatology.* Oxford: Blackwell Publishing, 2006.

Mulliken JB, Glowacki J. Haemangiomas and vascular malformations in infants and children: a classification based on endothelial characteristics. *Plast Reconstr Surg* 1982;**69**:412–22.

Spring MA, Bentz ML. Cutaneous vascular lesions. *Clin Plastic Surg* 2005;**32**:171–86.

Sundine MJ, Wirth GA. Hemangiomas: an overview. *Clin Pediatr* 2007;**46**:206–21.

Neurosurgery

Ventricular shunts

Effective treatment for hydrocephalus began with the development of an implantable silicone tube and one-way valve device in the 1950s (Spitz–olter valve (Box 11.2). Ventriculoperitoneal (VP) shunts are devices which consist of a ventricular catheter, reservoir, valve, and a distal catheter placed in the peritoneal or pleural cavity. Ventriculoatrial (VA) shunts (rarely indicated nowadays) have a distal catheter in the right atrium via the internal jugular vein.

Box 11.2 Spitz–Holter valve

John Holter was a hydraulics technician who had a son, Casey, with hydrocephalus due to spina bifida and who had sustained complications due to the devices available at the time. He therefore designed the first workable, implantable VA shunt in conjunction with American neurosurgeon Eugene Spitz in Philadelphia in 1956. It was implanted first into another patient – but was later used in his son.

Shunt failure rate has been reported as 38% in the first year, 48% after 2 years, and 54% at 3 years after placement.

Shunt blockage

Infants
- Irritability, vomiting, lethargy, 'sunsetting' appearance of the eyes, enlarging head circumference, tense fontanelle, splayed sutures (infants)

Children
- Headache, nausea and vomiting, lethargy, diplopia, papilloedema, abducens (VI) nerve palsy (children)

Investigations
- CT head, x-ray of shunt tubing, FBC, U&E, CRP.
- Aspiration of the shunt reservoir may be performed by a neurosurgeon to establish patency and exclude infection

Management
Early consultation with a neurosurgeon is recommended. If the above investigations are normal then a period of inpatient observation may be warranted. Shunt obstruction requires urgent exploration with replacement of the malfunctioning component or replacement of the entire shunt.

Shunt infection
- Infection complicates 2–15% of shunt placements.
- Most occur within 3 months of placement and 90% within 1 year.
- Risk of complication is increased in premature and neonatal infants.
- Commonest organisms are *Staph. epidermidis* (coagulase –ve *Staph.*) and *Staph. aureus*, which are responsible for one-third of infections each. The remaining third consists of a mixed variety of organisms including *Acinetobacter* spp. and *E. coli*.

Clinical features
- Headache, lethargy, photophobia, pyrexia, raised ICP (cranial nerve palsy, papilloedema), meningism (Kernig's sign – knee extension with flexed hips provokes pain).

Investigations
- CT head, FBC, U&E, CRP
- CSF may be sent for microscopy and cell counts.

Management
Externalization or removal of the shunt and replacement with an external ventricular catheter. Initial treatment involves empirical intravenous (e.g. cefotaxime) and/or intrathecal antibiotics (e.g. vancomycin) with modification once sensitivities become available.

Aim for shunt replacement once infection is treated with return of cell counts to normal and sterile CSF on culture.

Head injury

May be classified by morphology:
- skull fractures (linear, depressed, basilar)
- intracranial haematomas (extradural, subdural, intracerebral)
- diffuse brain injury.

Always think about the mechanism of injury when assessing a patient with a head injury. The possibility of a C-spine, thoracic, visceral, or limb injury must be considered especially in high-velocity accidents. Non-accidental injury should be suspected with unexplained events or multiple unexplained injuries.

Peri-orbital haematomas, retro-auricular haematomas (Battle's sign), or CSF leak indicate a base of skull fracture.

Investigations
- CT head/C-spine/chest/abdomen
- FBC, U&E, X match.
- Glasgow Coma Scale (Table 11.5)

Management
- Priorities for resuscitation follow APLS guidelines (ABC)
- Depressed fractures if compound may require debridement and elevation. Patients with a persistent CSF leak require referral to a neurosurgeon.

If the patient has a deteriorating conscious level or focal signs related to the mass effect of the lesion, then urgent evacuation is required. Patient with a GCS ≤8 or less will require intubation and sedation. Mannitol (1–2 mg/kg body weight) may be given on the advice of the neurosurgeon.

Of patients with a GCS ≤8 at 6 h post injury, ~50% will die.

Table 11.5 Paediatric Glasgow Coma Scale range (3–15) – use if <2 years (i.e. preverbal)

		SCORE
Best eye opening	Spontaneously	4
	To speech	3
	To pain	2
	No response	1
Best verbal response	Coos/babbles 'normal'	5
	Irritable/cries continuously	4
	Cries to pain	3
	Moans to pain	2
	No response	1
Best motor response	Spontaneous /purposeful movements	6
	Withdraws from touch	5
	Withdraws from pain	4
	Abnormal flexion	3
	Abnormal extension	2
	No response	1

Paediatric brain tumours

Commonest solid tumours in children comprising 22% of all childhood malignancy up to age 14 years and 10% of all tumours in 15–19-year age group. Most are located in the posterior fossa (e.g. pilocytic astrocytoma, medulloblastoma, and ependymoma).

Clinical features

May present with posterior fossa syndrome (headache, vomiting, ataxia and nystagmus) and/or symptoms of hydrocephalus (see above). Persistent vomiting may be misdiagnosed as gastroenteritis, leading to a delayed presentation. Infants may present with progressively enlarging head circumference.

Investigations

- CT/MRI brain and spine with contrast
- FBC, U&E, G&S.
- Tumour markers (e.g. α-fetoprotein, β-HCG) may be raised in pineal germinomas

Management

Dexamethasone, antiemetics, analgesia, intravenous fluids. Surgery may be required as an emergency or at next available elective list, depending on clinical condition of child.

Treatment of hydrocephalus may require external ventricular drainage, endoscopic third ventriculostomy, or urgent surgery for tumour removal.

Five-year survival for all brain tumours is ~60%.

Brain abscess and subdural/extradural empyema

May be due to direct extension (sinus infection), iatrogenic (following neurosurgical procedures), penetrating head trauma, haematogenous dissemination (congenital cyanotic heart disease, pulmonary AV fistula), or as sequlae of meningitis

Clinical features

Headache, vomiting, seizures, focal neurological signs, papilloedema, depressed conscious level, menigismus, tenderness over paranasal sinus. Always have a low index of suspicion as the actual findings may be minimal.

Investigations

FBC, U&E, CRP, G&S, CT/MRI with contrast. Lumbar puncture is usually contraindicated.

Management

Patients can deteriorate rapidly, therefore early referral to a neurosurgeon is recommended. Anticonvulsants (e.g. phenytoin) are recommended as seizures can occur in up to 45% of patients. Broad-spectrum antibiotics based on local microbiology policy should be instituted until specifc sensitivities are known. The role of steroids remains controversial but they should be considered for significant mass effect from abscesses. Fungal abscesses should be considered in iummunocompromised children.

Early surgery (burrhole drainage or craniotomy) is usually indicated.

Early involvement of an ENT surgeon is essential in those with a sinus infection.

Further reading

May PL. Paediatric neurosurgery. *Curr Opin Neurol Neurosurg* 1999;**5**:25–9.

Pizer B, May PL. Central nervous system tumours in children. *Eur J Surg Oncol* 1997;**23**:559–64.

Teasdale G, Jennett B. Assessment of coma and impaired consciousness. A practical scale. *Lancet* 1974;**2**:81–4 (original GCS for use in adults and older children).

Index

Illustrations, tables, book titles and boxed text are in italics.